The British Medical Association

CHILDREN'S
MEDICAL GUIDE

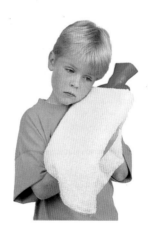

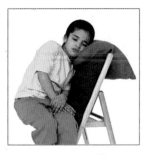
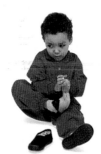
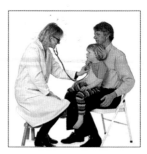
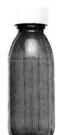
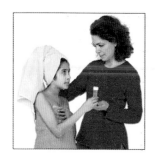
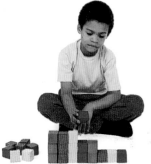
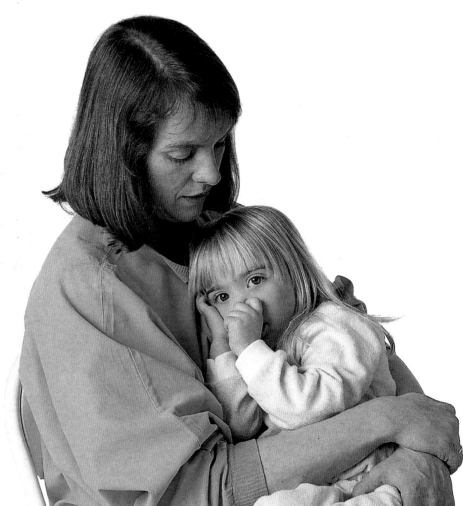
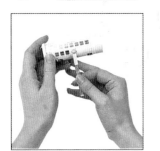
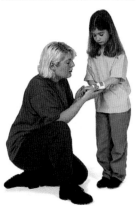
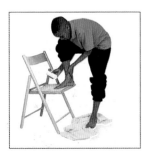
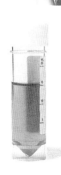
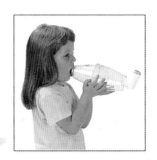
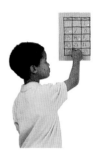
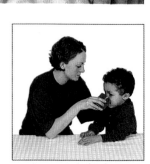

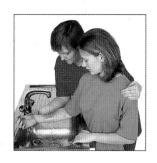
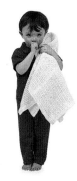
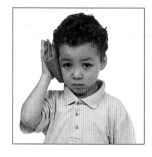
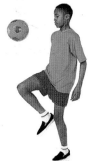
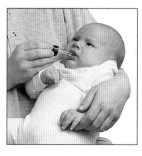

The British Medical Association
CHILDREN'S MEDICAL GUIDE

Dr. Bernard Valman

MEDICAL EDITOR
Dr. Tony Smith

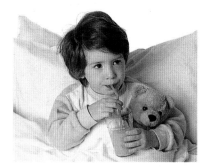

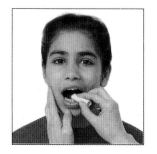

DORLING KINDERSLEY
LONDON · NEW YORK · SYDNEY · MOSCOW

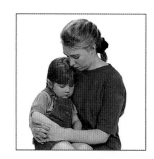

A DORLING KINDERSLEY BOOK

BRITISH MEDICAL ASSOCIATION
Chairman of the Council Dr. A.W. Macara
Treasurer Dr. W.J. Appleyard
Chairman of the BMA Journal Committee Sir Anthony Grabham
Associate Editor, British Medical Journal Dr. Tony Smith

DORLING KINDERSLEY
Senior Editors Andrea Bagg, Mary Lindsay
Editors Louise Clairmonte, Jill Hamilton

Project Art Editor Chris Walker
Art Editor Rachel Gibson
Designers Mark J. Wilde, Philip Ormerod, Nicola Hampel

Managing Editor Martyn Page
Managing Art Editor Bryn Walls
Senior Managing Editor Krystyna Mayer
Senior Managing Art Editor Lynne Brown

Illustrators Joanna Cameron, Tony Graham, Halli Verrinder
DTP Designer Jason Little
Production Alison Jones

The British Medical Association Children's Medical Guide
provides information on a wide range of health and medical topics.
The book is not a substitute for medical diagnosis, however,
and you are advised always to consult your doctor for specific
information on personal health matters. The naming of any organization,
product, or alternative therapy in this book does not imply BMA endorsement;
the omission of any such names does not indicate BMA disapproval.

First published in Great Britain in 1998
by Dorling Kindersley Limited,
9 Henrietta Street,
London WC2E 8PS

2 4 6 8 10 9 7 5 3 1

First published in hardback as The British Medical Association Children's Symptoms

Visit us on the World Wide Web at
http://www.dk.com

Reproduced by GRB Editrice, Italy
Printed and bound by Graphicom, Italy

FOREWORD

Children become ill more frequently than adults. Although they gradually acquire immunity to the common viruses causing colds, coughs, sore throats, and diarrhoea, children have repeated minor illnesses. Their activity and their physical immaturity result in frequent injuries.

In children, illness or injury may happen very quickly, but recovery may be just as fast. In these circumstances, parents want to know when to get medical help. The symptom charts will help you to differentiate between minor problems and those that need immediate attention. The charts are not a substitute for your own doctor but they should enable you to decide when to let nature take its course or use home remedies, and to recognize warning signs that require urgent medical help.

If symptoms do need medical assessment, more questions follow. What are the causes? How serious is the condition? How is it treated? All of these questions should be answered by the doctors looking after your child. This book is intended to back up your doctor by explaining the main features of the more common childhood disorders and to reassure you that most of these illnesses have a good outlook.

Dr. Tony Smith
Associate Editor
British Medical Journal

CONTENTS

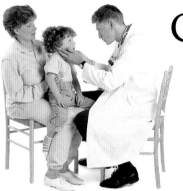

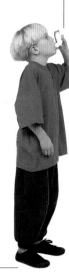

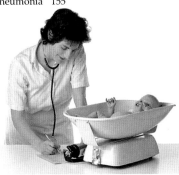

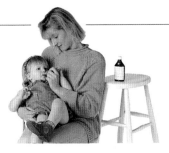

FIRST AID & NURSING A SICK CHILD 202

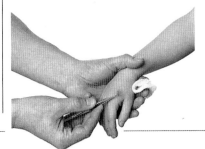

HOW TO USE THIS BOOK

The book is divided into four sections that provide information on the child's body and how it works, and what can go wrong. The first section, Your Child's Body, concentrates on the basics of anatomy, growth, and development. The second section, which is the core of the book, comprises Symptom Charts. When your child is ill, the question-and-answer charts will help you to determine the possible cause and decide whether medical attention is required. The third section, Diseases and Disorders, provides details of more than 140 conditions. The final section covers essential first-aid techniques and emergency procedures.

Your Child's Body
The first section of the book describes the anatomy, growth, and development of children. Following on from this general introduction are guidelines for safe and healthy living for children of all ages. Problems in babies, being different from those that affect older children, are covered in the final part of this opening section.

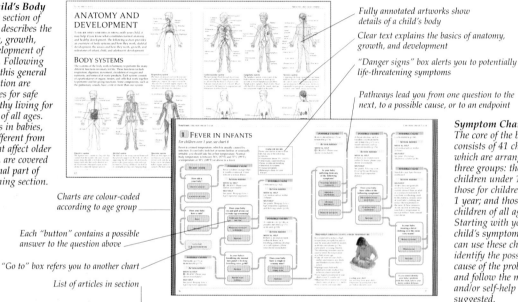

Charts are colour-coded according to age group

Each "button" contains a possible answer to the question above

"Go to" box refers you to another chart

List of articles in section

Fully annotated artworks show details of a child's body

Clear text explains the basics of anatomy, growth, and development

"Danger signs" box alerts you to potentially life-threatening symptoms

Pathways lead you from one question to the next, to a possible cause, or to an endpoint

Symptom Charts
The core of the book consists of 41 charts, which are arranged in three groups: those for children under 1 year; those for children over 1 year; and those for children of all ages. Starting with your child's symptoms you can use these charts to identify the possible cause of the problem and follow the medical and/or self-help action suggested.

Diseases and Disorders
Arranged by body system, each of the articles in this section describes a disease or disorder. The articles include information about the symptoms and causes of the problem, whether and when you should seek medical help, what the doctor might do, self-help measures you can follow at home, and the outlook.

Photograph illustrates the cause or appearance of the disease

Clear, step-by-step photographs show first-aid techniques

Boxes highlight special information or alternative methods or situations

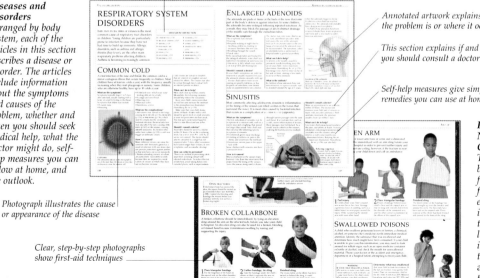

Annotated artwork explains what the problem is or where it occurs

This section explains if and when you should consult a doctor

Self-help measures give simple remedies you can use at home

First Aid and Nursing a Sick Child
The final part of the book demonstrates first-aid methods for life-threatening emergencies. Also included is first-aid treatment for broken limbs and some other injuries before going to hospital. Nursing a Sick Child gives the basic instructions for looking after a child who is unwell.

HOW TO USE THE CHARTS

Find the chart that matches your child's main symptom. Beginning at the box labelled "Start here", follow the pathway to the first question. Choose the appropriate answer, and take the pathway leading from that answer. It may go to another question; a possible cause, which directs you to information elsewhere in the book and also tells you what action to take –

whether to obtain medical help and what self-help measures might be helpful; a reference to another symptom chart; or an endpoint.

CAUTION Remember that the charts provide only likely diagnoses. If you have any doubts about either the diagnosis or the treatment of any symptoms, always consult your doctor.

"Go to" box
You may look up your child's symptoms on one chart but find that the pathway leads to one of these boxes, referring you to another chart that is more appropriate for your child's illness

Question box
Each question is followed by two or more possible answers. Choose the one that most closely matches your child's symptoms, and follow the pathway leading from it to another location on the chart

"Danger signs" box
Symptoms that may indicate a serious condition are listed in these boxes. If you notice any of these symptoms, follow the instructions to call an ambulance or phone your doctor at once

Possible causes
The possible causes of your child's symptoms are given here. They are usually accompanied by cross-references to further information given in other sections of the book

Action needed
The necessary medical and self-help measures are described under the heading "Action needed". You may be instructed to obtain medical help (see below) and/or use self-help procedures

Self-help panel
These panels describe in detail various self-help measures that you can use to help relieve your child's symptoms. Some charts have assessment panels, which show you how to evaluate your child's breathing rate, growth, vision, and hearing ability

Endpoint box
Some pathways may lead to an endpoint, rather than a possible cause. This endpoint tells you when you should seek medical assistance if it is not possible to identify your child's problem from the symptom chart

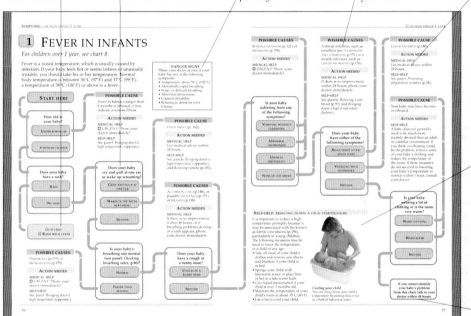

MEDICAL HELP

There are five levels of medical help, depending on the severity of your child's condition. If a problem can be remedied by self-help measures alone, the medical help category is omitted.

⊕ EMERGENCY! Call an ambulance!
Your child's condition may be life-threatening or lead to permanent disability. Get medical help immediately, by calling an ambulance. In some cases, you may prefer to call your doctor or take your child to hospital yourself.

⊕ URGENT! Phone your doctor immediately!
Your child may have a serious illness that requires prompt medical treatment. Phone your doctor or an accident and emergency department without delay.

Get medical advice within 24 hours.
Your child may be suffering from a condition that requires urgent medical assessment and should be seen by a doctor within 24 hours. If you cannot see the doctor, you should speak to him or her on the phone.

Make an appointment to see your doctor.
Your child's condition requires medical treatment, but your child will not be adversely affected if the next available appointment is not for 3 or 4 days.

Consult your doctor.
There is no need for you to make a special appointment or to contact the doctor with any haste; discuss your child's symptoms at the next appointment, or phone your doctor sooner if you become concerned.

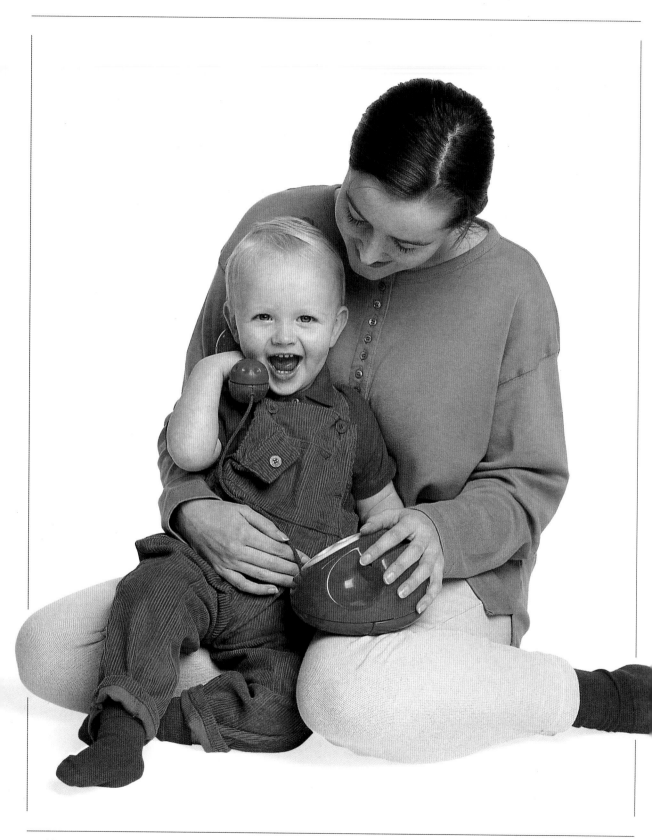

YOUR CHILD'S BODY

EARLY STIMULATION MAY PROMOTE
MENTAL DEVELOPMENT

A BASIC KNOWLEDGE of a child's anatomy and normal physical, emotional, and mental development gives parents a clearer understanding of the many common problems or illnesses that tend to affect children. This section begins with a brief look at the development of children from birth to adolescence. The section continues with advice on infant feeding and weaning, and provides nutritional guidelines for growing children. To maximize a child's chance of a safe, healthy life, information about immunization, prevention of accidents, and care in the sun is also included. Babies tend to have a different set of problems from toddlers and older children and some of these, such as feeding and sleeping problems, are covered at the end of the section.

SECTION THROUGH THE EYE

ANATOMY AND DEVELOPMENT

TO DECIDE WHEN SOMETHING IS WRONG with your child, it may help if you know what constitutes normal anatomy and healthy development. The following section provides an overview of body systems and how they work, skeletal development, the senses and how they work, growth, and milestones of infant, child, and adolescent development.

BODY SYSTEMS

The systems of the body work in harmony to perform the many different functions necessary for life. These functions include respiration, digestion, movement, circulation of oxygen and nutrients, and removal of waste products. Each system consists of a particular set of organs, tissues, and cells that work together to perform vital life-giving functions. Some components, such as the pulmonary vessels, have a role in more than one system.

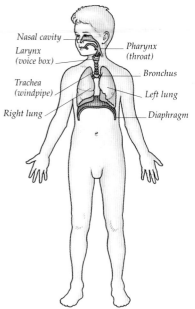

Respiratory system
The lungs, air passages such as the nose and trachea, and breathing muscles, including the diaphragm, comprise the respiratory system. Associated blood vessels supply oxygen to the body tissues and remove waste carbon dioxide and take it to the lungs for exhalation.

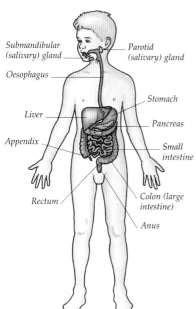

Digestive system
The digestive tract consists of a long tube that extends from the mouth to the anus. As food passes along this tube, it is broken down into minute molecules that can be absorbed into the bloodstream. Associated organs secrete chemicals to assist the digestive process.

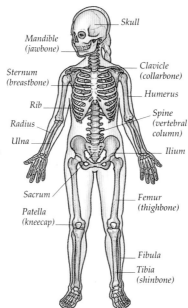

Skeletal system
The skeleton is the strong internal framework that provides support for the body. As well as supporting the soft tissues, the skeleton also protects the organs and provides anchorage for muscles. During childhood, the skeleton is continually growing and changing shape.

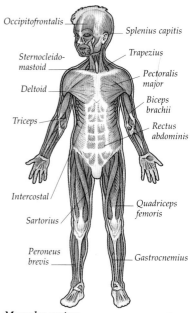

Muscular system
There are three types of muscle: voluntary, involuntary, and cardiac. Voluntary muscles (above) work with the skeleton to enable the body to move. Involuntary muscles surround hollow organs, such as the intestines and stomach. The heart is made of cardiac muscle.

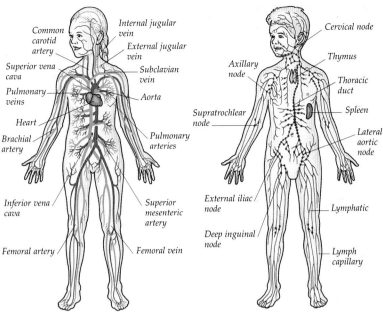

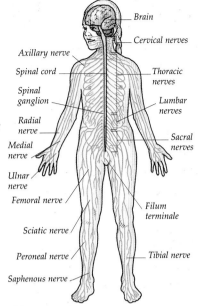

Cardiovascular system
The heart pumps blood through the arteries, veins, and capillaries. Oxygen and nutrients are delivered by the blood to all parts of the body and waste products are removed. Blood is returned to the lungs for reoxygenation and elimination of carbon dioxide.

Lymphatic system
The lymphatic system, a major part of the body's immune system, is made up of a network of vessels (lymphatics) and filters (lymph nodes). Lymph, a fluid of white blood cells that flows through the vessels, destroys microorganisms trapped in the nodes.

Nervous system
Comprising the brain, spinal cord, and many millions of nerve cells, the nervous system is the control centre for all voluntary activities and involuntary bodily functions. Nerves are responsible for perception of sensations, such as touch, taste, smell, vision, and hearing.

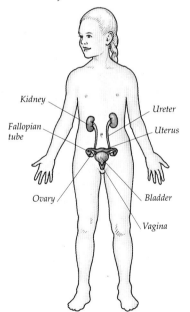

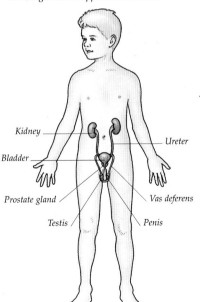

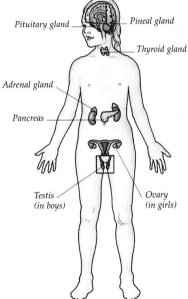

Girl's genitourinary system
The urinary system – kidneys, ureters, and bladder – filters waste products, surplus water, and excess salts from the blood. The genital system, composed of two ovaries, the uterus, and various ducts, produces hormones and, from puberty, one or more eggs every month.

Boy's genitourinary system
As in a girl, a boy's urinary system comprises kidneys, ureters, and bladder. Urine and, after puberty, semen pass out of the body through the urethra and penis. The testes produce hormones that are responsible for the male characteristics that appear at puberty.

Endocrine system
The endocrine glands manufacture hormones, the body's chemical messengers. Hormones are distributed to all parts of the body by the blood and help to regulate internal processes, such as growth. Some glands, such as the testis and ovary, are inactive until puberty.

SKELETAL DEVELOPMENT

At birth most of a baby's skeleton is composed of bone but some parts, notably the ends of the arm, leg, hand, and foot bones, are made of cartilage and do not ossify (turn into bone) until late adolescence. The cartilage continues to grow before ossifying, which allows the rapid growth of childhood to take place; this process continues through childhood until adult size is reached. The number of individual bones in the body decreases as adulthood approaches: a newborn baby may have over 300 distinct bones, but many of these fuse together as the child grows, resulting in an adult skeleton of 206 bones.

GROWTH OF THE SKULL

At birth, a baby's skull is not fully ossified – the individual bones making up the cranium (brain case) are joined by flexible bands of fibrous tissue. These areas allow the skull to change shape during childbirth and enable rapid growth of the brain during the first year or two of life. The anterior fontanelle towards the front of the skull is the largest band of fibrous tissue and it is clearly visible through the skin.

The bones of the face enlarge at the same rate as the rest of the skull so that when growth is complete, the head is in proportion to the rest of the body.

DEVELOPMENT OF THE TEETH

At birth, the primary teeth are already developing in the jaws. The first of these erupt by about 6 months, and by the age of 3 years the entire set of 20 primary teeth has come through. Meanwhile, the secondary set of 32 teeth is developing in the jaws and will appear between the ages of 6 and 16 years. As these teeth erupt, the primary teeth are displaced and fall out. The third molars (wisdom teeth) usually break through at 16 or older, although sometimes they never appear.

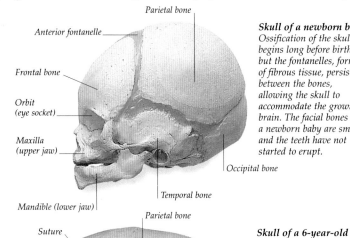

Skull of a newborn baby
Ossification of the skull begins long before birth, but the fontanelles, formed of fibrous tissue, persist between the bones, allowing the skull to accommodate the growing brain. The facial bones of a newborn baby are small and the teeth have not started to erupt.

Parietal bone
Anterior fontanelle
Frontal bone
Orbit (eye socket)
Maxilla (upper jaw)
Occipital bone
Temporal bone
Mandible (lower jaw)

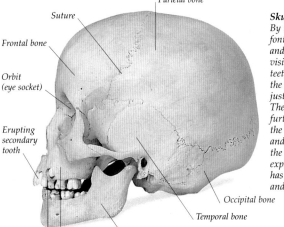

Skull of a 6-year-old
By the age of 6 years, the fontanelles have ossified, and they are no longer visible. All the primary teeth have erupted and the secondary teeth are just beginning to emerge. The maxilla is lower and further forwards than in the newborn baby's skull and the eye sockets and the nasal region have expanded. The mandible has grown downwards and forwards.

Parietal bone
Suture
Frontal bone
Orbit (eye socket)
Erupting secondary tooth
Primary tooth
Maxilla (upper jaw)
Mandible (lower jaw)
Temporal bone
Occipital bone

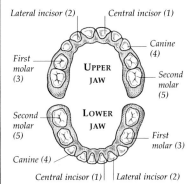

Lateral incisor (2)
Central incisor (1)
Canine (4)
First molar (3)
UPPER JAW
Second molar (5)
Second molar (5)
LOWER JAW
First molar (3)
Canine (4)
Central incisor (1)
Lateral incisor (2)

Primary teeth
Deciduous, or primary, teeth erupt between the ages of 6 months and 3 years in a specific order (as shown in brackets, above). The pattern is the same in upper and lower jaws.

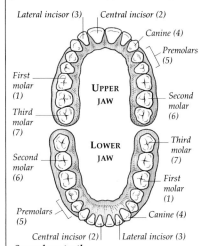

Lateral incisor (3)
Central incisor (2)
Canine (4)
Premolars (5)
First molar (1)
UPPER JAW
Second molar (6)
Third molar (7)
Second molar (6)
LOWER JAW
Third molar (7)
First molar (1)
Premolars (5)
Canine (4)
Central incisor (2)
Lateral incisor (3)

Secondary teeth
Permanent, or secondary, teeth erupt between the ages of 6 and 16 years in the order shown in brackets (above). The premolars, canines, and incisors directly replace primary teeth.

MAIN AREAS OF BONE GROWTH

In childhood, most of the long bones contain cartilage, which allows the bones to grow. The cartilage in these areas grows and absorbs calcium to develop into bone. Limb, hand, and foot bones, the areas in which most growth occurs, are made up of a diaphysis (shaft), which is the main part of the bone, and an epiphysis (growing region) at either one or both ends. During the course of a child's growing years, the epiphyses gradually ossify, leaving a cartilage plate where growth continues until adult height and size is reached in late adolescence.

Bony and ossifying areas are clearly visible on an X-ray, whereas cartilage does not show up very clearly. X-rays, therefore, can be used by a doctor to tell the age of a child and also to decide whether his or her growth is normal. This type of assessment is possible because the areas of ossification appear in a particular sequence in every child. For example, at the age of 1 year, a child will develop areas of ossification in the shoulder, hand, hip, and foot. From the age of 2 years, additional areas of ossification are formed in the shoulder, elbow, hand, hip, knee, and foot bones. Additional ossification centres are established each year and growth continues in the old areas as well as in the new ones.

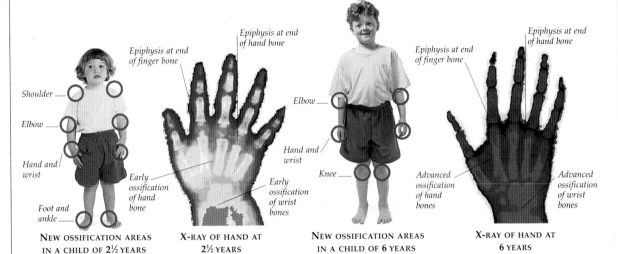

Shoulder
Elbow
Hand and wrist
Foot and ankle

Epiphysis at end of finger bone
Epiphysis at end of hand bone
Early ossification of hand bone
Early ossification of wrist bones

Elbow
Hand and wrist
Knee

Epiphysis at end of finger bone
Advanced ossification of hand bones

Epiphysis at end of hand bone
Advanced ossification of wrist bones

NEW OSSIFICATION AREAS IN A CHILD OF 2½ YEARS

X-RAY OF HAND AT 2½ YEARS

NEW OSSIFICATION AREAS IN A CHILD OF 6 YEARS

X-RAY OF HAND AT 6 YEARS

Bone growth in a 2½-year-old
New areas of ossification include bones in the shoulder, elbow, wrist, hand, foot, and ankle; areas of ossification established earlier continue to grow. The X-ray of the hand shows the shafts of the bones (opaque areas) have ossified but the ends (transparent areas) are still growing.

Bone growth in a 6-year-old
By the age of 6 years, ossification sites in other elbow, hand, and wrist bones have formed; a new site appears in the knee. The hand X-ray shows many ossified wrist bones (opaque areas) but there are still growing centres at the top ends of the hand bones (transparent areas).

BONE REPAIR

Children are naturally curious and adventurous, with the result that they are particularly prone to falls and dislocated and broken bones. When a bone is fractured, the natural healing process begins immediately and, in children, the whole sequence takes only a few weeks. To prevent a broken bone from reforming in a misaligned position – thus leaving a crooked, unstable bone that is liable to further injury – the displaced edges of bone must be lined up and fixed promptly. A fracture at the growing end of a bone may disrupt growth, causing the bone to be shorter than it should be.

Repair and regeneration of bone following a break is a type of ossification. It differs from the formation of completely new bone from cartilage in that the damaged area has to be cleared of wound debris before new bone can grow. This process is carried out by specialized blood cells and connective tissue cells, which invade the site and absorb the debris. New bone is laid down between the bone ends, and after a few weeks the bone is repaired.

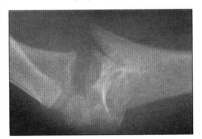

Fractured humerus
The humerus in the upper part of the picture has broken close to the elbow joint. This is one type of fracture that very commonly affects children of all ages.

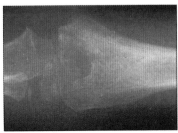

Healed fracture
A few weeks later the bone has reformed and is correctly positioned for optimum mobility of the elbow. The repaired site is as strong as the original bone prior to the injury.

THE SENSES

The five senses – sight, hearing, touch, smell, and taste – are responsible for giving your child vital information about his or her surroundings. The eyes and ears are the most important of the sensory organs. Touch relies on receptors in the skin that detect temperature, pressure, and pain. The related senses of smell and taste, as detected by the nose and tongue, differentiate the main tastes and warn against potentially noxious substances in food and air. Smell also activates secretion of saliva for digesting food.

All senses are normally present at birth, but they need adequate stimulation to develop fully. Taste and smell are often more acute in children than in adults because they have not been subjected to pollutants, such as smoke.

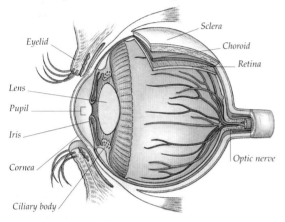

SECTION THROUGH THE EYE

Eye structure and vision
Sight is the most complex of the senses. Light rays enter through the pupil at the front of the eye and register on the retina at the back. The light rays are converted to nerve impulses that are passed, via the optic nerve, to the brain, where they are interpreted as images.

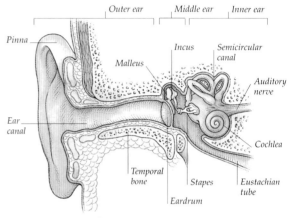

SECTION THROUGH THE EAR

Ear structure and hearing
The ears are the organs of hearing. Sound waves pass from the outer to the middle ear. From there, a system of membranes and tiny bones conveys vibrations to the inner ear. Vibrations are converted to nerve impulses in the cochlea and passed, via the auditory nerve, to the brain.

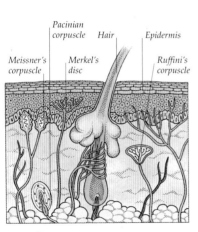

SECTION THROUGH THE SKIN

Skin structure and touch
Specialized skin cells, which detect pressure, pain, and temperature, are free nerve endings or bulb-like structures. These receptors are not related exclusively to one touch sensation.

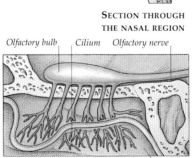

SECTION THROUGH THE NASAL REGION

ENLARGED NASAL REGION

Nose structure and smell
Smells dissolve in mucus in the nasal cavity and stimulate the hair-like cilia of specialized nerve cells. The nerve impulses generated travel along the olfactory nerve to the brain.

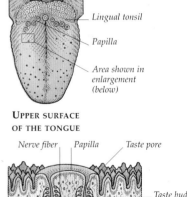

UPPER SURFACE OF THE TONGUE

SECTION THROUGH A PAPILLA

Tongue structure and taste
Taste buds are located mainly within papillae on the surface of the tongue. Different types of papillae arranged over the tongue can detect bitter, sour, salty, or sweet tastes.

GROWTH CHARTS

The growth charts on the following pages allow you to record and plot your child's growth. By plotting head circumference, weight, and height against age, you can compare your child's growth with the normal range for that age. Growth in babies should be monitored by regular attendance at a baby clinic so that any growth problems are picked up early. If any of your child's measurements fall outside the shaded area, or if the growth curve is erratic, make an appointment to see your doctor.

HOW TO USE THE CHARTS

First, measure your child using the illustrations in the box below as a guide. Use the weight measurements recorded at the clinic if your child is too young or too small to be weighed on your bathroom scales.

The charts on the following pages cover all the measurements and ages required to track your child's growth: head circumference and weight for boys and girls from birth to 2 years, and height and weight for boys and girls between 2 and 18 years. Find your child's age along the bottom of the chart and draw an imaginary vertical line until it meets head circumference, height, or weight, found on the side of the chart. Note the measurement; plot the point first with a pencil dot and then overwrite with a pen once you are sure the point is in the correct place.

Take measurements regularly and draw a line connecting the dots to form a "growth curve". The charts will show you how your child compares to the average for all children of the same age, which is represented by the 50th centile line. If the curve does not run parallel to the 50th centile line, or fails to keep within the shaded area, make an appointment to see your doctor.

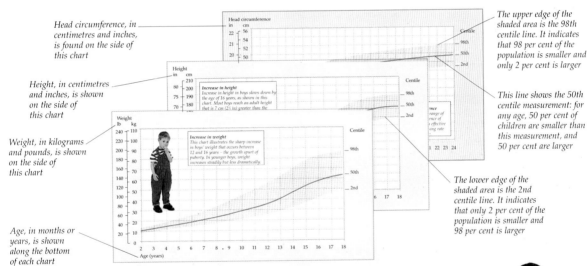

Head circumference, in centimetres and inches, is found on the side of this chart

Height, in centimetres and inches, is shown on the side of this chart

Weight, in kilograms and pounds, is shown on the side of this chart

Age, in months or years, is shown along the bottom of each chart

The upper edge of the shaded area is the 98th centile line. It indicates that 98 per cent of the population is smaller and only 2 per cent is larger

This line shows the 50th centile measurement: for any age, 50 per cent of children are smaller than this measurement, and 50 per cent are larger

The lower edge of the shaded area is the 2nd centile line. It indicates that only 2 per cent of the population is smaller and 98 per cent is larger

Increase in height
Increase in height in boys slows down by the age of 16 years, as shown in this chart. Most boys reach an adult height that is 7 cm (2⅔ in) greater than the

Increase in weight
This chart illustrates the sharp increase in boys' weight that occurs between 12 and 16 years, at the growth spurt of puberty. In younger boys, weight increases steadily but less dramatically.

MEASURING YOUR CHILD

These illustrations show you how to measure your child's height and head circumference. If your child is too small to be weighed accurately on bathroom scales, measure him or her on the special infants' scales at the clinic. If you want to weigh an older child using domestic bathroom scales, ensure that they are accurate or have been recently calibrated. Keep a written record of the actual measurements and the dates on which they were taken. They may be an invaluable record of your child's physical development.

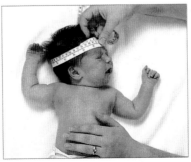

Measuring a child's head circumference
Wrap a paper or plastic tape measure around the largest part of the head, from a point midway between the hairline and eyebrows at the front to the bony protuberance at the back.

Measuring a child's height
Stand your child, in bare feet, against a wall or door. Lower a book, with the spine against the wall, or a cereal or similar packet, narrow side on to the wall, on to his or her head. Mark with a pencil the position where the base of the book's spine or lower edge of the packet meets the wall. Measure the distance from the floor with a metal tape measure that can be locked to ensure that an accurate reading is taken.

BOYS' GROWTH CHARTS

BOYS' HEAD CIRCUMFERENCE FROM BIRTH TO 2 YEARS

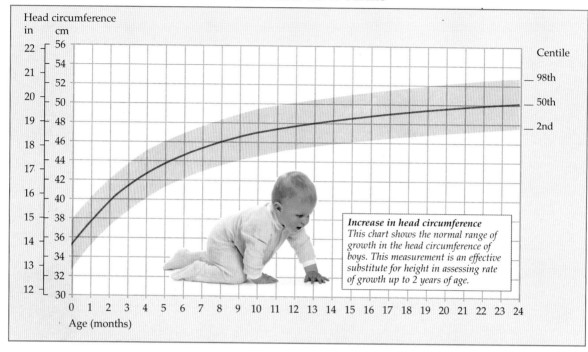

Increase in head circumference
This chart shows the normal range of growth in the head circumference of boys. This measurement is an effective substitute for height in assessing rate of growth up to 2 years of age.

BOYS' WEIGHT FROM BIRTH TO 2 YEARS

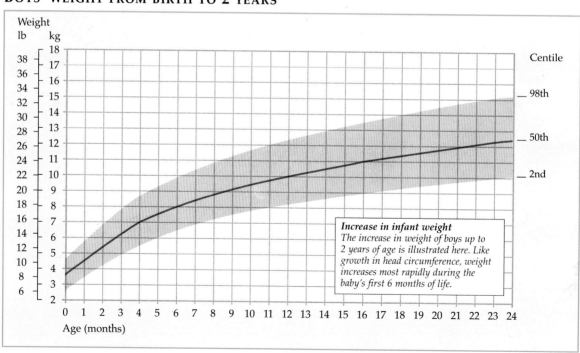

Increase in infant weight
The increase in weight of boys up to 2 years of age is illustrated here. Like growth in head circumference, weight increases most rapidly during the baby's first 6 months of life.

BOYS' HEIGHT FROM 2 TO 18 YEARS

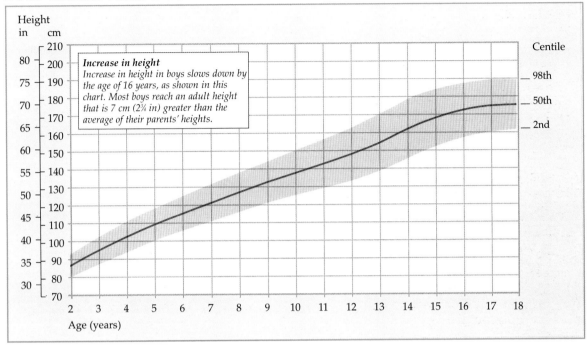

Height
in   cm

Increase in height
Increase in height in boys slows down by the age of 16 years, as shown in this chart. Most boys reach an adult height that is 7 cm (2¾ in) greater than the average of their parents' heights.

Centile
98th
50th
2nd

Age (years)

BOYS' WEIGHT FROM 2 TO 18 YEARS

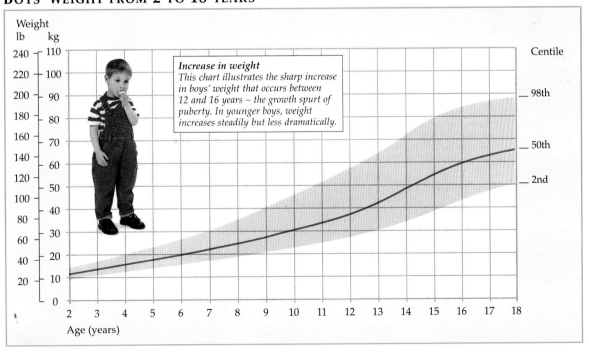

Weight
lb   kg

Increase in weight
This chart illustrates the sharp increase in boys' weight that occurs between 12 and 16 years – the growth spurt of puberty. In younger boys, weight increases steadily but less dramatically.

Centile
98th
50th
2nd

Age (years)

GIRLS' GROWTH CHARTS

GIRLS' HEAD CIRCUMFERENCE FROM BIRTH TO 2 YEARS

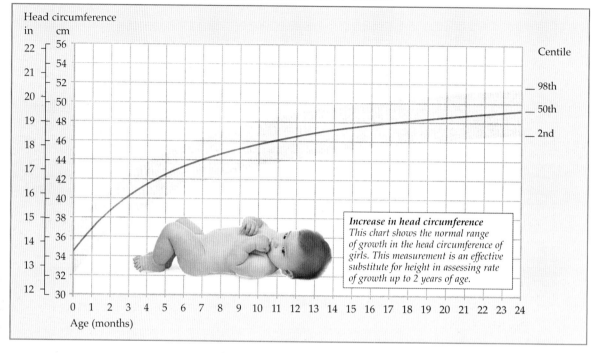

Increase in head circumference
This chart shows the normal range of growth in the head circumference of girls. This measurement is an effective substitute for height in assessing rate of growth up to 2 years of age.

GIRLS' WEIGHT FROM BIRTH TO 2 YEARS

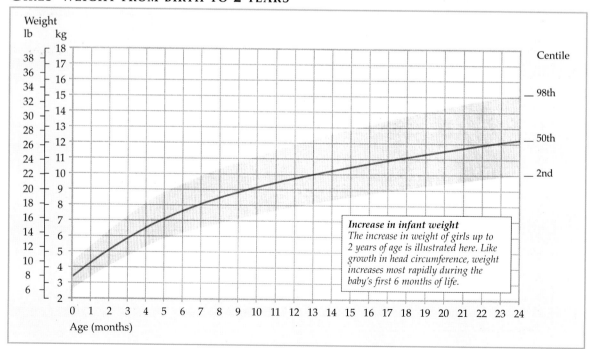

Increase in infant weight
The increase in weight of girls up to 2 years of age is illustrated here. Like growth in head circumference, weight increases most rapidly during the baby's first 6 months of life.

GIRLS' HEIGHT FROM 2 TO 18 YEARS

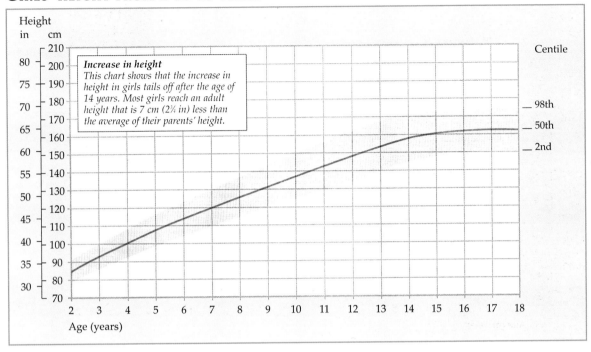

Height
in   cm

Centile

— 98th

— 50th

— 2nd

Increase in height
This chart shows that the increase in
height in girls tails off after the age of
14 years. Most girls reach an adult
height that is 7 cm (2¾ in) less than
the average of their parents' height.

Age (years)

GIRLS' WEIGHT FROM 2 TO 18 YEARS

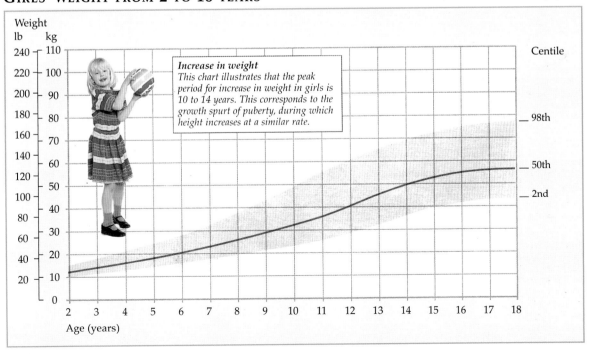

Weight
lb   kg

Centile

— 98th

— 50th

— 2nd

Increase in weight
This chart illustrates that the peak
period for increase in weight in girls is
10 to 14 years. This corresponds to the
growth spurt of puberty, during which
height increases at a similar rate.

Age (years)

THE NEWBORN BABY

A newborn baby is not merely a passive bundle of reflexes and random movements. From birth, a baby is aware of sights, sounds, smells, and touch; in fact, an infant only a few hours old can recognize a human face and his or her mother's smell, and reacts to loud, sudden noise and the gentle tones of a human voice. All babies are very responsive to touch and various touch reflexes are present from birth. A newborn baby is a highly receptive human being full of potential.

APPEARANCE OF THE NEWBORN BABY

At birth, many babies have a number of blemishes or irregularities, which, while perfectly normal, may cause the parents some concern. Examples of these peculiarities are: an asymmetrical or lumpy head; puffy, sticky eyes; drooping eyelids; squint; wrinkled, hairy, red, and greasy skin; dry and peeling skin on hands and feet; spots and small areas of discoloured skin; yellow skin, caused by jaundice; and disproportionately large genitals in both boys and girls. Most of these disappear in a few weeks.

Rarely, however, there may be a more serious problem, such as an infection, which requires treatment (see INFANT PROBLEMS, p.31).

Newborn peculiarities
All newborn babies have numerous variations in appearance, many of which are caused by the process of birth and the transition from a sterile, liquid environment to air. Although parents may be alarmed by the apparent imperfections in their child, most of these have gone within a few weeks.

Asymmetrical head

Puffy, sticky eyes

Wrinkled, greasy skin

Peeling skin on hand

Red patch on skin

Peeling skin on foot

Enlarged genitals

BEHAVIOUR OF THE NEWBORN BABY

A baby's behaviour in the newborn period is designed to maximize the chances of survival; it ensures that the baby's basic needs – food, cleanliness, warmth, affection, stimulation, and protection – are met. Some of the reflexes present at birth, for example the rooting and sucking reflexes (see opposite), are concerned with feeding. Others, such as the startle reflex, are relics of a more primitive past and these disappear after a few weeks. All the reflexes are eventually replaced by voluntary, controlled movements and actions as the baby's muscles and nervous system mature.

From the moment of birth, a baby communicates by crying. Over the first few weeks of life you will begin to distinguish the different types of crying caused, for example, by hunger, pain, or tiredness.

Gradually, a pattern of behaviour emerges and your baby becomes a more predictable individual.

LOCOMOTION REFLEXES

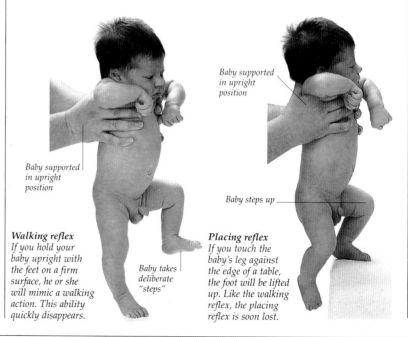

Baby supported in upright position

Baby supported in upright position

Baby steps up

Baby takes deliberate "steps"

Walking reflex
If you hold your baby upright with the feet on a firm surface, he or she will mimic a walking action. This ability quickly disappears.

Placing reflex
If you touch the baby's leg against the edge of a table, the foot will be lifted up. Like the walking reflex, the placing reflex is soon lost.

SURVIVAL REFLEXES

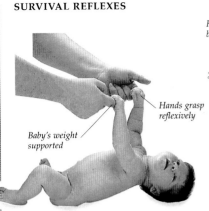

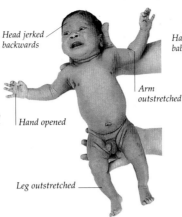

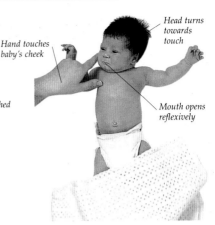

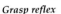

Baby's weight supported

Hands grasp reflexively

Head jerked backwards

Hand opened

Arm outstretched

Leg outstretched

Hand touches baby's cheek

Head turns towards touch

Mouth opens reflexively

Grasp reflex
If you touch your baby's palm with your finger, his or her hand will close around it. The clenched fist is surprisingly strong and it can even support the baby's entire body weight. This ability, soon lost, is probably a remnant from our evolutionary past.

Startle (or Moro) reflex
Whenever your baby is startled or feels that he or she might fall or be dropped, a violent reaction ensues. The arms are flung out as if clutching for support, the hands open wide, and the head jerks back. This reflex sometimes indicates incorrect handling of your baby.

Rooting and sucking reflex
If you stroke or touch your baby's cheek, he or she will turn towards you with an open mouth. Placing a finger, nipple, or teat in your baby's mouth will elicit sucking. This behaviour is a combination of the most basic reflexes that allows the newborn baby to feed.

STIMULATION OF THE NEWBORN BABY

Visual and auditory stimulation is essential for the normal development of sight and hearing. The eye-to-eye contact between mother and baby provides the infant's first means of communication; even a few days after birth an infant may mimic gestures, such as tongue protrusion, mouth opening, and head movements. Talk to your baby at every opportunity, and you will eventually be rewarded with gurgles and smiles.

The newborn baby can see clearly objects that are at a distance of about 20–25 cm (8–10 in). Arrangements of lines and shapes can be discriminated from a young age. It has been observed that newborn babies prefer patterns to bright, solid colours, and stripes and angles to circular patterns. Exposure to such visual stimuli can be increased by providing pictures and toys at the optimum distance for focusing.

Physical contact is also essential for healthy development. A newborn baby is accustomed to the noise and feel of a heartbeat and the motion of walking. A baby who is carried in a sling during early life will be less fretful than one who does not have such close physical contact with a parent.

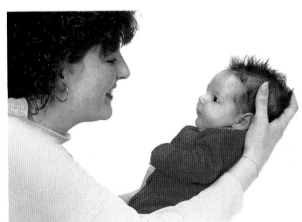

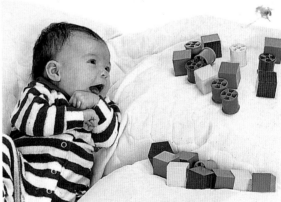

Early communication
Your face will prove irresistible to your baby and eye-to-eye contact is an essential part of the bonding process, which, like stimulation, is essential for healthy physical and emotional development. Talking and singing to your baby will elicit a range of responses, such as movements of the head and sticking out the tongue, and he or she will stop feeding or crying if you speak in a soothing voice. Close physical contact while caring for your baby helps to strengthen bonding.

A stimulating environment
Although your newborn baby will spend most of the day asleep, the waking hours provide many opportunities for stimulation. A mobile hanging within focusing range provides an excellent form of visual stimulation. In your baby's cot or pram, you can place pictures of faces or abstract patterns cut out of magazines for your baby to focus on. Musical toys may calm your baby while you are out of sight. Such early stimulation will help the brain and nervous system to develop.

DEVELOPMENTAL MILESTONES

The ages at which children acquire various physical, mental, and social skills vary from one child to another. The chart below shows when the main skills, or developmental milestones, are achieved. The abilities appear in a specific order that depends on the maturation of the nervous system and the acquisition of preceding skills. Failure to achieve an individual skill in the time span shown on the chart is not in itself a cause for concern.

Your child's development can be assessed using the chart below. The chart can be used in two ways. First, you can check the normal age range for the acquisition of a particular ability. To do this, find the skill in the chart; the red rule indicates the range of ages at which the ability is usually

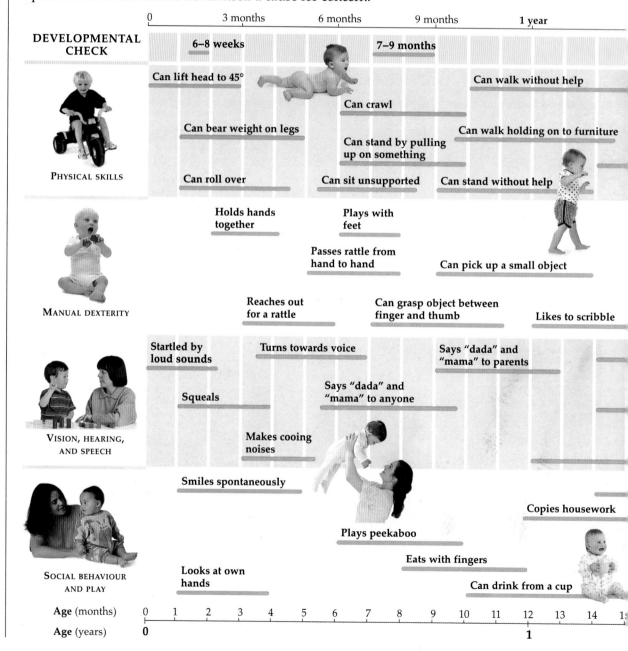

DEVELOPMENTAL CHECK

6–8 weeks

7–9 months

PHYSICAL SKILLS

Can lift head to 45°

Can crawl

Can bear weight on legs

Can stand by pulling up on something

Can roll over

Can sit unsupported

Can walk without help

Can walk holding on to furniture

Can stand without help

MANUAL DEXTERITY

Holds hands together

Plays with feet

Passes rattle from hand to hand

Can pick up a small object

Reaches out for a rattle

Can grasp object between finger and thumb

Likes to scribble

VISION, HEARING, AND SPEECH

Startled by loud sounds

Turns towards voice

Says "dada" and "mama" to parents

Squeals

Says "dada" and "mama" to anyone

Makes cooing noises

Smiles spontaneously

SOCIAL BEHAVIOUR AND PLAY

Copies housework

Plays peekaboo

Eats with fingers

Looks at own hands

Can drink from a cup

Age (months)	0	1	2	3	4	5	6	7	8	9	10	11	12	13	14	15
Age (years)	0												1			

Chart timeline top: 0 | 3 months | 6 months | 9 months | 1 year acquired. For example, the majority of babies learn to stand unaided between the ages of 9 and 14 months.

Alternatively, the chart can be used to determine the range of skills that might be expected of a baby or child of a particular age. Find your child's age along the bottom of the chart. Then follow that age up the grid to discover which rules cross or end just to the left of that age. For example, in terms of physical skills, a 4-month-old baby can probably lift his or her head, roll over, and support body weight on his or her legs. A 2-year-old child's verbal skills typically include putting two words together and being able to identify parts of the body by pointing at them.

Although all children acquire skills in much the same order, occasionally a stage is missed out; for example, children may walk without having learned to crawl. At certain ages up to 5 years, your doctor should carry out developmental checks on your child (see top of chart). These checks provide good opportunities to discuss any general or specific concerns you may have about your child's development. As well as assessing the acquisition of skills, the doctor will test your child's sight and hearing, and also check his or her height and weight.

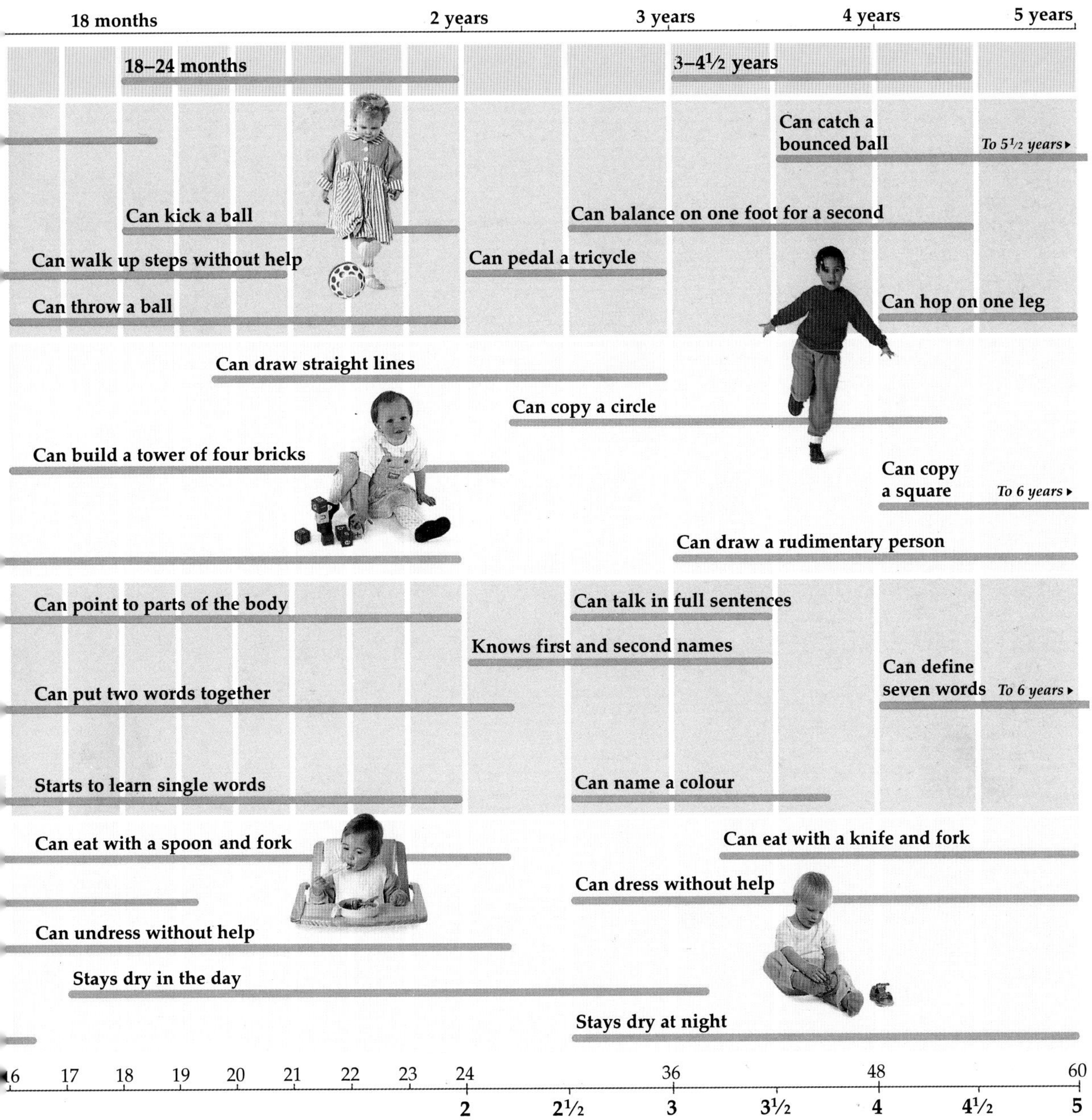

18 months	2 years	3 years	4 years	5 years

18–24 months

3–4½ years

Can catch a bounced ball   *To 5½ years ▶*

Can kick a ball

Can balance on one foot for a second

Can walk up steps without help

Can pedal a tricycle

Can throw a ball

Can hop on one leg

Can draw straight lines

Can copy a circle

Can build a tower of four bricks

Can copy a square   *To 6 years ▶*

Can draw a rudimentary person

Can point to parts of the body

Can talk in full sentences

Knows first and second names

Can put two words together

Can define seven words   *To 6 years ▶*

Starts to learn single words

Can name a colour

Can eat with a spoon and fork

Can eat with a knife and fork

Can dress without help

Can undress without help

Stays dry in the day

Stays dry at night

16	17	18	19	20	21	22	23	24		36		48		60
								2	2½	3	3½	4	4½	5

25

ADOLESCENT DEVELOPMENT

Adolescence marks the change from childhood to adulthood – usually considered the age of 18. The physical changes (puberty) begin in boys at an average age of 12 years, when the testes begin to grow, and in girls at an average age of 11½ years, when the breasts start to develop. Puberty is initiated by hormones, produced by the pituitary and adrenal glands, which stimulate the secretion of oestrogen in girls and testosterone in boys. These hormones trigger the physical changes, such as increase in height and weight (known as the growth spurt), and also the emotional changes. The age at which puberty starts varies but there is no need for concern unless it is before 8 years or after 14 in girls or before 9 years or after 15 in boys.

EMOTIONAL DEVELOPMENT

Adolescence can be a difficult time for both youngsters and parents. It is a period of testing in which your child will try to establish and redefine a sense of identity, both within and outside the family unit. An adolescent may demand independence that is inappropriate for the teenage years. He or she may behave in a manner that is contrary to guidelines and values instilled in childhood, and may seem overly confrontational and critical of you and other adults.

Your child's emotional development will not proceed at the same rate as physical development. Adolescents who look grown up and demand adult privileges may still be emotionally immature, confused, and lacking in confidence. It is important that adults do not have unreasonable expectations of adolescents during this time. The period of maturation should not be viewed too negatively because it is an essential part of growing up and most adolescents turn into responsible adults.

PHYSICAL CHANGES IN GIRLS

The growth spurt may begin before there are any other signs of physical development. During growth in height, breast buds and pubic hair appear, followed by underarm hair and sweat glands. Menstruation begins between 11 and 14 years, and ovulation follows at varying times afterwards.

PHYSICAL CHANGES IN BOYS

The growth spurt in boys occurs later than in girls. The first sign of puberty is enlargement of the testes; darkening of the scrotum, appearance of pubic hair, and lengthening of the penis follow. Body hair appears next and the voice deepens when the growth spurt is well established.

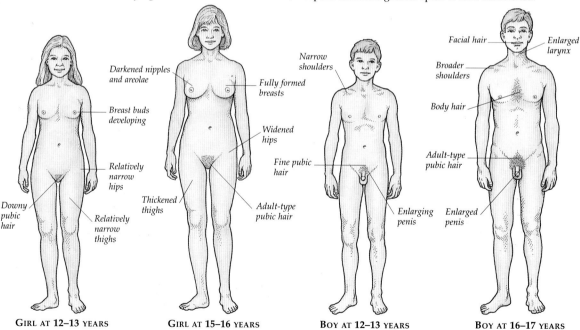

Darkened nipples and areolae

Breast buds developing

Relatively narrow hips

Downy pubic hair

Relatively narrow thighs

Fully formed breasts

Widened hips

Thickened thighs

Adult-type pubic hair

Narrow shoulders

Fine pubic hair

Enlarging penis

Facial hair

Enlarged larynx

Broader shoulders

Body hair

Adult-type pubic hair

Enlarged penis

GIRL AT **12–13** YEARS   GIRL AT **15–16** YEARS   BOY AT **12–13** YEARS   BOY AT **16–17** YEARS

Stages of development in girls
In girls, puberty is heralded by emerging breast buds and growth of downy pubic hair. By 15 or 16 years, a girl will have reached adult proportions, with wider hips, fat deposits in the abdomen and thighs, fully developed breasts, and adult-type pubic and underarm hair.

Stages of development in boys
In early puberty, the testes and scrotum start to enlarge. By the age of about 17 years, a boy's penis will have reached its maximum size and hair will have grown under the arms and on the face, legs, chest, and abdomen. The voice deepens as the larynx and vocal cords enlarge.

HEALTHY LIVING

THE FOUNDATIONS OF A HEALTHY LIFE are laid down in childhood by sensible eating, immunization against the major childhood illnesses, and taking precautions against accidents at home, school, and on the road. Adequate mental and physical stimulation is also essential. Breast-feeding provides the ideal balance of nutrients for the best start in life. When weaning your baby, you should use fresh foods, keeping sugary, salty, and fried foods to a minimum.

To grow and develop normally, your child needs a safe environment. You can help to achieve this by removing hazards, teaching your child to recognize and avoid danger, and ensuring that supervision is at hand.

INFANT FEEDING

How you decide to feed your baby is your choice entirely. Breast-feeding has many advantages over bottle-feeding: human milk provides the correct proportion of nutrients for a growing infant and antibodies to boost the immune system. However, some women cannot or choose not to breast-feed, and for their babies formula milk in a bottle is an acceptable alternative.

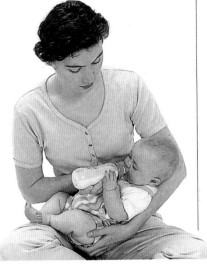

Bottle-feeding your baby
With your baby cradled in one arm, use the other to hold the bottle firmly and at an angle so that no air is allowed to enter the teat and milk is delivered at a constant rate.

BREAST-FEEDING

If you decide to breast-feed, you can be sure you are giving your baby the best start in life. Breast milk contains the right proportions of nutrients essential for early growth and development; it is also readily available, easily digested, virtually sterile, cheap, comes at the right temperature, and contains the mother's antibodies, which offer some protection against disease. Breast-feeding can be a very rewarding experience for both mother and baby.

Some women experience problems, particularly when trying to establish breast-feeding, but with perseverance, help, and time, such early difficulties can usually be overcome. Common problems are latching-on difficulty, engorged or infected breasts or sore nipples, and inadequate milk supply (see FEEDING PROBLEMS, p.32).

Breast-feeding works by supply and demand, so the more a baby sucks, the more milk is produced. After the first few days of feeding, a pattern will emerge that ensures the baby receives enough milk. Supplementary bottles can upset this balance and should only be given with advice from a professional; if your baby's hunger is satisfied by a bottle, your breasts will not receive the stimulation they need to produce sufficient milk.

To maintain a good supply of milk, you should eat a well-balanced diet and drink plenty of fluids. Ensure that the extra energy you need in order to feed your baby is obtained from healthy foods, such as fruit, vegetables, and dairy products, rather than sugary carbohydrates.

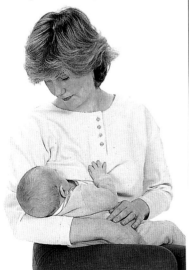

Breast-feeding your baby
Sitting in a comfortable upright position, you should maintain eye contact as your baby feeds. This is part of the bonding process.

BOTTLE-FEEDING

Bottle-feeding has the advantage of being less physically demanding on the mother; also, other adults can help with feeds. There may be different FEEDING PROBLEMS (p.32), including intolerance to the protein in cow's milk (see FOOD INTOLERANCE, p.182).

Different makes of milk formula are available, although all are of similar composition. Infants who are allergic to cow's milk can be given an alternative.

Boiled water should always be used for mixing feeds and manufacturer's instructions regarding proportions of powder to water must be followed strictly. All bottles, teats, and other feeding equipment should be sterilized before every use to prevent infection.

WEANING

Weaning is the gradual transition from a diet of milk to mixed feeding. Before the age of 4 months, milk provides all of the nutrients required by a baby. Between 4 and 6 months your baby's digestive system will have developed sufficiently to cope with more complex food and there will be signs, such as still being hungry after a feed or demanding more frequent feeds, that he or she is ready to be weaned.

FIRST FOODS

Weaning your baby off milk on to solid food is a gradual process that can take 3 or 4 months or longer to complete. Some babies take to solids immediately while others are fussy and take longer to adapt. The chart (below) is one way to approach weaning but this can be adapted to suit your needs and your way of life. There are no hard and fast rules about when to start, how long the process should take, or which foods to offer; more important is a positive and flexible attitude.

During the first few weeks that you are weaning your baby, your job is to introduce the idea of solid food and eating from a spoon. Your baby will not be receiving any nourishment from the small amount of food you offer in the initial stages.

Choose a time to start when both you and your baby are relaxed. Often, lunchtime is the best time of day to introduce solids. Your baby may be more willing to try something new then than at breakfast, when hunger may be acute, or teatime, when he or she may be tired. Start with half a milk feed; with your baby still on your lap, offer a spoon of food, then more milk.

Baby rice or puréed vegetables or fruit (not citrus) are the best foods to start with because they are unlikely to cause an adverse reaction. If your child rejects a food or develops diarrhoea, vomiting, or a rash avoid the food for a few weeks. Gradually reduce milk intake and use only formula or breast milk until your baby is 1 year old.

HEALTHY WEANING

It is important to wean your baby on to the healthy foods you would like him or her to eat when older. Try to offer home-prepared foods using fresh ingredients. Avoid adding salt to your cooking. Sugary foods, such as rusks and sweet biscuits, should be restricted to avoid obesity and DENTAL CARIES (p.177) later in life. Try to vary the tastes and textures you offer so that your baby samples a wide range of different foods; this may prevent your baby growing into a fussy eater.

SUGGESTED WEANING SCHEDULE					
STAGE	EARLY MORNING/ THROUGHOUT DAY	BREAKFAST	LUNCH	TEA	BEDTIME
Weeks 1–2	Milk feed. Offer cooled, boiled water outside mealtimes.	Milk feed.	Half a milk feed. Then 1 to 2 teaspoons of baby cereal mixed with milk, or vegetable or fruit purée. Rest of milk feed.	Milk feed.	Milk feed.
Weeks 3–4	Milk feed. Offer cooled, boiled water outside mealtimes.	1 teaspoon of gluten-free cereal. Give milk feed before, during, or after cereal.	3 to 4 teaspoons of baby cereal, vegetable, or fruit purée. Give milk feed before, during, or after solids.	Milk feed.	Milk feed.
Weeks 5–6	No early milk feed. Offer cooled, boiled water or diluted fruit juice outside mealtimes.	1 to 2 teaspoons of cereal. Give milk feed before, during, or after cereal.	2 to 3 teaspoons of a protein (puréed cheese, vegetable, fish, or meat), then 2 to 3 teaspoons of a sweet. Give milk feed before, during, or after solids.	1 to 2 teaspoons of baby cereal, vegetable, or fruit purée. Give milk feed before, during, or after solids.	Milk feed.
Weeks 7–8	Offer non-milk drinks in a beaker. Your baby's food can be mashed.	5 to 6 dessertspoons of cereal. Give milk feed before, during, or after cereal.	2 to 3 dessertspoons of a protein followed by the same amount of a sweet (yoghurt or mashed fruit). Half a milk feed.	A protein followed by a sweet. Give milk feed before, during, or after solids.	Milk feed.
Weeks 9–10	Offer non-milk drinks in a beaker.	Cereal, with the milk feed given before, during, or after.	A protein followed by a sweet. Offer milk in a beaker.	A protein followed by a sweet. Half a milk feed.	Milk feed.
Week 11 onwards	Your baby should drink about ½ litre (1 pint) of milk each day.	Cereal and milk feed. From 13 weeks, milk at breakfast can be given in a beaker.	A protein followed by a sweet. Offer milk in a beaker.	A protein followed by a sweet. Milk in a beaker.	Milk feed.

HEALTHY EATING

By the time your child is 1 year old, he or she should have tried a wide variety of foods. At this stage, definite likes and dislikes in food are common and you may worry that the diet is lacking in variety and nutritional value. You can encourage healthy eating by offering nutritious meals made from fresh ingredients. Processed and convenience foods are not inherently unhealthy provided they are not always given in preference to fresh foods. Sensible eating habits established in childhood will improve your child's chance of a healthy life.

NUTRIENT REQUIREMENTS

Children need more food than adults in proportion to their size because they are more active and need fuel for growth. Food intake peaks in the teenage years – a time of great physical growth and bodily change. Over the age of 5 years, the recommended daily energy requirements should come from the following sources: carbohydrates, 50 per cent; fats, 35 per cent; proteins, 15 per cent. In younger children, fats should not be restricted to adult levels since they provide energy in a more concentrated form than carbohydrates.

Energy requirements
This chart compares daily energy intake for boys and girls of different ages. Over the age of 5 years, most energy should come from starchy foods, such as bread, rice, and pasta.

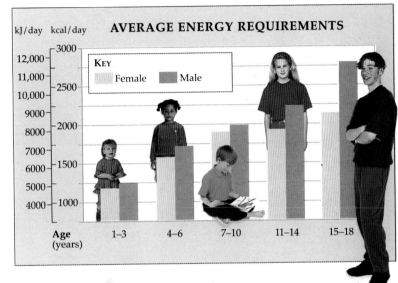

AVERAGE ENERGY REQUIREMENTS

KEY
☐ Female ■ Male

kJ/day: 4000, 5000, 6000, 7000, 8000, 9000, 10,000, 11,000, 12,000
kcal/day: 1000, 1500, 2000, 2500, 3000

Age (years): 1–3, 4–6, 7–10, 11–14, 15–18

A BALANCED DIET

You can provide your child with a healthy diet and encourage sensible eating by following a few basic rules. Offer food from the main food groups in the following ratio: six servings of starchy foods, five of fruit or vegetables, and four of protein foods – two of dairy products (milk included) and two of non-dairy protein foods – each day. Aim for variety within each group, such as different vegetables each day. Keep sugary and fried foods to a minimum. Vitamins and minerals are provided by a balanced diet but if your child is a fussy eater, a supplement may be required.

The food pyramid
A simple guide to the nutrients required each day is illustrated by the food pyramid, which shows sample foods from each food group. Even though your child's activity levels and requirements for growth may vary, the ratio of food from each of the main groups should remain approximately the same. Starchy foods, fruit, and vegetables should be the main components. A small portion of a protein food – fish, lean meat, eggs, and milk or other dairy products – should be eaten daily. Sugary and fried foods are not an essential food group and their intake should be kept as low as possible.

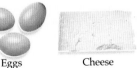

Sugar   Oil
SUGARY AND FRIED FOODS

Eggs   Cheese   Tuna
DAIRY AND OTHER PROTEIN FOODS

Banana   Strawberries   Broccoli   Apple   Sweetcorn
FRUIT AND VEGETABLES

Cornflakes   Rice   Bread   Potatoes   Pasta   Wholegrain cereal
STARCHY FOODS

SAFETY AND HEALTH

Although it is not possible to protect your child from every accident or illness, you can take certain precautions to reduce the possibility of a serious illness or life-threatening emergency. Immunization is very effective at preventing a number of childhood diseases, such as measles and pertussis. Protection from sunlight is particularly important since a child's skin is very susceptible to burning, which can lead to skin cancer in adulthood. Use a high-factor sun cream and make sure that your child wears a hat and other protective clothing; exposure to the sun should be increased gradually day by day. Choking in a small child can be avoided if you make sure that nuts and toys with small parts are kept out of reach. Keep all hazardous items, including plastic bags, medicines, and garden and household chemicals, locked away. Teach your child what to do in the event of a fire and install smoke detectors in every room.

IMMUNIZATION

Certain infectious diseases can be prevented by having your child vaccinated according to the schedule below. Serious adverse reactions to vaccines are extremely rare but you should talk to your doctor if you are concerned.

AGE	DISEASE
2 months	Diphtheria, pertussis, and tetanus (DPT), polio, Hib*
3 months	Diphtheria, pertussis, and tetanus (DPT), polio, Hib*
4 months	Diphtheria, pertussis, and tetanus (DPT), polio, Hib*
12–18 months	Measles, mumps, rubella (MMR)
3–5 years	Diphtheria, tetanus, polio, MMR
10–14 years	Rubella (girls only): to be phased out
13 years	Tuberculosis (BCG)
15–19 years	Diphtheria, tetanus, polio boosters

* Hib: *Haemophilus influenzae* type b, a bacterium that can cause meningitis.

PREVENTING ACCIDENTS

Between the ages of 1 and 15 years, more children are killed by accidents than by illness. Many accidents can be prevented if you follow certain safety procedures, such as teaching your child how to avoid danger on the road and in the playground and by keeping your home as hazard-free as possible.

Road traffic accidents are responsible for the majority of deaths. Approved restraints in the car are essential for the prevention of death or serious injury in the event of an accident.

Children are naturally curious. Even the home environment contains many potential sources of danger, such as electric sockets and wires, razors, glass doors, open windows, baths, garden ponds or swimming pools, and DIY home and garden equipment.

As your child grows up, the safety requirements will change; for example, a toddler must be protected from stairs and sharp table corners while an older child needs to be taught about bicycle and road safety.

Storing medicines
Medicines should be stored in child-proof containers out of your child's reach, preferably in a locked medicine cabinet. Prescribed drugs should not be kept beyond the course of an illness nor over-the-counter drugs after their expiry date. Always discard drugs in a place where they will not be accessible to your child.

Safety in the kitchen
Burns and scalds are the main causes of accidental death in the home. Teach your child to stay away from the cooker. A hob guard minimizes the chance of a young child knocking over a hot pan. Handles should point towards the centre or back of the hob. Always keep noxious household chemicals locked away.

Safety in the garden
There are many substances in the garden that are harmful if swallowed. Remove poisonous species, such as fungi or yew. Always store garden chemicals in a locked cupboard or shed. You should warn your child not to eat leaves or berries but if accidental ingestion occurs, see FIRST AID: Swallowed poisons *(p.211).*

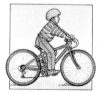

Safety in the playground
Teach your child to play safely. Only allow him or her to use a slide that is on a soft surface, such as grass. Roundabouts are a potential source of danger as hands and feet can get caught underneath. Swings should be used only by the age group for which they were designed, and by only one child at a time.

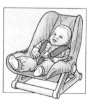

Riding a bicycle
When your child is riding a bicycle, make sure that he or she wears a protective helmet and fluorescent clothing and reflectors to make him or her easily visible. Children under the age of 14 or 15 years should not cycle in traffic or at night. Ensure that the bicycle is maintained in good working order.

Safety in the car
A baby of less than 10 kg (22 lb) should travel in a rear-facing car seat, strapped into the front or back seat of the car. However, never put a child in the front seat if the car has air bags. Toddlers weighing less than 18 kg (40 lb) should use a moulded car seat and older children should have a booster seat in the back.

INFANT PROBLEMS

MANY INFANTS – NEWBORN AND OLDER – have irregularities in appearance and behaviour patterns that may concern the parents. A squint or skin discoloration, such as birthmarks, are common in newborn babies and usually disappear in time without treatment. Many difficulties that affect older infants, such as feeding and sleeping problems, can be solved by the parents themselves using self-help measures.

THE NEWBORN BABY

A newborn baby must adapt quickly to a world dramatically different from the uterus out of which he or she has emerged. Many body systems, such as the respiratory and digestive systems, are not fully functional when the baby is born, and take minutes, days, months, or even years to mature.

SKIN PROBLEMS

Many minor problems characteristic of newborn babies affect the skin, and most disappear without treatment.

Birthmarks rarely cause discomfort, but they may be unsightly. Among the most common birthmarks are port-wine stain and strawberry naevus. A port-wine stain, which is flat and purplish red, does not disappear but it can often be covered with a cream or may be reduced by laser treatment.

A strawberry naevus grows rapidly over the first few weeks. Treatment is not required unless it is on an eyelid; most disappear by the age of 7 years.

For the first few days after birth, babies are unable to excrete wastes efficiently; this causes a build-up of yellow pigment in the skin (jaundice). Many newborn babies have a mild form of jaundice that usually clears up without treatment. Some babies require light treatment, also called phototherapy.

OTHER PROBLEMS

Newborn babies may have other minor problems, such as an umbilical HERNIA (p.187), SQUINT (p.166), or infections. Most disappear spontaneously.

An umbilical hernia forms when a gap in the muscles of the abdominal wall allows a loop of intestine to bulge out near the navel. The hernia usually disappears before the age of 2 years.

Babies often appear cross-eyed because eye muscle control is poor. A persistent problem or one existing after the age of 4 months may need treatment.

During birth, infections such as ORAL THRUSH (p.176) or CONJUNCTIVITIS (p.165), may be picked up from the mother. Other minor infections of the mouth, eyes, skin, and navel are also common in the first few weeks of life.

SOME MINOR PROBLEMS OF THE NEWBORN BABY

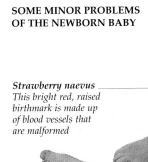

Port-wine stain
This purple-red area does not usually fade but it can be concealed with a special cream or reduced by laser

Sticky eye
Mild conjunctivitis in a newborn baby may be caused by a blocked tear duct or by bacteria in the birth canal

Strawberry naevus
This bright red, raised birthmark is made up of blood vessels that are malformed

Urticaria
Unlike urticaria in older children, this type of rash disappears in the first week of life

Jaundice
Yellow skin is caused by a build-up of pigment as the immature liver is unable to excrete wastes at a fast enough rate

Sucking blisters
Vigorous sucking from the breast or bottle can cause one or more large blisters to appear on the upper lip

Milia
Small white spots that occur mainly around the nose, these clear up without any special treatment

THE OLDER INFANT

Infants commonly suffer from a range of minor problems, which include teething, feeding problems, and sleeping difficulties. Although most of these problems disappear as the baby grows older, they can cause considerable anxiety and tension in both parents, particularly if several problems occur simultaneously. For most of these problems there are self-help measures that may alleviate them. However, if the difficulties cannot be cured by self-help alone, it is important to seek professional advice before resentment or feelings of inadequacy set in.

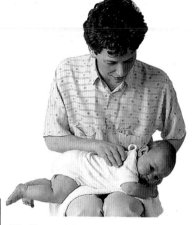

Winding position
After every feed, move your baby into another position so that any swallowed air will be released from the stomach.

FEEDING PROBLEMS

Before a baby is weaned (see p.28), the most common type of feeding problem is the mother's anxiety about whether the baby is getting enough milk. If you are bottle-feeding, it is easy to measure how much milk is being taken, but with breast-feeding this is difficult and you have to rely on the baby's weight gain as a gauge of intake. If you are worried about this aspect of feeding, you should discuss it with your health visitor or doctor.

With bottle-feeding it is important to make up the feeds correctly to avoid overfeeding or underfeeding your baby. Check the size of the teat opening: one that is too large can cause wind and one that is too small will make feeding difficult. Feeding equipment must always be sterilized to protect against infection, such as gastroenteritis.

A few feeding problems and possible solutions are shown in the chart below.

WIND

Whether your baby is breast-fed or bottle-fed, wind is distressing and may prevent an adequate intake of nutrients because your baby's stomach will feel full and feeding will stop. During and after a feed you should help your baby to bring up any air that has been taken in with the milk. The best way to wind your baby is to move him or her from a feeding to a sitting position or to an upright position against your shoulder. Laying your baby stomach-down on your lap also releases wind. Rubbing your baby's back at the same time provides comfort and reassurance.

COLIC

Infants between the ages of about 2 weeks and 3 months are commonly affected by a type of inconsolable crying known as colic. Your baby may

BREAST-FEEDING PROBLEMS

PROBLEM	SOLUTION	PROBLEM	SOLUTION
Mastitis (infected, blocked milk duct)	Continue to breast-feed. Get medical advice within 24 hours.	Latching-on difficulty	Ensure baby takes nipple and areola into mouth. If breasts are full, express a little milk.
Sore nipples	Ensure baby latches on correctly. Prevent breasts from becoming overfull. Keep nipples dry. Use a nipple cream.	"Evening colic"	Offer more frequent feeds in the evening. Try to rest during the day to avoid becoming overtired in the evening.
Engorged breasts	Feed frequently. Express milk if baby is not ready to feed. Place warm flannels on breasts.	Inadequate milk supply	Eat a healthy diet (800 kcal / 3,345 kJ a day more than usual). Do not get overtired. Offer a feed when your baby wants one.

BOTTLE-FEEDING PROBLEMS

PROBLEM	SOLUTION
Infection	Always sterilize all feeding equipment. Wash hands before giving feeds. Store made-up milk in refrigerator. Throw away any milk after a feed.
Overfeeding	Never add more powder or less water than the instructions recommend. Never add cereal to feeds.
Teat opening too small	Use a sterilized needle or knife to make a bigger opening in teat.

draw up his or her legs as if in extreme pain and become very red in the face. A common cause is failure to bring up wind that enters the stomach during feeding or crying, with the result that air passes into the small intestine and causes pain and excessive contractions.

In "evening colic", the baby cries as if in great pain for a few hours in the early evening. This condition tends to affect breast-fed babies mainly and hunger may be a contributing factor. Even if it is not long since you last fed your baby, it is worth offering another feed. If you breast-feed, your milk supply may be reduced in the evening when you are tired and your baby will need to feed more often; tension, such as that caused by the baby's incessant crying, may further reduce the milk and perpetuate the problem.

Rocking or walking with your baby, going for a ride in the car, or rubbing his or her abdomen, may calm and comfort your baby temporarily. If you are breast-feeding, try to rest during the day so that your evening milk supply is plentiful. Although many products are available that claim to alleviate evening colic, no medical evidence supports these claims.

FAILURE TO THRIVE

Gaining insufficient weight according to the standardized baby growth charts (see pp.17–21) is called failure to thrive. However, most babies who put on weight slowly are perfectly healthy and you should not be anxious if your baby is putting on weight slowly. A mother's expectations about weight gain may be unrealistic and not take into account factors such as birth weight or parental size.

You should attend a baby clinic or doctor's surgery on a regular basis to have your baby weighed so that the actual weight change can be plotted and monitored by an expert. If it is established that your baby's weight gain is abnormal, the doctor will look for a physical cause, such as feeding problems or MALABSORPTION (p.183) or an emotional or social problem.

TEETHING

You can expect your baby's first teeth to appear around the age of 6 months and the last of the primary teeth to come through by about 3 years (see DEVELOPMENT OF TEETH, p.14). The incisors often arrive with little upset to the baby but eruption of the canines and molars can cause considerable discomfort. The first signs of teething are dribbling, redness of the gum at the site of the new tooth, and a flushed cheek; your baby will probably be fretful and may have problems feeding. Some babies are helped by biting on a hard object, such as a rusk or teething ring. Liquid paracetamol can be given to relieve the pain.

You should not attribute symptoms such as fever or diarrhoea to teething since there is no medical evidence of any connection.

SLEEPING PROBLEMS

Like adults, babies vary widely in sleep requirements so do not conclude that there is a problem if your infant sleeps less or more than another baby of the same age. Sleeping problems include not settling at bedtime to waking in the night, or not sleeping during the day. A sleep pattern only becomes a problem if it is unduly disruptive to the parents or child.

By the age of 3 or 4 months, most babies no longer need frequent night feeds and may not wake up at night. If your baby wakes and cries, wait a little while before responding. Establish a routine with a consistent bedtime and a definite order of events leading up to this, such as a bath and a feed.

Temporary sleeping problems often occur with illness or any disruption to the routine, such as a weekend away.

Teething aids
Various hard or cold objects, such as rusks or teething rings, can sometimes ease the pain and distress caused by teething.

FLEXIBLE TEETHING RING   **SUGAR-FREE RUSKS**

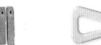

TEETHING BISCUITS   **COOLED TEETHING RING**

PREVENTION OF SUDDEN INFANT DEATH

Although sudden infant death is very rare, it is important to follow the latest guidelines for prevention. These are:
- Put your baby to sleep on his or her back.
- Do not smoke; keep your baby out of smoky atmospheres.
- Do not let your baby get too warm (see below).
- Put your baby at the foot of the cot so that he or she cannot wriggle under the covers.
- Contact your doctor if you think your baby is unwell.

Temperature and bedding
This diagram shows the amount of bedding that is required for a range of room temperatures in order to keep your baby's body temperature at the optimum level.

ROOM	°C	°F	BEDDING
	27	80	*Sheet only*
Too hot	24	75	*Sheet + 1 blanket**
	21	70	*Sheet + 2 blankets**
Just right	18	65	*Sheet + 3 blankets**
	15	60	
Too cold	13	55	*Sheet + 4 blankets**
	10	50	

*A double layer of blankets counts as two blankets.

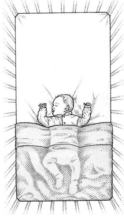

Correct sleeping position
A baby should sleep on his or her back, with the feet at the bottom of the cot.

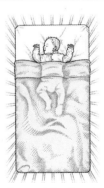

Incorrect sleeping position
A baby put to sleep at the head of the cot is at risk of moving down under the covers and either overheating or suffocating.

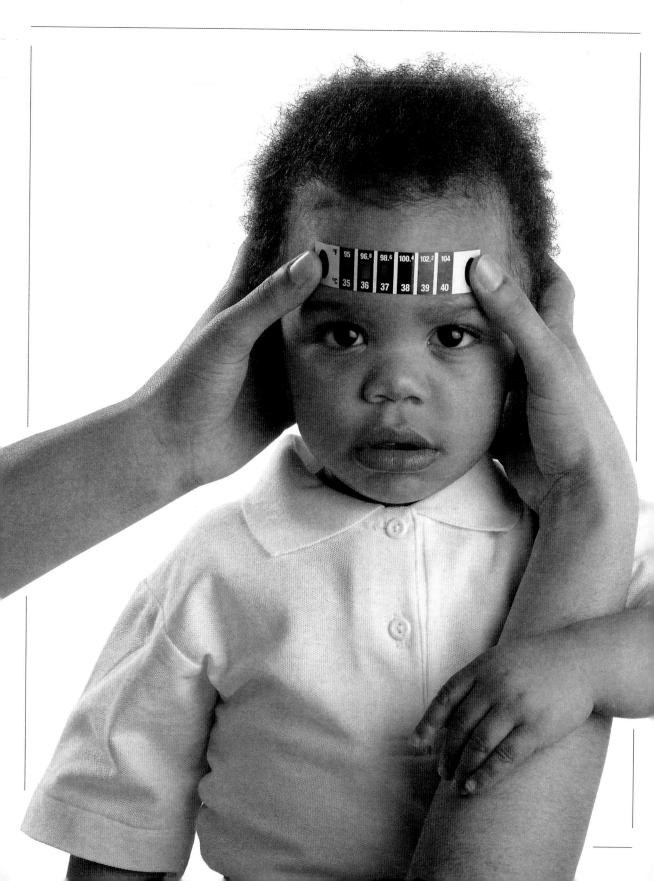

SYMPTOM CHARTS

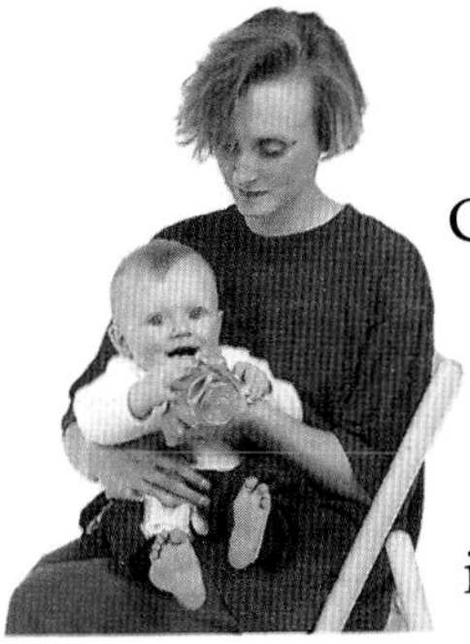

BOTTLE-FEEDING A BABY

CHILDREN OFTEN SUFFER from minor ailments, most of which are not serious and disappear within a few days. Sometimes, however, a symptom might indicate a more serious problem. The charts in this section aim to help parents and other carers decide whether a child's symptom or set of symptoms require medical assessment and, if so, the urgency with which a diagnosis should be sought. By following the questions and answers you will arrive at one or more possible causes of your child's symptoms. The causes refer you to DISEASES AND DISORDERS (p.116) where the problems are discussed in greater detail. Also included are measures that can be taken at home to help relieve the symptoms. For instructions on using the charts, see HOW TO USE THE CHARTS (p.9).

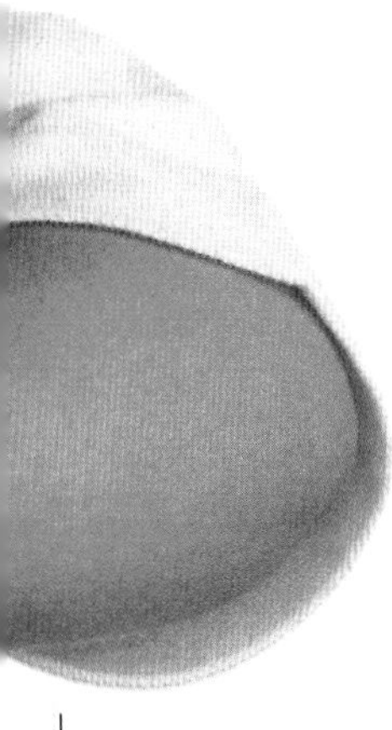

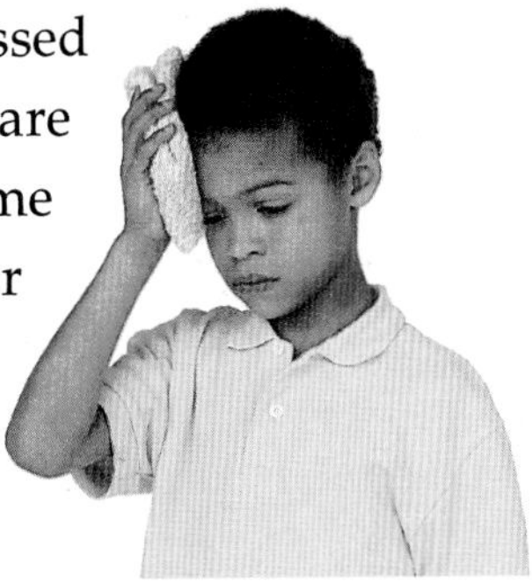

RELIEF FOR A HEADACHE

1 FEVER IN INFANTS

For children over 1 year, see chart 8

Fever is a raised temperature; it is usually caused by infection. If your baby feels hot or seems listless or unusually irritable, take his or her temperature (see NURSING A SICK CHILD, p.212). Normal body temperature is between 36°C (97°F) and 37°C (99°F); a temperature of 38°C (100°F) or above is a fever.

DANGER SIGNS
Phone your doctor at once if your baby has any of the following symptoms:
- Temperature above 39°C (102°F).
- Abnormally rapid breathing.
- Noisy or difficult breathing.
- Abnormal drowsiness.
- Unusual irritability.
- Refusing to drink for over 6 hours.

START HERE

How old is your baby?
- UNDER 6 MONTHS
- 6 MONTHS OR OVER

Does your baby have a rash?
- RASH
- NO RASH

Go to chart
22 RASH WITH FEVER

POSSIBLE CAUSE
Fever in babies younger than 6 months is unusual; it may indicate a serious illness.

ACTION NEEDED
MEDICAL HELP
✚ URGENT! Phone your doctor immediately!

SELF-HELP
See panel: *Bringing down a high temperature* (opposite).

Does your baby cry and pull at one ear or wake up screaming?
- CRIES AND PULLS AT ONE EAR
- WAKES IN THE NIGHT SCREAMING
- NEITHER

POSSIBLE CAUSE
OTITIS MEDIA (p. 162).

ACTION NEEDED
MEDICAL HELP
Get medical advice within 24 hours.

SELF-HELP
See panels: *Bringing down a high temperature* (opposite) and *Relieving earache* (p.101).

POSSIBLE CAUSES
A COMMON COLD (p.148), or possibly INFLUENZA (p.151) or MEASLES (p.118).

ACTION NEEDED
MEDICAL HELP
If there is no improvement within 48 hours, or if breathing problems develop or a rash appears, phone your doctor immediately.

POSSIBLE CAUSES
PNEUMONIA (p.155) or BRONCHIOLITIS (p.155).

ACTION NEEDED
MEDICAL HELP
✚ URGENT! Phone your doctor immediately!

SELF-HELP
See panel: *Bringing down a high temperature* (opposite).

Is your baby's breathing rate normal (see panel: *Checking breathing rates*, p.90)?
- NORMAL
- FASTER THAN NORMAL

Does your baby have a cough or a runny nose?
- COUGH OR A RUNNY NOSE
- NEITHER

POSSIBLE CAUSES

ROSEOLA INFANTUM (p.121) or MENINGITIS (p.158).

ACTION NEEDED

MEDICAL HELP
✚ URGENT! Phone your doctor immediately!

POSSIBLE CAUSES

A throat infection, such as tonsillitis (see PHARYNGITIS AND TONSILLITIS, p.151) or a mouth infection, such as GINGIVOSTOMATITIS (p.176).

ACTION NEEDED

MEDICAL HELP
If there is no improvement within 24 hours, phone your doctor immediately.

SELF-HELP
See panels: *Relieving a sore throat* (p.91) and *Bringing down a high temperature* (below).

POSSIBLE CAUSE

GASTROENTERITIS (p.180).

ACTION NEEDED

MEDICAL HELP
Get medical advice within 24 hours.

SELF-HELP
See panel: *Preventing dehydration in babies* (p.38).

POSSIBLE CAUSE

Your baby may have become overheated.

ACTION NEEDED

SELF-HELP
A baby does not usually need to be much more warmly dressed than an adult in a similar environment. If you think overheating might be the problem, remove some of your baby's clothing and reduce the room temperature. If your baby's temperature is not normal within 1 hour, or if your baby exhibits any of the DANGER SIGNS (opposite), consult your doctor.

Is your baby suffering from any of the following symptoms?

- VOMITING WITHOUT DIARRHOEA
- ABNORMAL DROWSINESS
- UNUSUAL IRRITABILITY
- NONE OF THE ABOVE

Does your baby have either of the following symptoms?

- RELUCTANCE TO EAT SOLID FOOD
- VOMITING WITH DIARRHOEA
- NEITHER

Is your baby wearing a lot of clothing or is the room very warm?

- WARM CLOTHING
- WARM ROOM
- NEITHER

SELF-HELP: BRINGING DOWN A HIGH TEMPERATURE

Reducing a high temperature makes a child feel more comfortable, and decreases the possibility of FEBRILE CONVULSIONS (p.156) in children of 3 months to 5 years old. The following steps may be taken to lower a temperature in a child of any age:

- Take off most of your child's clothes and remove any sheets and blankets if your child is in bed.
- Sponge your child with lukewarm water or place him or her in a lukewarm bath.
- Give liquid paracetamol if your child is over 3 months old.
- Maintain the temperature of your child's room at about 15°C (60°F).
- Use a fan to cool your child.

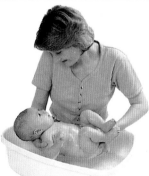

Cooling your child
You can bring down your child's temperature by putting him or her in a bath of lukewarm water.

If you cannot identify your baby's problem from this chart, talk to your doctor within 24 hours.

2 DIARRHOEA IN INFANTS

For children over 1 year, see chart 9

Diarrhoea is the passage of runny faeces more frequently than normal. However, babies who are entirely breast-fed pass semi-fluid faeces that should not be confused with diarrhoea. Any baby who has diarrhoea must be given plenty of fluids in order to prevent dehydration.

DANGER SIGNS

Phone your doctor at once if your baby has any of the following symptoms:
- Vomiting for 6 hours.
- Sunken fontanelle.
- Passing very small amounts of dark, concentrated urine.
- Sunken eyes.
- Loose skin.
- Abnormal drowsiness or irritability.

START HERE

Does your baby have a fever – a temperature of 38°C (100°F) or above?

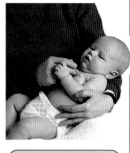

- **FEVER**
- **NO FEVER**

POSSIBLE CAUSE

GASTROENTERITIS (p.180),

ACTION NEEDED

MEDICAL HELP
Get medical advice within 24 hours.

SELF-HELP
See panels: *Preventing dehydration in babies* (below) and *Bringing down a high temperature* (p.37).

How long has the diarrhoea lasted?

- **2 WEEKS OR MORE**
- **LESS THAN 2 WEEKS**

Has your baby had any of the following symptoms in the past few days?

- **VOMITING**
- **POOR FEEDING**
- **LETHARGY**
- **NONE OF THE ABOVE**

SELF-HELP: PREVENTING DEHYDRATION IN BABIES

If your baby is in danger of becoming dehydrated – a condition that might result from persistent diarrhoea, a fever, or vomiting – it is important to give extra fluids. The best form in which to give your baby extra fluids is as an oral electrolyte rehydrating solution, such as Dioralyte or Rehidrat, which can be purchased without a prescription. If a rehydrating solution is not available, you can prepare a rehydrating solution by dissolving 2 level teaspoons of sugar in 200 ml (7 fl.oz) of cooled, boiled water.

All babies should receive between 500 and 1500 ml (18 and 53 fl.oz) per day; the exact amount varies according to the baby's weight. The table (right) is a guide to the amount of fluid your baby should be given each day. For the duration of your baby's symptoms, make sure that he or she drinks small amounts of the rehydrating solution every 2 to 3 hours.

If your baby is vomiting, you should give him or her a smaller amount of fluid every hour as larger amounts may just be vomited back.

BABY'S WEIGHT		DAILY FLUID INTAKE	
kg	lb	ml	fl.oz
Under 4	Under 9	500	18
4	9	600	21
5	11	750	26
6	13	900	32
7	15	1050	37
8	18	1200	42
9	20	1350	48
Over 10	Over 22	1500	53

Daily fluid intake requirements
To prevent dehydration, follow the chart above to determine the appropriate daily fluid intake for your baby.

POSSIBLE CAUSES

Persistent diarrhoea in infants most often occurs after, or as a complication of, a viral infection. Other possible causes include FOOD INTOLERANCE (p.182), GIARDIASIS (p.187), COELIAC DISEASE (p.183), and CYSTIC FIBROSIS (p.201), but these disorders are much less common.

ACTION NEEDED

MEDICAL HELP
Make an appointment to see your doctor.

SELF-HELP
See panel: *Preventing dehydration in babies* (opposite).

POSSIBLE CAUSE

GASTROENTERITIS (p.180).

ACTION NEEDED

MEDICAL HELP
Get medical advice within 24 hours.

SELF-HELP
See panel: *Preventing dehydration in babies* (opposite).

Have you been giving your baby prescribed medicine for any other disorder?

- NO MEDICINE
- MEDICINE

Is the amount of fruit juice or squash in your baby's diet more or less than usual?

- MORE THAN USUAL
- LESS THAN USUAL
- NO CHANGE

POSSIBLE CAUSE

New foods may cause diarrhoea.

ACTION NEEDED

MEDICAL HELP
Such episodes are usually short-lived. However, if your baby's diarrhoea persists or if the diarrhoea seems to be associated with particular foods, make an appointment to see your doctor.

SELF-HELP
Make sure your baby does not become dehydrated (see panel: *Preventing dehydration in babies*, opposite). If you can identify the food that is causing your baby's diarrhoea, stop offering the food until you have seen your doctor.

POSSIBLE CAUSE

Your baby's diarrhoea could possibly be a side effect of the medicine that he or she is taking.

ACTION NEEDED

MEDICAL HELP
Phone your doctor to find out whether the medicine may be causing your baby's symptoms and whether you should stop giving it.

POSSIBLE CAUSE

In large quantities, the sugar in fruit juice or squash can lead to diarrhoea.

ACTION NEEDED

SELF-HELP
Always mix fruit juice with an equal quantity of cooled, boiled water. Try giving your baby cooled, boiled water instead of fruit juice. Avoid giving squash.

When was a new solid introduced into your baby's diet?

- LESS THAN 24 HOURS AGO
- MORE THAN 24 HOURS AGO
- BABY HAS NOT YET BEEN WEANED

POSSIBLE CAUSES

FOOD INTOLERANCE (p.182) or mild GASTROENTERITIS (p.180).

ACTION NEEDED

MEDICAL HELP
Get medical advice within 24 hours.

SELF-HELP
Stop offering any solid food to your baby until you have seen your doctor. Make sure, however, that your baby does not become dehydrated by giving plenty of liquids (see panel: *Preventing dehydration in babies*, opposite).

3 VOMITING IN INFANTS

For children over 1 year, see chart 10

In young babies, it is important not to confuse vomiting, which might indicate an illness, with posseting, which is the effortless regurgitation of small amounts of milk. However, a single episode of vomiting is common in infants and is unlikely to have a serious cause.

DANGER SIGNS
Phone your doctor at once if your baby has any of the following symptoms:
• Vomiting for 6 hours.
• Sunken fontanelle.
• Passing very small amounts of dark, concentrated urine.
• Sunken eyes.
• Loose skin.
• Abnormal drowsiness or irritability.

START HERE

Does your baby seem well and is he or she taking feeds normally?

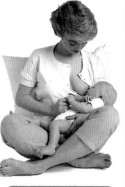

SEEMS WELL AND IS FEEDING NORMALLY

SEEMS UNWELL OR IS NOT FEEDING NORMALLY

Was milk brought up effortlessly?

NO

YES

How much milk did your baby bring up?

LARGE AMOUNT

SMALL AMOUNT

POSSIBLE CAUSE

GASTRO-OESOPHAGEAL REFLUX (p.186).

ACTION NEEDED

MEDICAL HELP
Get medical advice within 24 hours.

POSSIBLE CAUSE

PYLORIC STENOSIS (p.186).

ACTION NEEDED

MEDICAL HELP
Get medical advice within 24 hours.

How old is your baby?

UNDER 2 MONTHS

2 MONTHS OR OVER

When does your baby vomit?

AFTER EVERY FEED

AT UNPREDICTABLE TIMES

Does your baby have a fever – a temperature of 38°C (100°F) or above?

FEVER

NO FEVER

POSSIBLE CAUSE

Posseting (regurgitation) is the most likely cause. It is usually due to wind and is seldom serious.

ACTION NEEDED

SELF-HELP
See panel: *Dealing with wind* (p.47).

POSSIBLE CAUSES

ROSEOLA INFANTUM (p.121) or MENINGITIS (p.158).

ACTION NEEDED

MEDICAL HELP
✚ URGENT! Phone your doctor immediately!

POSSIBLE CAUSES

BRONCHIOLITIS (p.155) or PERTUSSIS (p.123).

ACTION NEEDED

MEDICAL HELP
Get medical advice within 24 hours.

SELF-HELP
See panels: *Bringing down a high temperature* (p.37) and *Relieving a cough* (p.90).

Does your baby have any of the following symptoms?

- ABNORMAL DROWSINESS
- REFUSING TO EAT OR DRINK
- DIARRHOEA
- COUGH
- NONE OF THE ABOVE

POSSIBLE CAUSE

GASTROENTERITIS (p.180).

ACTION NEEDED

MEDICAL HELP
✚ URGENT! Phone your doctor immediately!

SELF-HELP
See panel: *Preventing dehydration in babies* (p.38).

POSSIBLE CAUSE

GASTROENTERITIS (p.180).

ACTION NEEDED

MEDICAL HELP
✚ URGENT! Phone your doctor immediately!

SELF-HELP
See panel: *Preventing dehydration in babies* (p.38).

Go to chart
1 FEVER IN INFANTS

POSSIBLE CAUSES

BRONCHIOLITIS (p.155) or PERTUSSIS (p.123).

ACTION NEEDED

MEDICAL HELP
Get medical advice within 24 hours.

SELF-HELP
See panels: *Bringing down a high temperature* (p.37) and *Relieving a cough* (p.90).

Does your baby have any of the following symptoms?

- DIARRHOEA
- COUGH
- GREENISH-YELLOW VOMIT
- NONE OF THE ABOVE

POSSIBLE CAUSE

INTESTINAL OBSTRUCTION (p.185).

ACTION NEEDED

MEDICAL HELP
✚ EMERGENCY! Call an ambulance! While waiting, do not give your baby anything to eat or drink.

If your baby has vomited only once and otherwise seems quite well, he or she is unlikely to be seriously ill. However, if your baby vomits again or if any other symptoms develop, talk to your doctor.

4 FEEDING PROBLEMS

For children over 1 year, see chart 11

Problems with feeding can be distressing for the parents and the child. Breast-feeding problems are common, especially in the first few weeks after birth. However, if your baby is gaining weight at the expected rate and otherwise seems well, there is usually no need to be concerned.

START HERE

Does your baby seem willing to feed?
- WILLING
- UNWILLING

How is your baby fed?
- MAINLY BREAST-FED
- MAINLY BOTTLE-FED
- HAS STARTED ON SOLIDS

Does your baby feed more often than other babies?
- ABOUT THE SAME
- MORE OFTEN

POSSIBLE CAUSE

Frequent feeding, as often as once every 2 hours, is normal in breast-fed babies, particularly in the first few weeks of life (see INFANT FEEDING, p.27).

ACTION NEEDED

SELF-HELP
Even though your baby is probably well, you may be tired yourself. Have a break from night-time feeds by expressing breast milk for your partner to feed to your baby. If you are depressed or irritable, consult your doctor.

Was your baby previously eager to feed?
- PREVIOUSLY EAGER
- NOT PREVIOUSLY EAGER

POSSIBLE CAUSES

Suddenly refusing to feed may be a sign of a COMMON COLD (p.148), but it could be caused by a more serious illness.

ACTION NEEDED

MEDICAL HELP
✚ URGENT! Phone your doctor immediately!

Is your baby gaining weight normally (see GROWTH CHARTS, pp.17–21)?
- GAINING WEIGHT NORMALLY
- NOT GAINING WEIGHT NORMALLY

POSSIBLE CAUSE

Some babies need to be coaxed to feed and may even fall asleep while feeding. If your baby seems well, there is no cause for concern.

ACTION NEEDED

MEDICAL HELP
If other symptoms develop, make an appointment to see your doctor.

POSSIBLE CAUSE

FAILURE TO THRIVE (p.33).

ACTION NEEDED

MEDICAL HELP
Make an appointment to see your doctor.

Are you worried that you are not producing sufficient milk for your baby?

WORRIED

NOT WORRIED

Is your baby gaining weight normally (see GROWTH CHARTS, pp.17–21)?

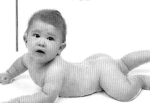

NOT GAINING WEIGHT NORMALLY

GAINING WEIGHT NORMALLY

POSSIBLE CAUSE

FAILURE TO THRIVE (p.33).

ACTION NEEDED

MEDICAL HELP
Make an appointment to see your doctor.

POSSIBLE CAUSE

Mothers quite commonly feel that they are not producing sufficient milk if their baby cries a lot and seems difficult to satisfy. However, if your baby is gaining weight at the normal rate, there is no doubt that he or she is receiving enough milk.

ACTION NEEDED

MEDICAL HELP
If your baby continues to cry and you are concerned, consult your doctor.
See also chart 6, EXCESSIVE CRYING.

Does your baby often cry during or after a feed?

CRIES AT THE BEGINNING OF A FEED

CRIES AFTER A FEED

DOES NOT CRY

Go to chart
6 EXCESSIVE CRYING

POSSIBLE CAUSE

The breasts may not release milk immediately, or the flow may be too forceful.

ACTION NEEDED

SELF-HELP
If milk is not released at once, try to be more relaxed when you feed your baby. If the flow is too forceful, express some milk before your baby starts to feed.

If you cannot identify your baby's problem from this chart, talk to your doctor within 48 hours.

POSSIBLE CAUSE

Children have strong likes and dislikes in food from a very young age. Unfamiliar foods and textures may be rejected and even foods that were accepted initially may later be refused.

ACTION NEEDED

SELF-HELP
During your baby's first year, food and eating are new experiences. If he or she rejects foods, appears not to be interested, or likes only sweet foods, continue to offer a varied diet so that your baby has the best chance of receiving sufficient healthy nutrients (see WEANING, p.28).

Does your baby often cry after he or she has had a feed?

DOES NOT CRY

CRIES

Go to chart
6 EXCESSIVE CRYING

Does your baby often reject certain foods that you offer?

REJECTS CERTAIN FOODS

EATS MOST FOODS READILY

If you cannot identify your baby's problem from this chart, talk to your doctor within 48 hours.

5 SLOW WEIGHT GAIN

For growth problems in children over 1 year, see chart 12

A close check can be kept on your baby's weight gain by regular attendance at a baby clinic and by using the charts on pp.17–21. If you are concerned about your baby's failure to put on weight as expected and there is no obvious reason for it, you should consult this symptom chart.

START HERE

How is your baby's general health?

- SEEMS UNWELL
- IS ALERT AND FEEDING NORMALLY

POSSIBLE CAUSE

An underlying disorder may be responsible for your baby's failure to gain weight normally (see FAILURE TO THRIVE, p.33).

ACTION NEEDED

MEDICAL HELP
Make an appointment to see your doctor.

How do you decide when to feed your baby?

- FEED WHENEVER BABY CRIES
- FEED ACCORDING TO A ROUTINE

POSSIBLE CAUSE

Insufficient milk may be responsible for your baby's failure to gain weight normally.

ACTION NEEDED

MEDICAL HELP
If your baby does not start to put on weight normally within 2 weeks, make an appointment to see your health visitor or doctor.

SELF-HELP
Offer your baby a feed when he or she cries, rather than according to a strict routine (see INFANT FEEDING, p.27 and FEEDING PROBLEMS, p.32).

How is your baby being fed?

- MAINLY BREAST-FED
- MAINLY BOTTLE-FED
- HAS STARTED ON SOLIDS

POSSIBLE CAUSE

You may be giving your baby foods that do not meet all his or her nutritional needs.

ACTION NEEDED

MEDICAL HELP
Talk to your health visitor or doctor, who may recommend that you adjust your baby's diet (see also WEANING, p.28).

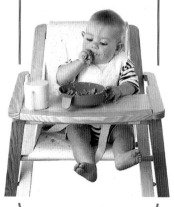

How do you decide when to feed your baby?

- FEED ACCORDING TO A ROUTINE
- FEED WHENEVER BABY CRIES

POSSIBLE CAUSE

You may not be producing enough milk to provide your baby with all the nutrients he or she needs. If your baby is over 3 months old, he or she may be ready to start on solids.

ACTION NEEDED

MEDICAL HELP
Talk to your health visitor or doctor, who may recommend that you offer supplementary bottles to your baby or start him or her on solids (see WEANING, p.28).

Does your baby always finish the entire contents of the bottle?

- ALWAYS DRINKS EVERY DROP
- SOMETIMES LEAVES SOME OF THE FEED

POSSIBLE CAUSE

If feeds are too diluted, your baby may not be receiving enough nutrients.

ACTION NEEDED

MEDICAL HELP
If your baby does not start to put on weight normally within 2 weeks, make an appointment to see your health visitor or doctor.

SELF-HELP
Always follow instructions for making up feeds. You can offer additional cooled, boiled water if the weather is warm or if your baby has a fever.

POSSIBLE CAUSE

Your baby may need more food than the amount you have been offering.

ACTION NEEDED

MEDICAL HELP
If your baby does not start to put on weight normally within 2 weeks, make an appointment to see your health visitor or doctor.

SELF-HELP
Let your baby have as much milk as he or she wants. If your baby is over 3 months old, it may be time to start him or her on solids (see WEANING, p.28).

If you cannot identify your baby's problem from this chart, talk to your doctor within 48 hours.

Could you possibly be making up your baby's feeds in the wrong proportions?

- UNLIKELY
- COULD BE ADDING TOO MUCH WATER
- COULD BE ADDING TOO LITTLE MILK FORMULA

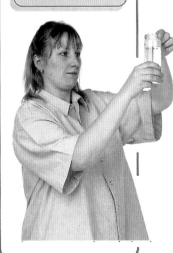

ASSESSMENT: GROWTH PATTERNS IN INFANCY

Most babies follow the standard growth curves but there may be variations that give the impression that a baby's growth is abnormal:
- If a parent is shorter than average, the baby may also be small.
- Breast-fed babies have a dramatic weight gain in their first few months, which then tails off.
- The baby of a diabetic mother is heavy at birth but then fails to gain weight for a few months.
- Premature babies appear light for their age.

A small baby
These charts show a hypothetical growth pattern for a baby whose parents are small. The starting points on both the head size and weight charts are near the bottom of the normal range. This trend continues as the baby grows older, indicating that the baby's growth, as recorded by head circumference, is in proportion to his or her weight gain.

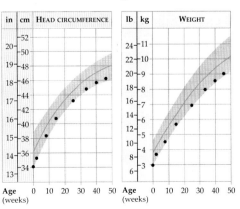

6 EXCESSIVE CRYING

All babies cry because it is the only way in which they can communicate. Crying usually indicates hunger, thirst, tiredness, or discomfort. However, if your baby's crying is inconsolable, more persistent than usual, or sounds different from normal, he or she may require medical attention.

START HERE

Is your baby crying in a way that is unusual for him or her?

UNUSUAL

NO DIFFERENT

Was your baby reluctant to take the last feed?

RELUCTANT

WILLING

POSSIBLE CAUSE

Your baby may be in pain as a result of a disorder, such as OTITIS MEDIA (p.162).

ACTION NEEDED

MEDICAL HELP
✚ URGENT! Phone your doctor immediately!

POSSIBLE CAUSES

COLIC (p.32), TEETHING (p.33), or NAPPY RASH (p.136).

ACTION NEEDED

MEDICAL HELP
If your baby develops further symptoms or is still distressed after 24 hours, make an appointment to see your doctor.

Does feeding your baby stop the crying?

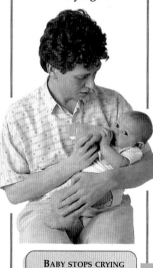

BABY STOPS CRYING

BABY CONTINUES CRYING

POSSIBLE CAUSE

Hunger is one of the most common causes of crying in a young baby.

ACTION NEEDED

SELF-HELP
If your baby stops crying after a feed, you may need to reduce the intervals between feeds to keep up with the demand.

When you burp your baby, does he or she stop crying?

CONTINUES CRYING

STOPS CRYING

Is your baby comforted by a drink of cooled, boiled water?

BABY NOT COMFORTED

BABY COMFORTED

POSSIBLE CAUSE

Thirst may be causing your baby to cry, especially if he or she is bottle-fed or if the weather is particularly hot.

ACTION NEEDED

SELF-HELP
Give your baby extra drinks of cooled, boiled water from a sterilized bottle or spoon.

**How old is
your baby?**

- UNDER 3 MONTHS
- 3 MONTHS OR OVER

**When does the
crying occur?**

- LATE AFTERNOON OR
EARLY EVENING
- AT OTHER TIMES

POSSIBLE CAUSE

Evening COLIC (p.32).

ACTION NEEDED

SELF-HELP
Feed your baby first. You can
then try to calm him or her by
rocking, by patting his or her
back, or by massaging his or
her abdomen.

**If you pick up
your baby and give
your full attention,
does this have any
effect on the crying?**

- STOPS THE CRYING
- NO EFFECT

**Has there been a
change in household
routine or increased
tension at home ?**

- CHANGE IN
HOUSEHOLD ROUTINE
- TENSION AT HOME
- NEITHER

POSSIBLE CAUSE

Your baby may be unsettled
because of the change in
routine or increased tension.

ACTION NEEDED

SELF-HELP
During a period of domestic
upheaval, give your baby
extra attention. If your own
tension could be upsetting
your baby, try to eliminate
the cause. Having more time
to yourself, using relaxation
techniques, or talking over
problems with friends or
relatives may be helpful. If
you are feeling angry or
resentful at your baby's
crying, consult your doctor.

**If you cannot identify
your baby's problem
from this chart, talk to your
doctor within 48 hours.**

POSSIBLE CAUSE

Your baby may need more
comforting and parental
reassurance than other babies
of the same age.

ACTION NEEDED

SELF-HELP
Cuddle your baby as often as
he or she wants; there is no
risk of "spoiling" your child
at such a young age.

POSSIBLE CAUSE

WIND (p.32).

ACTION NEEDED

SELF-HELP
See panel: *Dealing with
wind* (right).

SELF-HELP: DEALING WITH WIND

A baby who cries just before a feed
or who feeds greedily is likely to
swallow air, which gets trapped in
the baby's intestine and causes
discomfort. The following tips may
prevent wind from occurring or
may help to release the wind:
- Ensure that the hole in the teat is
the right size and is not blocked.
- Feed your baby in a semi-upright
position, so that the milk falls to
the bottom of the stomach.
- Try burping your baby after each
feed. Holding him or her against
your shoulder or sitting or lying
face down on your lap will
release any trapped air. Rub or
pat the back to calm your baby.

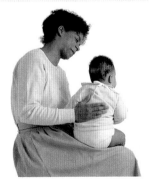

Burping position
*After every feed, put your baby into a
position such as that shown above, in
which burping is made easy.*

7 SKIN PROBLEMS IN INFANTS

For other spots and rashes, see chart 23

Young babies have very sensitive skin that can be irritated easily. Rashes confined to the nappy area are particularly common and can be distressing for your baby. If the skin inflammation or irritation is persistent or accompanied by other symptoms, your baby should be seen by a doctor.

START HERE

How old is your baby?

- UNDER 3 MONTHS
- 3 MONTHS OR OVER

Does your baby have a scaly, itchy rash in any of the following places?

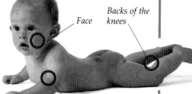

Face
Backs of the knees
Insides of the elbows

- FACE
- INSIDES OF THE ELBOWS
- BACKS OF THE KNEES
- NONE OF THE ABOVE

Does your baby have either of the following skin problems?

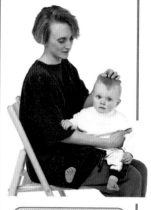

- INFLAMED, SCALY RASH
- CRUSTY YELLOW PATCHES ON SCALP
- NEITHER

POSSIBLE CAUSE

ATOPIC ECZEMA (p.135).

ACTION NEEDED

MEDICAL HELP
If the rash is extensive, very itchy, or weeping, or if it is upsetting your baby, make an appointment to see your doctor.

SELF-HELP
See panel: *Relieving itchiness* (opposite).

POSSIBLE CAUSE

NAPPY RASH (p.136).

ACTION NEEDED

MEDICAL HELP
If the rash persists for more than 10 days or if your baby's skin is broken or ulcerated, make an appointment to see your doctor.

If you cannot identify your baby's problem from this chart, talk to your doctor within 48 hours.

Is the rash in any of the following places?

NECK

BEHIND THE EARS

FACE

GROIN

ARMPITS

TWO OR MORE

ONE OR NONE

How is your baby's general health?

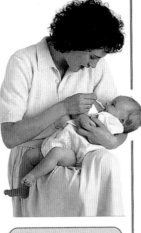

BABY IS WELL AND FEEDING NORMALLY

BABY SEEMS UNWELL WITH A FEVER

BABY SEEMS UNWELL WITHOUT A FEVER

POSSIBLE CAUSE

SEBORRHOEIC DERMATITIS (p.134).

ACTION NEEDED

MEDICAL HELP
If the rash does not clear up within a few weeks or if it is extensive or weeping, make an appointment to see your doctor.

POSSIBLE CAUSE

A minor skin irritation.

ACTION NEEDED

MEDICAL HELP
If the rash persists for more than a day or if your baby becomes generally unwell, make an appointment to see your doctor.

SELF-HELP
See panel: *Relieving itchiness* (below).

Go to chart
22 RASH WITH FEVER

Go to chart
23 SPOTS AND RASHES

POSSIBLE CAUSE

Cradle cap (see SEBORRHOEIC DERMATITIS, p.134).

ACTION NEEDED

MEDICAL HELP
If the crusts are extensive or if your baby develops any other symptoms, make an appointment to see your doctor.

Does your baby have either of the following symptoms?

INFLAMED SPOTS ON THE GENITALS OR ANUS

SPOTS OR BLOTCHES ANYWHERE ON THE BODY

NEITHER

SELF-HELP: RELIEVING ITCHINESS

Try to discourage your child from scratching since this may lead to infection. The following tips may help:

- Use a non-irritating substance, such as a water-based cream or a baby soap, for bathing. Make sure that the water is not too hot.
- If your child's skin is very dry, itchiness may be more severe. Try to keep the skin well moisturized by using an emollient, such as petroleum jelly or a water-based cream, several times a day.

Bathing a baby
You can use a mild cleanser such as baby soap or aqueous cream, or add a specially formulated oil when bathing your child.

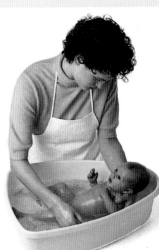

8 FEVER IN CHILDREN

For children under 1 year, see chart 1

Fever – a temperature above 38°C (100°F) – is usually an indication of viral or bacterial infection; however, fever can also be caused by overheating. If your child seems unwell, take his or her temperature and note any other symptoms that might help the doctor to make a diagnosis.

POSSIBLE CAUSE

MENINGITIS (p.158).

ACTION NEEDED

MEDICAL HELP
✚ EMERGENCY! Call an ambulance!

START HERE

Does your child have a rash?

RASH

NO RASH

Go to chart
22 RASH WITH FEVER

Does your child seem very unwell and does he or she also have any of the following symptoms?

STIFF NECK

HEADACHE

ABNORMAL DROWSINESS

UNUSUAL IRRITABILITY

NONE OF THE ABOVE

How would you describe your child's breathing?

UNUSUALLY NOISY

UNUSUALLY RAPID

NORMAL

Does your child have any of the following symptoms?

SORE THROAT OR REFUSING SOLID FOOD

COUGH

RUNNY NOSE

NONE OF THE ABOVE

POSSIBLE CAUSE

Tonsillitis (see PHARYNGITIS AND TONSILLITIS, p.151).

ACTION NEEDED

MEDICAL HELP
If your child is no better after 24 hours, consult your doctor.

SELF-HELP
See panels: *Bringing down a high temperature* (p.37) and *Relieving a sore throat* (p.91).

POSSIBLE CAUSES

A COMMON COLD (p.148) or INFLUENZA (p.151). MEASLES (p.118) is also a possibility.

ACTION NEEDED

MEDICAL HELP
If there is no improvement within 48 hours, if symptoms worsen, or if other symptoms develop, phone your doctor immediately.

SELF-HELP
See panels: *Bringing down a high temperature* (p.37) and *Relieving a cough* (p.90).

POSSIBLE CAUSES

CROUP (p.150), ASTHMA (p.153), or BRONCHITIS (p.154).

ACTION NEEDED

MEDICAL HELP
✚ URGENT! Phone your doctor immediately!

SELF-HELP
See panel: *Easing breathing in an asthma attack* (p.87).

POSSIBLE CAUSE

PNEUMONIA (p.155).

ACTION NEEDED

MEDICAL HELP
✚ URGENT! Phone your doctor immediately!

SELF-HELP
See panels: *Bringing down a high temperature* (p.37) and *Relieving a cough* (p.90).

POSSIBLE CAUSE

MUMPS (p.122).

ACTION NEEDED

MEDICAL HELP
Make an appointment to see your doctor.

SELF-HELP
See panel: *Bringing down a high temperature* (p.37).

Does your child have a swelling between the ear and the angle of the jaw on one or both sides?

- SWELLING
- NO SWELLING

Does your child have any of the following symptoms?

- PASSES URINE MORE FREQUENTLY THAN USUAL
- PAIN OR BURNING SENSATION WHEN PASSING URINE
- VOMITING WITH OR WITHOUT DIARRHOEA
- NONE OF THE ABOVE

Does your child have any of the following problems?

- EARACHE OR PULLING AT EITHER EAR
- WAKES UP SCREAMING DURING THE NIGHT
- NONE OF THE ABOVE

Has your child been outside in the sun or in a hot room for several hours?

- OUT IN THE SUN
- IN A HOT ROOM
- NEITHER

POSSIBLE CAUSE

URINARY TRACT INFECTION (p.193).

ACTION NEEDED

MEDICAL HELP
Get medical advice within 24 hours.

SELF-HELP
See panel: *Bringing down a high temperature* (p.37).

POSSIBLE CAUSE

GASTROENTERITIS (p.180).

ACTION NEEDED

MEDICAL HELP
Get medical advice within 24 hours.

SELF-HELP
See panel: *Preventing dehydration in children* (p.53).

POSSIBLE CAUSE

OTITIS MEDIA (p.162).

ACTION NEEDED

MEDICAL HELP
Get medical advice within 24 hours.

SELF-HELP
See panels: *Bringing down a high temperature* (p.37) and *Relieving earache* (p.101).

POSSIBLE CAUSE

Your child may have become overheated.

ACTION NEEDED

MEDICAL HELP
If the self-help measures do not succeed in lowering your child's temperature within 1 hour, phone your doctor immediately.

SELF-HELP
See panel: *Bringing down a high temperature* (p.37).

If you cannot identify your child's problem from this chart, phone your doctor at once.

9 DIARRHOEA IN CHILDREN

For children under 1 year, see chart 2

Frequent, loose stools are usually caused by infection and do not normally continue for more than a few days. If your child drinks plenty of clear fluids while the diarrhoea lasts, there should be no ill effects. If the diarrhoea recurs or persists for over a week, your child should see a doctor.

DANGER SIGNS
Phone your doctor at once if your child has any of the following symptoms:
- Abdominal pain for 3 hours.
- Vomiting for 12 hours.
- Refusing to drink for 6 hours.
- Sunken eyes.
- Abnormal drowsiness.
- Passing no urine for more than 6 hours during the day.

START HERE

When did the diarrhoea start?

WITHIN THE PAST 3 DAYS

OVER 3 DAYS AGO

Has your child been constipated and had diarrhoea at the same time?

CONSTIPATED

NOT CONSTIPATED

Does your child have any of the following symptoms?

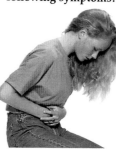

ABDOMINAL PAIN

VOMITING

FEVER

NONE OF THE ABOVE

POSSIBLE CAUSE
GASTROENTERITIS (p.180).

ACTION NEEDED
MEDICAL HELP
Get medical advice within 24 hours.

SELF-HELP
See panel: *Preventing dehydration in children* (opposite).

POSSIBLE CAUSE
Your child's diarrhoea could possibly be a side effect of the medicine he or she is taking.

ACTION NEEDED
MEDICAL HELP
Phone your doctor to find out whether the medicine may be causing your child's symptoms and whether you should stop giving it.

POSSIBLE CAUSE
Overflow soiling as a result of chronic CONSTIPATION (p.181).

ACTION NEEDED
MEDICAL HELP
Make an appointment to see your doctor.

SELF-HELP
See panel: *Preventing constipation* (p.109).

Have you been giving your child any medicine?

MEDICINE

NO MEDICINE

Did the diarrhoea start just before an exciting or stressful event or period of time?

- EXCITING EVENT OR PERIOD OF TIME
- STRESSFUL EVENT OR PERIOD OF TIME
- NEITHER

POSSIBLE CAUSE

Children may suffer from diarrhoea in response to excitement or emotional stress. The diarrhoea is likely to clear up quickly.

ACTION NEEDED

MEDICAL HELP
If the diarrhoea continues or is distressing to your child, consult your doctor.

POSSIBLE CAUSE

GASTROENTERITIS (p.180).

ACTION NEEDED

MEDICAL HELP
Get medical advice within 24 hours.

SELF-HELP
See panel: *Preventing dehydration in children* (below).

POSSIBLE CAUSE

TODDLER'S DIARRHOEA (p.181).

ACTION NEEDED

MEDICAL HELP
Make an appointment to see your doctor.

How old is your child?

- UNDER 3 YEARS
- 3 YEARS OR OVER

What are the features of your child's faeces?

- CONTAIN RECOGNIZABLE MORSELS OF FOOD
- UNIFORMLY RUNNY

SELF-HELP: PREVENTING DEHYDRATION IN CHILDREN

If your child has persistent diarrhoea or a fever, or if he or she is vomiting, it is important to give extra fluids as a prevention against dehydration. The best form in which to give your child fluids is as an oral rehydrating solution, such as Dioralyte or Rehidrat, which can be purchased without a prescription. If these solutions are not available, you can make up a rehydrating solution at home by dissolving 2 level teaspoons of sugar in 200 ml (7 fl.oz) of cooled, boiled water. Unsweetened fruit juice may be substituted for the sugar solution, but you should avoid milk for the first day.

All children should drink between 1 and 1.5 litres (35 and 53 fl.oz) per day. For the duration of the diarrhoea, make sure you offer your child some liquid or rehydrating solution every 2 to 3 hours. If your child is vomiting as well, give small sips every hour.

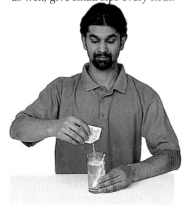

Rehydrating solution
Encourage your child to remain adequately hydrated by offering special ready-made or home-prepared fluids.

POSSIBLE CAUSES

In children, chronic (long-lasting) diarrhoea is most likely to be caused by either FOOD INTOLERANCE (p.182) or GIARDIASIS (p.187). Some other possibilities include COELIAC DISEASE (p.183) and CYSTIC FIBROSIS (p.201) but these are rare. Crohn's disease (see INFLAMMATORY BOWEL DISEASE, p.184) is a less likely cause because it is very rare for this disease to affect children under the age of about 7 years.

ACTION NEEDED

MEDICAL HELP
Make an appointment to see your doctor.

SELF-HELP
See panel: *Preventing dehydration in children* (left).

10 VOMITING IN CHILDREN

For children under 1 year, see chart 3

In children, an episode of vomiting without other symptoms is unlikely to indicate a serious disorder; it may be a result of overeating or excitement. Repeated vomiting is often caused by infection of the digestive tract, but infection anywhere else in the body can also be responsible.

DANGER SIGNS

Call an ambulance at once if your child has any of the following symptoms:
- Greenish-yellow vomit.
- Abdominal pain for 6 hours.
- Flat, pink or purple spots that do not disappear when pressed.

Phone your doctor at once if your child has any of the following symptoms:
- Vomiting for 12 hours.
- Abnormal drowsiness.
- Refusing to drink for 6 hours.
- Sunken eyes.
- Dry tongue.
- Passing no urine for more than 6 hours during the day.

START HERE

What colour is your child's vomit?
- GREENISH-YELLOW
- ANY OTHER COLOUR

Does your child have any of the following symptoms?
- DIARRHOEA
- CONTINUOUS ABDOMINAL PAIN FOR 6 HOURS
- ABNORMAL DROWSINESS
- PALE FAECES AND DARK URINE
- NONE OF THE ABOVE

POSSIBLE CAUSE

INTESTINAL OBSTRUCTION (p.185).

ACTION NEEDED

MEDICAL HELP
✚ EMERGENCY! Call an ambulance! While waiting, do not give your child anything to eat or drink.

POSSIBLE CAUSE

GASTROENTERITIS (p.180).

ACTION NEEDED

MEDICAL HELP
Get medical advice within 24 hours.

SELF-HELP
See panel: *Preventing dehydration in children (p.53).*

POSSIBLE CAUSE

APPENDICITIS (p.179).

ACTION NEEDED

MEDICAL HELP
✚ EMERGENCY! Call an ambulance! While waiting, do not give your child anything to eat or drink.

POSSIBLE CAUSE

HEPATITIS (p.188).

ACTION NEEDED

MEDICAL HELP
Get medical advice within 24 hours.

Has your child recently suffered a blow to the head?
- POSSIBLY
- UNLIKELY

Does your child have any of the following symptoms?

FEVER

PAIN ON PASSING URINE

ABDOMINAL PAIN

BEDWETTING

- ONE OR NONE
- TWO OR MORE

POSSIBLE CAUSE

HEAD INJURY (p.159).

ACTION NEEDED

MEDICAL HELP
✚ **EMERGENCY!** Call an
ambulance! While waiting, do
not give your child anything
to eat or drink.

SELF-HELP: DEALING WITH VOMITING

When your child vomits, the
following measures may help:
• Support your child's head during
  vomiting. When the vomiting has
  stopped, sponge your child's face
  and give sips of water to rinse
  out his or her mouth.
• Reassure your child, who might
  be upset or frightened.
• Make your child take small
  drinks of water or rehydrating
  solution (30 ml / 1 fl.oz) every
  hour to replace the fluids lost by
  vomiting (see panel: *Preventing
  dehydration in children*, p.53).
• Encourage your child to lie down
  and rest. Put a bowl by the bed in
  case vomiting starts again.

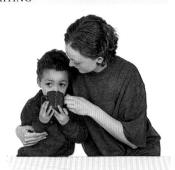

Preventing dehydration
*Encourage your child to drink plenty of
water or rehydrating solution to avoid
the danger of dehydration.*

**Does your child
have any of the
following symptoms?**

- HEADACHE
- STIFF NECK
- FLAT SPOTS THAT DO NOT DISAPPEAR WHEN PRESSED
- NONE OF THE ABOVE

If you cannot identify
your child's problem
from this chart, talk to your
doctor within 48 hours.

POSSIBLE CAUSE

MENINGITIS (p.158).

ACTION NEEDED

MEDICAL HELP
✚ **EMERGENCY!** Call an
ambulance!

**Did the vomiting
occur in any of the
following situations?**

- FOLLOWING A BOUT OF COUGHING
- BEFORE OR AFTER AN EXCITING OR STRESSFUL EVENT
- DURING A JOURNEY
- NONE OF THE ABOVE

If you cannot identify
your child's problem
from this chart, talk to your
doctor within 48 hours.

POSSIBLE CAUSE

URINARY TRACT INFECTION
(p.193).

ACTION NEEDED

MEDICAL HELP
Get medical advice within
24 hours.

SELF-HELP
See panel: *Bringing down a
high temperature* (p.37).

POSSIBLE CAUSE

PERTUSSIS (p.123).

ACTION NEEDED

MEDICAL HELP
Get medical advice within
24 hours.

SELF-HELP
See panels: *Dealing with
vomiting* (above) and *Relieving
a cough* (p.90).

POSSIBLE CAUSE

Children often vomit in
reaction to an exciting event
or to stress.

ACTION NEEDED

MEDICAL HELP
If the vomiting persists,
consult your doctor.

POSSIBLE CAUSE

Travel sickness.

ACTION NEEDED

SELF-HELP
For any journey, you can give
your child a travel sickness
remedy. In a car, try to travel
when there is little traffic.
Opening the car windows to
improve ventilation may help.

11 LOSS OF APPETITE

For children under 1 year, see chart 4

A child's appetite increases or decreases according to energy requirements and periods of growth. Provided there are no other symptoms and growth is in the normal range for your child's age (see GROWTH CHARTS, pp.17–21), you need not be concerned about any temporary loss of appetite.

START HERE

When did you notice your child's loss of appetite?

- LESS THAN A WEEK AGO
- OVER A WEEK AGO

Does your child have a fever – a temperature of 38°C (100°F) or above?

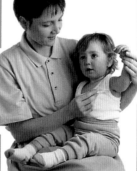

- FEVER
- NO FEVER

Go to chart
8 FEVER IN CHILDREN

Is your child gaining weight normally (see GROWTH CHARTS, pp.17–21)?

- NOT GAINING WEIGHT NORMALLY
- GAINING WEIGHT NORMALLY

POSSIBLE CAUSE

FAILURE TO THRIVE (p.33).

ACTION NEEDED

MEDICAL HELP
Make an appointment to see your doctor.

Is your child also suffering from either of the following symptoms?

- SORE THROAT
- RASH
- NEITHER

Go to chart
23 SPOTS AND RASHES

Does your child have any of the following symptoms?

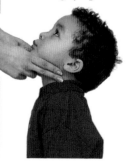

- SWOLLEN GLANDS IN THE NECK
- PALE FAECES AND DARK URINE
- NONE OF THE ABOVE

Go to chart
28 SORE THROAT

Go to chart
28 SORE THROAT

SELF-HELP: STIMULATING YOUR CHILD'S APPETITE

A child who is reluctant to eat or who has lost his or her appetite may need some encouragement.

- If the loss of appetite is caused by illness, do not force your child to eat. A sick child may only want liquids; ice cream and yoghurt will soothe a painful throat and provide some nutrients.
- If your child is very young, you can make eating fun by making pizza faces or playing an eating game like "trains" or "planes".
- Do not expect your child to eat as much as you do at mealtimes; five or six smaller meals or snacks may be more suitable for a child's immature digestive system and active metabolism.
- Try to ensure that your child eats the appropriate quantities of each food group (see HEALTHY EATING, p.29). "Junk" foods need not be dismissed provided they are not eaten on a regular basis.
- You may be able to tempt a fussy eater by offering small portions of a wide range of foods.

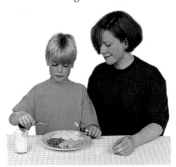

Tempting a fussy eater
Helpings of favourite foods, particularly if they are nutritious, can be offered to a fussy eater or a child who has lost his or her appetite, whatever the reason.

POSSIBLE CAUSES

Your child may be eating between meals or exercising less than usual, resulting in reduced energy requirements. As long as your child seems well otherwise, there is no cause for concern.

ACTION NEEDED

MEDICAL HELP
If your child complains of feeling ill, get medical advice within 24 hours.

SELF-HELP
See HEALTHY EATING (p.29) and panel: *Stimulating your child's appetite* (right).

POSSIBLE CAUSE

INFECTIOUS MONONUCLEOSIS (p.124).

ACTION NEEDED

MEDICAL HELP
Make an appointment to see your doctor.

POSSIBLE CAUSE

Viral HEPATITIS (p.188).

ACTION NEEDED

MEDICAL HELP
Make an appointment to see your doctor.

POSSIBLE CAUSE

URINARY TRACT INFECTION (p.193).

ACTION NEEDED

MEDICAL HELP
Get medical advice within 24 hours.

Does your child have either of the following symptoms?

- **PASSING URINE MORE FREQUENTLY**
- **BEDWETTING (AFTER BEING DRY AT NIGHT)**
- **NEITHER**

POSSIBLE CAUSES

A number of factors could cause a temporary loss of appetite. For instance, your child may be having snacks between meals or taking less exercise than usual, which results in reduced energy requirements. As long as your child seems well otherwise, there is no cause for concern.

ACTION NEEDED

MEDICAL HELP
If your child complains of feeling ill, get medical advice within 24 hours.

SELF-HELP
See HEALTHY EATING (p.29) and panel: *Stimulating your child's appetite* (above).

12 GROWTH PROBLEMS

For slow weight gain in children under 1 year, see chart 5

Some children are naturally smaller or larger than their peers, and there is wide variation in what is considered normal for height, weight, and rate of growth at any age. In most children, growth occurs in irregular spurts; if you are concerned about your child, consult the charts on pp.17–21.

START HERE

In what way does your child's growth seem abnormal?

- **INCREASE IN HEIGHT SEEMS SLOW**
- **WEIGHT GAIN IS SLOW COMPARED TO INCREASE IN HEIGHT**

Is your child's height normal for his or her age (see GROWTH CHARTS, pp.17–21)?

- **NORMAL**
- **BELOW NORMAL**

POSSIBLE CAUSES

Very short stature is usually inherited. A long illness, GROWTH HORMONE DEFICIENCY (p.189), or HYPOTHYROIDISM (p.189) are other possibilities.

ACTION NEEDED

MEDICAL HELP
Make an appointment to see your doctor.

How is your child's health in general?

- **SEEMS UNWELL OR IS NOT EATING NORMALLY**
- **SEEMS WELL AND IS EATING NORMALLY**

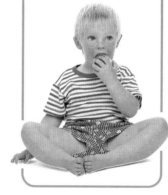

How much has your child grown in height during the last 6 months?

- **LESS THAN 2.5 CM (1 IN)**
- **2.5 CM (1 IN) OR MORE**

POSSIBLE CAUSES

Loss of appetite because of an underlying disorder such as an infection is the most likely explanation. Rarely, an inability to absorb nutrients as a result of COELIAC DISEASE (p.183), CYSTIC FIBROSIS (p.201), or Crohn's disease (see INFLAMMATORY BOWEL DISEASE, p.184) may be responsible.

ACTION NEEDED

MEDICAL HELP
Make an appointment to see your doctor.

POSSIBLE CAUSE

Slow growth during any 6-month period is not abnormal if your child seems healthy and grows normally during the next 6 months.

ACTION NEEDED

MEDICAL HELP
If your child seems unwell or grows less than 2.5 cm (1 in) during the next 6 months, make an appointment to see your doctor.

SELF-HELP
See HEALTHY EATING (p.29) and panel: *Growth patterns in childhood* (opposite).

Has your child had a prolonged illness since he or she was last measured and weighed?

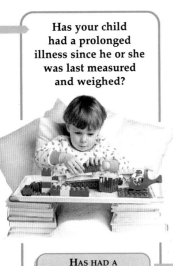

HAS HAD A PROLONGED ILLNESS

HAS BEEN GENERALLY HEALTHY

POSSIBLE CAUSE

A prolonged period of illness, particularly one in which your child is confined to bed for any length of time or has to undergo extensive hospital treatment, can interrupt normal growth.

ACTION NEEDED

MEDICAL HELP
If your child does not start to put on weight normally within the next 4 weeks, make an appointment to see your doctor.

SELF-HELP
See HEALTHY EATING (p.29) and panel: *Growth patterns in childhood* (below).

POSSIBLE CAUSE

There are certain times in all children's development when either their weight gain or their increase in height is slow. At other times they may have a growth spurt – for instance, during puberty. Such an irregular growth pattern is normal, and should not be a cause for concern.

ACTION NEEDED

MEDICAL HELP
If your child does not start to put on weight normally within the next 4 weeks, make an appointment to see your doctor.

SELF-HELP
See HEALTHY EATING (p.29) and panel: *Growth patterns in childhood* (below).

POSSIBLE CAUSE

Many children have irregular growth patterns but these rarely indicate an underlying problem. Your child may grow relatively slowly at certain times and more rapidly at others. Around puberty, both boys and girls have a growth spurt.

ACTION NEEDED

MEDICAL HELP
If your child seems unwell or grows less than 2.5 cm (1 in) during the next 6 months, make an appointment to see your doctor.

SELF-HELP
See HEALTHY EATING (p.29) and panel: *Growth patterns in childhood* (right).

ASSESSMENT: GROWTH PATTERNS IN CHILDHOOD

Although most children follow the standard growth curves (pp.17–21), there are a number of variations that may give the impression that a child is not growing normally:
• A naturally slim child may appear to gain weight slowly relative to his or her height.
• An overweight child may appear to increase relatively slowly in height compared to his or her weight gain.

• A child whose mother or father is shorter than average may grow slowly and be smaller than his or her classmates.
• An overweight toddler will grow faster in height than in weight as he or she grows older.
• An adolescent who is late reaching puberty may be shorter and lighter than his or her classmates. However, most late developers catch up eventually.

A slender child
These charts show a hypothetical growth pattern for a naturally slim, but perfectly fit and healthy, child. The points plotted for height are near the top of the curve while weight is closer to average (shown by the 50th centile line). As long as both height and weight increase in proportion, and weight gain is only slightly less than expected, you need not be concerned.

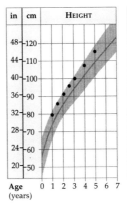
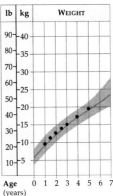

13 SPEECH PROBLEMS

When your child is learning to talk, it is normal for his or her speech to be both hesitant and repetitive. If the stammering persists or if the acquisition and use of new words is slow, there may be a physical cause. Individual variation is normal, and boys are often slower than girls at learning verbal skills.

START HERE

Does your child have any of the following speech difficulties?

- TALKS LITTLE OR NOT AT ALL
- HAS A LISP OR OTHER SPEECH DEFECT
- STAMMERS OR SPEAKS HESITANTLY
- NONE OF THE ABOVE

How old is your child?

- 2 YEARS OR OVER
- UNDER 2 YEARS

How is your child affected by the speech difficulty?

- IS EMBARRASSED
- HAS DIFFICULTY BEING UNDERSTOOD
- NEITHER

How would you describe your child's development in other areas (see DEVELOPMENTAL MILESTONES, pp.24–25)?

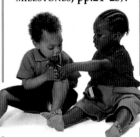

- NORMAL
- SLOWER THAN NORMAL

POSSIBLE CAUSE

Hesitancy and stammering (see SPEECH PROBLEMS, p.171) are normal in young children, and most children outgrow them within a few years.

ACTION NEEDED

MEDICAL HELP
If hesitancy and stammering persist after the age of 5 years or if they recur, make an appointment to see your doctor.

If you cannot identify your child's problem from this chart, talk to your doctor.

POSSIBLE CAUSE

Minor speech defects (see SPEECH PROBLEMS, p.171) are common and are usually outgrown.

ACTION NEEDED

MEDICAL HELP
If the speech defect affects your child's ability to communicate, or his or her performance in school, make an appointment to see your doctor.

POSSIBLE CAUSE

If the speech defect (see SPEECH PROBLEMS, p.171) is minor, it is unlikely to have any physical cause. Speech that is difficult for other people to understand may have a physical cause, such as impaired hearing.

ACTION NEEDED

MEDICAL HELP
Make an appointment to see your doctor.
See also chart 34, HEARING PROBLEMS.

How many words can your child say?

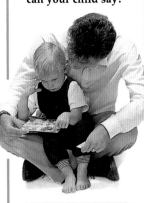

MORE THAN FIVE

FIVE OR FEWER

POSSIBLE CAUSE

Late speech development (see SPEECH PROBLEMS, p.171) is not likely to be a cause for concern if your child is developing normally in most other areas and has normal hearing.

ACTION NEEDED

MEDICAL HELP
If you are worried, make an appointment to see your doctor.

SELF-HELP
Encourage your child to talk by speaking to him or her often and by providing frequent opportunities to play with other children.

POSSIBLE CAUSES

A physical abnormality or slow mental development may affect your child's speech development.

ACTION NEEDED

MEDICAL HELP
Make an appointment to see your doctor.

SELF-HELP
Speak to your child often and and encourage him or her to respond to you. Providing frequent opportunities for your child to play with other children is also helpful.

POSSIBLE CAUSES

Delayed speech development (see SPEECH PROBLEMS, p.171) may be caused by a variety of factors, including lack of stimulation, emotional stress, impaired hearing, or slow mental development. It may also result from the normal variation in development.

ACTION NEEDED

MEDICAL HELP
Make an appointment to see your doctor.

SELF-HELP
Encourage your child to talk by speaking to him or her often and by providing frequent opportunities for your child to play with other children.

POSSIBLE CAUSE

A child who is reluctant to speak but is capable of pronouncing words clearly and using them meaningfully is unlikely to have a physical defect that affects either speaking or hearing (see SPEECH PROBLEMS, p.171). An emotional problem may be responsible for your child's reluctance to speak.

ACTION NEEDED

MEDICAL HELP
Make an appointment to see your doctor.

How do the words sound?

CLEAR AND DISTINCT

DIFFICULT TO UNDERSTAND

POSSIBLE CAUSE

Unclearly spoken words are often a result of a physical defect, such as impaired hearing. When a hearing-impaired child learns speech from parents, teachers, and siblings, the words are heard indistinctly and are then pronounced unclearly when repeated by the child.

ACTION NEEDED

MEDICAL HELP
Make an appointment to see your doctor.
See also chart 34, HEARING PROBLEMS.

SELF-HELP
Always try to speak clearly to your child and emphasize the pronunciation of any new words. Make sure your child can see your lips as you talk.

14 TOILET-TRAINING PROBLEMS

Most children achieve bladder and bowel control between the ages of 2 and 5 years, although older children may have the occasional "accident". Unless there is a physical problem, toilet-training occurs naturally and the process cannot be hastened by pressure from parents.

START HERE

How old is your child?
- 2 YEARS OR OVER
- UNDER 2 YEARS

Is your child able to control defecation?
- HAS CONTROL
- LACKS CONTROL

How long have you been trying to toilet-train your child?
- LESS THAN A YEAR
- MORE THAN A YEAR

Has your child ever achieved bowel control?
- NEVER HAD CONTROL
- PREVIOUSLY HAD CONTROL

What kind of faeces does your child pass?
- LIQUID FAECES THAT OFTEN SOIL HIS OR HER UNDERCLOTHES
- NORMAL FAECES

POSSIBLE CAUSE

At this age, a child's nervous system is not yet sufficiently developed for complete bowel or bladder control to be achieved.

ACTION NEEDED

SELF-HELP
There is no point in trying to toilet-train your child before he or she is ready. Wait until your child is older and begins to show signs that he or she can exercise some voluntary control over bowel and bladder functions. See panel: *Toilet-training tips* (opposite).

POSSIBLE CAUSE

Late bowel control may be your child's way of rebelling against your efforts at toilet-training. Rarely, there may be a physical cause.

ACTION NEEDED

MEDICAL HELP
Make an appointment to see your doctor.

SELF-HELP
See panel: *Toilet-training tips* (opposite).

POSSIBLE CAUSE

Overflow soiling as a result of chronic CONSTIPATION (p.181).

ACTION NEEDED

MEDICAL HELP
Make an appointment to see your doctor.

SELF-HELP
See panel: *Preventing constipation* (p.109).

Does your child have bladder control?

- NO CONTROL DAY OR NIGHT
- CONTROL DURING THE DAY BUT NOT AT NIGHT

How old is your child?

- BETWEEN 2 AND 3 YEARS
- 3 YEARS OR OVER

POSSIBLE CAUSE

Few children have reliable control over their bowel or bladder functions before they are 3 years old. This is normal and is not a cause for concern.

ACTION NEEDED

SELF-HELP
See panel: *Toilet-training tips* (below).

Might your child be worried or anxious about something?

- POSSIBLY
- UNLIKELY

Has your child ever been dry at night for periods of a week or more?

- NO
- YES

POSSIBLE CAUSE

Delayed maturation of the nervous system is the most likely explanation. However, it is unlikely that the delay is a sign of a physical disorder (see ENURESIS, p.192).

ACTION NEEDED

MEDICAL HELP
If your child is over 5 years old, make an appointment to see your doctor.

POSSIBLE CAUSE

URINARY TRACT INFECTION (p.193).

ACTION NEEDED

MEDICAL HELP
Get medical advice within 24 hours.

POSSIBLE CAUSES

Emotional stress or anxiety (see ANXIETY AND FEARS, p.170) may sometimes result in your child temporarily losing bowel or bladder control.

ACTION NEEDED

MEDICAL HELP
If the problem persists or recurs, make an appointment to see your doctor.

SELF-HELP: TOILET-TRAINING TIPS

Achieving bowel and bladder control is as natural a part of a child's development as learning to walk; your role is to make the process as easy and relaxed as possible. Bowel control is usually achieved before bladder control, and night-time bladder control is the last to occur. It is advisable to leave toilet-training until your child is physiologically and mentally ready, which is unlikely to be before the age of about 18 months. The earlier you start, the longer it will take. The following tips may help:
- Familiarize your child with the potty.
- Help and encourage your child to use the potty but avoid making it a source of tension.
- Sit your child on the potty at specific times of the day when you know success is likely.

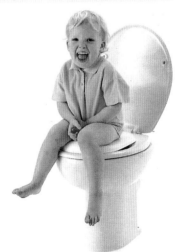

Second stage of toilet-training
A child who has mastered the use of the potty can progress to using the toilet with a child seat.

15 HEADACHE

Headaches may accompany any acute infection with fever. They may also occur on their own or, more seriously, with a variety of other symptoms. You should consult your doctor if a headache is severe, persistent, or recurrent, or if it is the first time your child has had a particular type of headache.

START HERE

How does your child seem?

- GENERALLY WELL
- UNWELL
- EXTREMELY UNWELL

POSSIBLE CAUSE

Tension headaches (see RECURRENT HEADACHES, p.161) may be caused by anxiety.

ACTION NEEDED

MEDICAL HELP
If such headaches occur regularly and cause distress to your child, consult your doctor.

SELF-HELP
See panel: *Relieving a headache* (opposite).

Might your child be worried or anxious about something?

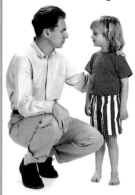

- POSSIBLY
- UNLIKELY

Does your child have any of the following symptoms?

| DROWSINESS |
| STIFF NECK |
| FEVER |
| VOMITING |
| REFUSAL TO DRINK |

- TWO OR MORE
- ONE OR NONE

POSSIBLE CAUSE

SINUSITIS (p.149).

ACTION NEEDED

MEDICAL HELP
Make an appointment to see your doctor.

Go to chart
8 FEVER IN CHILDREN

Do any of the following apply to your child?

- HAS RECENTLY HAD A COLD
- HAS A FEVER
- HAS BEEN VOMITING
- NONE OF THE ABOVE

POSSIBLE CAUSE

MENINGITIS (p.158).

ACTION NEEDED

MEDICAL HELP
✚ EMERGENCY! Call an ambulance!

If you cannot identify your child's problem from this chart, or if the headache is severe, talk to your doctor at once.

Go to chart
10 VOMITING IN CHILDREN

How often does your child suffer from headaches?

- OCCASIONALLY
- FREQUENTLY

SELF-HELP: RELIEVING A HEADACHE

Most headaches can be treated simply and effectively at home. However, if a headache persists for more than 4 hours, if your child seems very unwell, or if other symptoms develop, phone your doctor at once. The following measures might help to relieve the pain:

- Give liquid paracetamol.
- Let your child lie down in a cool, dark room. If he or she can sleep, it might relieve the headache.
- If your child feels hungry, give him or her a drink of milk or a plain biscuit.

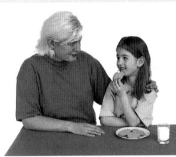

A light snack
Hunger is sometimes the cause of a headache. An easily digestible snack, such as a biscuit, might relieve it.

When has your child been getting headaches?

- EVERY DAY
- AFTER READING
- AFTER USING A COMPUTER OR WATCHING TELEVISION
- NONE OF THE ABOVE

POSSIBLE CAUSE

Frequent headaches (see RECURRENT HEADACHES, p.161), particularly those occurring at night or early in the morning, may be due to a brain abnormality.

ACTION NEEDED

MEDICAL HELP
Make an appointment to see your doctor.

POSSIBLE CAUSE

An occasional headache is rarely cause for concern.

ACTION NEEDED

SELF-HELP
See panel: *Relieving a headache* (above).

POSSIBLE CAUSE

Migraine (see RECURRENT HEADACHES, p.161).

ACTION NEEDED

MEDICAL HELP
For a first attack, if severe or prolonged, or for frequent attacks, make an appointment to see your doctor.

POSSIBLE CAUSE

Eyesight problems (see REFRACTIVE ERRORS, p.167) can sometimes cause headaches.

ACTION NEEDED

MEDICAL HELP
Make an appointment to see your doctor or optician.

Are the headaches accompanied or preceded by any of the following symptoms?

- ABDOMINAL PAIN
- NAUSEA OR VOMITING
- FLASHING LIGHTS OR OTHER VISUAL DISTURBANCES
- NONE OF THE ABOVE

Does anyone else in the family suffer from recurrent headaches?

- CLOSE RELATIVE, SUCH AS PARENT OR SIBLING
- DISTANT RELATIVE OR NO OTHER FAMILY MEMBER

If you cannot identify your child's problem from this chart, or if the headache is severe, talk to your doctor at once.

16 TOOTHACHE

The most likely cause of toothache in children is dental caries (tooth decay). Any child with pain that affects the teeth or gums should be seen by a dentist without delay. The key to preventing problems is to make sure your child has a healthy diet and cares properly for his or her teeth.

START HERE

Does your child have either of the following symptoms?

- CONTINUOUS, INTENSE PAIN
- FEVER
- NEITHER

What is the nature of the toothache?

- BOUTS OF THROBBING PAIN
- SHARP PAIN LASTING MINUTES, TRIGGERED BY HOT AND/OR COLD
- NEITHER

Has the tooth been filled recently?

- FILLED RECENTLY
- NOT FILLED RECENTLY

Is the pain brought on by eating hot, cold and/or sweet foods and does it last just a few seconds?

- YES
- NO

POSSIBLE CAUSE

DENTAL ABSCESS (p.178).

ACTION NEEDED

DENTAL HELP
✚ URGENT! Phone your dentist immediately!

SELF-HELP
See panel: *Relieving toothache* (below).

POSSIBLE CAUSES

DENTAL CARIES (p.177), a deep filling, or a tooth fracture may have caused inflammation of the tooth pulp (nerve tissue).

ACTION NEEDED

DENTAL HELP
Get dental advice within 24 hours.

SELF-HELP
See panel: *Relieving toothache* (below).

POSSIBLE CAUSES

The pain may be caused by DENTAL CARIES (p.177), a damaged filling, or a cracked or fractured tooth.

ACTION NEEDED

DENTAL HELP
Make an appointment to see your dentist.

SELF-HELP
See panels: *Relieving toothache* (left) and *How can I prevent dental caries?* (p.177).

SELF-HELP: RELIEVING TOOTHACHE

The following measures may help to relieve your child's pain:

- Give paracetamol syrup in the recommended dose. Do not apply it directly to the tooth as prolonged contact with the gums can result in a chemical burn.
- A young child may feel better if he or she is propped up against several pillows.

Easing toothache
A well-covered hot water bottle, held against the affected side of the face, may relieve your child's toothache.

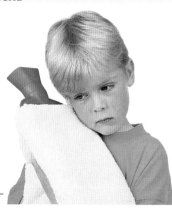

When is the tooth painful?

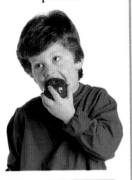

- **ON AND OFF, UNPREDICTABLY**
- **ONLY WHEN BITING OR CHEWING ON IT**

SELF-HELP: DEALING WITH A KNOCKED-OUT TOOTH

If a primary tooth is knocked out of your child's mouth, try to find it to ensure that it has not been inhaled or swallowed. A primary tooth cannot be reimplanted. However, a knocked-out secondary tooth can be grafted back into your child's gum by a dentist if this is done soon after the accident.

- Do not attempt to clean the tooth, which may damage the pulp (nerve tissue); put the tooth into a glass of milk, and take it, with your child, to the dentist.
- If a piece of a tooth crown has broken off, take it to the dentist, who may be able to bond it back into place.

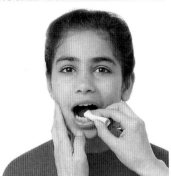

Treating a bleeding tooth socket
If the gum at the empty tooth socket is bleeding, place a gauze pad across it and tell your child to bite down hard.

POSSIBLE CAUSE

A filling that is uneven or higher than the level of the tooth's biting surface may cause pain when your child bites down on it.

ACTION NEEDED

DENTAL HELP
Make an appointment to see your dentist.

SELF-HELP
Until your child is able to see a dentist, give a diet of soft and liquid foods, and tell him or her to chew on the other side of the mouth.

Does your child have either of the following symptoms?

- **TENDER GUMS JUST BEHIND THE SECOND MOLARS**
- **CONTINUOUS, DULL PAIN IN SEVERAL UPPER BACK TEETH**
- **NEITHER**

POSSIBLE CAUSE

The wisdom teeth may be starting to emerge.

ACTION NEEDED

DENTAL HELP
Make an appointment to see your dentist.

SELF-HELP
See panel: *Relieving a sore mouth* (p.105).

POSSIBLE CAUSE

DENTAL CARIES (p.177).

ACTION NEEDED

DENTAL HELP
Make an appointment to see your dentist.

SELF-HELP
See panels: *Relieving toothache* (opposite) and *How can I prevent dental caries?* (p.177).

POSSIBLE CAUSE

A tooth that has been filled very recently is often slightly sensitive, particularly to cold. Sensitivity is especially likely after a deep filling.

ACTION NEEDED

DENTAL HELP
If sensitivity to heat develops or if pain intensifies or lasts for more than a few seconds, make an appointment to see your dentist. Such symptoms may indicate damage to the tooth pulp (nerve tissue).

POSSIBLE CAUSE

SINUSITIS (p.149).

ACTION NEEDED

MEDICAL HELP
Make an appointment to see your doctor.

17 FEELING GENERALLY UNWELL

If your child complains of feeling unwell, you should check his or her temperature and look for a rash. A symptom such as a headache may clear up with self-help measures, or it may be the first sign of an infection, such as influenza. If your child's condition worsens, consult your doctor.

DANGER SIGNS
Phone your doctor at once if your child has any of the following symptoms:
- Abnormal drowsiness or unresponsiveness.
- Temperature over 39°C (102°F).
- Vomiting for 12 hours.
- Fast or noisy breathing.
- Refusing to drink for 6 hours.
- Flat, pink or purple spots that do not disappear when pressed.

START HERE

Does your child have any of the following symptoms?

Does your child have a fever – a temperature of 38°C (100°F) or above?

FEVER

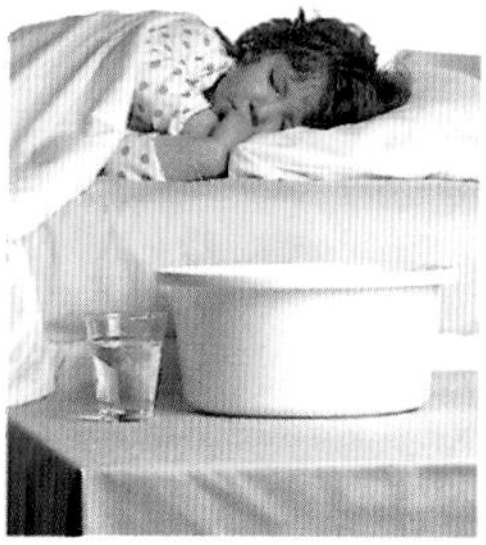

NO FEVER

VOMITING

DIARRHOEA

RASH

POSSIBLE CAUSE
GASTROENTERITIS (p.180).

ACTION NEEDED

MEDICAL HELP
Get medical advice within 24 hours.

SELF-HELP
See panel: *Preventing dehydration in babies* (p.38) or *Preventing dehydration in children* (p.53).

Go to chart
23 SPOTS AND RASHES

ABDOMINAL PAIN

NONE OF THE ABOVE

Go to chart
36 ABDOMINAL PAIN

Does your child have a rash?

RASH

NO RASH

How old is your child?

UNDER 1 YEAR

OVER 1 YEAR

Go to chart
1 FEVER IN INFANTS

Go to chart
22 RASH WITH FEVER

Go to chart
8 FEVER IN CHILDREN

Is your child interested in food and drink?

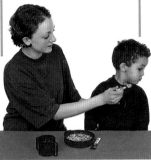

REFUSES TO EAT AND DRINK

REFUSES TO EAT

EATS AND DRINKS AS NORMAL

POSSIBLE CAUSE

Your child may be developing an infectious disease (see pp.118–125), particularly if he or she is listless or irritable or has other signs of illness.

ACTION NEEDED

MEDICAL HELP
If your child feels no better after 24 hours or develops other symptoms, make an appointment to see your doctor.

SELF-HELP
Try to make your child drink by offering his or her favourite liquid. See panel: *Preventing dehydration in babies* (p.38) or *Preventing dehydration in children* (p.53).

Go to chart
28 SORE THROAT

Might your child be worried or anxious about something?

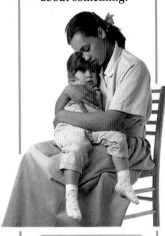

POSSIBLY

UNLIKELY

POSSIBLE CAUSES

Anxiety or problems at school can result in a child feeling unwell (see ANXIETY AND FEARS, p.170).

ACTION NEEDED

MEDICAL HELP
If your child still feels unwell after a day at home or if he or she regularly refuses to go to school, make an appointment to see your doctor.

In the past 3 weeks might your child have had contact with anyone who has an infectious disease?

NO CONTACT

CONTACT

If you cannot identify your child's problem from this chart, talk to your doctor within 48 hours.

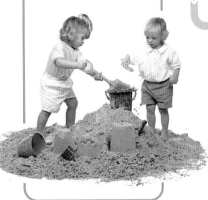

POSSIBLE CAUSE

One of the childhood infectious diseases (see pp.118–125), in its incubation period, might be causing your child to feel unwell.

ACTION NEEDED

MEDICAL HELP
If your child feels no better after 24 hours, or he or she develops other symptoms, make an appointment to see your doctor.

18 LUMPS AND SWELLINGS

Lumps and swellings occur on, or just below, the surface of the skin. Swellings may be lymph glands that have swollen to fight infection in a nearby part of the body. Injuries, bites, and stings can also cause lumps and swellings. A persistent or painful lump or swelling should be examined by a doctor.

START HERE

How would you describe your child's lump or swelling?

- PAINFUL RED LUMP
- SLIGHTLY RAISED, BRIGHT RED LUMP
- SOFT LUMP IN GROIN
- TENDER SWELLING NEAR AN INFECTED CUT OR GRAZE
- LARGE, TENDER LUMP ON HEAD
- NONE OF THE ABOVE

POSSIBLE CAUSES

A BOIL (p.137) or abscess.

ACTION NEEDED

MEDICAL HELP
If a lump is very painful or if more than one lump forms, make an appointment to see your doctor.

POSSIBLE CAUSE

The swelling is probably a nearby lymph gland, which has become swollen as it helps to fight the infection.

ACTION NEEDED

MEDICAL HELP
If your child's swelling or pain persists for more than a week, make an appointment to see your doctor.

POSSIBLE CAUSE

Your child may have been stung by an insect such as a bee or wasp (see INSECT BITES AND STINGS, p.138).

ACTION NEEDED

MEDICAL HELP
If your child has had an allergic reaction to an insect sting in the past, or if he or she shows any symptoms of ANAPHYLACTIC SHOCK (p.154), call an ambulance or take him or her to the nearest hospital accident and emergency department immediately.

SELF-HELP
If your child is not allergic to insect stings, you should try to remove the sting with eyebrow tweezers or your fingernail if it is still visible. Apply a cool compress to relieve any pain or irritation caused by the sting.

POSSIBLE CAUSE

HEAD INJURY (p.159).

ACTION NEEDED

MEDICAL HELP
✚ URGENT! Phone your doctor immediately!

Did your child have a recent accident or injury that involved banging the head?

- BLOW TO HEAD
- NO BLOW

If you cannot identify your child's problem from this chart, talk to your doctor within 48 hours.

POSSIBLE CAUSE

Inguinal hernia (see HERNIA, p.187).

ACTION NEEDED

MEDICAL HELP
Get medical advice within 24 hours.

POSSIBLE CAUSES

ATOPIC ECZEMA (p.135) or a viral infection, such as RUBELLA (p.119).

ACTION NEEDED

MEDICAL HELP
Make an appointment to see your doctor.

Does your child have any of the following symptoms?

- SORE THROAT
- RELUCTANCE TO EAT OR DRINK
- EARACHE
- NONE OF THE ABOVE

POSSIBLE CAUSE

Tonsillitis (see PHARYNGITIS AND TONSILLITIS, p.151).

ACTION NEEDED

MEDICAL HELP
If your child feels no better after 24 hours, consult your doctor.

SELF-HELP
See panel: *Relieving a sore throat (p.91).*

POSSIBLE CAUSE

OTITIS MEDIA (p.162).

ACTION NEEDED

MEDICAL HELP
Get medical advice within 24 hours.

SELF-HELP
See panel: *Relieving earache (p.101).*

What is the location of the lumps or swellings?

- BACK OF NECK
- SIDES OF NECK
- BETWEEN EAR AND JAW
- IN NECK AND ARMPIT AND/OR GROIN
- NONE OF THE ABOVE

If you cannot identify your child's problem from this chart, talk to your doctor within 48 hours.

POSSIBLE CAUSE

MUMPS (p.122).

ACTION NEEDED

MEDICAL HELP
Make an appointment to see your doctor.

POSSIBLE CAUSE

INFECTIOUS MONONUCLEOSIS (p.124).

ACTION NEEDED

MEDICAL HELP
Make an appointment to see your doctor.

Do any of the following apply?

- ANKLE IS SWOLLEN
- FOOT IS SWOLLEN
- SWELLING IN SCROTUM OR PENIS
- NONE OF THE ABOVE

Go to chart
21 FOOT PROBLEMS

Go to chart
40 GENITAL PROBLEMS IN BOYS

POSSIBLE CAUSES

STRAIN OR SPRAIN (p.127).

ACTION NEEDED

MEDICAL HELP
If pain is severe or there is no improvement after 24 hours, consult your doctor.

SELF-HELP
See panel: *Treating strains and sprains (p.73).*

If you cannot identify your child's problem from this chart, talk to your doctor within 48 hours.

19 PAINFUL LIMBS

Many children experience pain in an arm or leg; this pain is usually the result of a minor fall or injury and rarely requires medical attention. Sometimes a bone may be broken or a joint dislocated; these conditions need urgent treatment. Unexplained or persistent pain may also require attention.

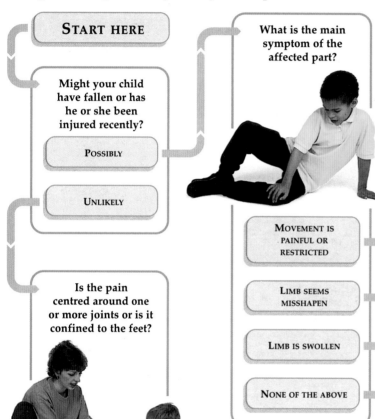

START HERE

Might your child have fallen or has he or she been injured recently?

POSSIBLY

UNLIKELY

Is the pain centred around one or more joints or is it confined to the feet?

What is the main symptom of the affected part?

MOVEMENT IS PAINFUL OR RESTRICTED

LIMB SEEMS MISSHAPEN

LIMB IS SWOLLEN

NONE OF THE ABOVE

POSSIBLE CAUSES

A broken bone or a dislocated joint (see FRACTURES AND DISLOCATIONS, p.128).

ACTION NEEDED

MEDICAL HELP
✚ EMERGENCY! Call an ambulance if the injury affects your child's leg or elbow. If an arm or shoulder is affected, immobilize the injury, then take your child to the nearest hospital accident and emergency department.

SELF-HELP
See FIRST AID: *Broken leg* (p.210) or *Broken arm* (p.211).

POSSIBLE CAUSES

Bruised or strained muscles or sprained ligaments (see STRAINS AND SPRAINS, p.127).

ACTION NEEDED

MEDICAL HELP
If the pain or swelling is severe or does not improve within 24 hours, consult your doctor.

SELF-HELP
See panel: *Treating strains and sprains* (opposite).

CONFINED TO FEET

Go to chart
21 FOOT PROBLEMS

CENTRED AROUND JOINTS

Go to chart
20 PAINFUL JOINTS

NEITHER

Does your child have a fever – a temperature of 38°C (100°F) or above – or does he or she seem unwell?

- FEVER
- SEEMS UNWELL
- NEITHER

Is your child suffering from any of the following symptoms?

- HEADACHE
- COUGH
- SORE THROAT
- RED OR TENDER AREA OVER A BONE
- NONE OF THE ABOVE

POSSIBLE CAUSE

INFLUENZA (p.151).

ACTION NEEDED

MEDICAL HELP
If there is no improvement within 48 hours, if breathing difficulties develop, or a rash appears, phone your doctor immediately.

SELF-HELP
See panel: *Bringing down a high temperature* (p.37).

POSSIBLE CAUSE

Bone infection (see BONE AND JOINT INFECTION, p.133).

ACTION NEEDED

MEDICAL HELP
✚ URGENT! Phone your doctor immediately!

Has your child been experiencing bouts of pain in the lower leg that persist for a few minutes?

- YES
- NO

POSSIBLE CAUSE

CRAMP (p.127).

ACTION NEEDED

MEDICAL HELP
If the problem persists, make an appointment to see your doctor.

SELF-HELP
Gently massage or stretch the affected leg.

If you cannot identify your child's problem from this chart or if the pain persists for over 24 hours, talk to your doctor.

POSSIBLE CAUSES

Bruised or strained muscles or sprained ligaments, possibly caused by an unnoticed injury (see STRAINS AND SPRAINS, p.127).

ACTION NEEDED

MEDICAL HELP
If your child is in severe pain, or he or she is reluctant to use the affected limb, or if there is no improvement within 24 hours, consult your doctor.

SELF-HELP
See panel: *Treating strains and sprains* (right).

SELF-HELP: TREATING STRAINS AND SPRAINS

If your child suffers a strain or sprain, the appropriate treatment is remembered as RICE – Rest, Ice, Compression, and Elevation. This treatment can also be used for deep bruising.

- Rest: tell your child to rest the affected part.
- Ice: apply a cold compress, such as ice or frozen peas wrapped in flannel, for 10–15 minutes.
- Compression: bandage a thick layer of cotton wool firmly around the injured area.
- Elevation: raise and support the affected part to minimize further swelling.

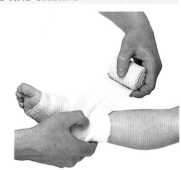

Compression
Wrap a pad of cotton wool around the affected area. Use a bandage to secure the cotton wool in place.

20 PAINFUL JOINTS

It is extremely rare for a child to be affected by a serious joint disorder. Usually, pain is caused by a minor strain or sprain of the muscles or ligaments around a joint. If your child's pain is persistent or if there are other symptoms, such as a fever, you should consult your doctor.

START HERE

Might your child have fallen or has he or she been injured recently?

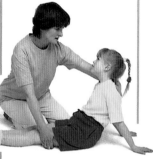

POSSIBLY

UNLIKELY

What is the main symptom of the affected joint?

RESTRICTED OR PAINFUL MOVEMENT

JOINT SEEMS MISSHAPEN

JOINT IS SWOLLEN

NONE OF THE ABOVE

How many joints are affected?

ONLY ONE JOINT

MORE THAN ONE JOINT

Does your child have any of the following symptoms?

FEVER

SEEMS UNWELL

RED, HOT, OR SWOLLEN JOINT

NONE OF THE ABOVE

POSSIBLE CAUSES

A dislocated joint or a break in a bone near the joint (see FRACTURES AND DISLOCATIONS, p.128).

ACTION NEEDED

MEDICAL HELP
✚ **EMERGENCY!** Call an ambulance if the injury affects your child's leg or elbow. If an arm, finger, or shoulder is affected, take your child to the nearest hospital accident and emergency department.

SELF-HELP
See FIRST AID: *Broken leg* (p.210) or *Broken arm* (p.211).

POSSIBLE CAUSE

Strained muscles or sprained ligaments near the joint (see STRAINS AND SPRAINS, p.127).

ACTION NEEDED

MEDICAL HELP
If the pain or swelling is severe or does not improve within 24 hours, consult your doctor.

SELF-HELP
See panel: *Treating strains and sprains* (p.73).

POSSIBLE CAUSE

Joint infection (see BONE AND JOINT INFECTION, p.133).

ACTION NEEDED

MEDICAL HELP
✚ **URGENT!** Phone your doctor immediately!

Does your child have a painful knee or hip joint or a limp?

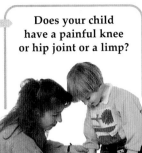

- LIMP
- PAINFUL HIP
- PAINFUL KNEE
- NONE OF THE ABOVE

POSSIBLE CAUSES

CONGENITAL HIP DISLOCATION (p.130) is a possibility in a child who is just learning to walk. An older child may be suffering from PERTHES' DISEASE (p.131) or SLIPPED FEMORAL EPIPHYSIS (p.131). Bone or joint infection (see BONE AND JOINT INFECTION, p.133), or IRRITABLE HIP (p.130) are possibilities in a child of any age. See also LIMPING (p.126).

ACTION NEEDED

MEDICAL HELP
Get medical advice within 24 hours.

POSSIBLE CAUSES

A minor STRAIN OR SPRAIN (p.127) is the most likely cause. Bone or joint infection (see BONE AND JOINT INFECTION, p.133) is also a possibility. If the knee is the joint affected, your child may have either chondromalacia patellae or Osgood-Schlatter disease (see KNEE DISORDERS, p.132). See also LIMPING (p.126).

ACTION NEEDED

MEDICAL HELP
If the pain is severe, is no better after 24 hours, or recurs, consult your doctor.

SELF-HELP
See panel: *Treating strains and sprains* (p.73).

POSSIBLE CAUSE

JUVENILE CHRONIC ARTHRITIS (p.132).

ACTION NEEDED

MEDICAL HELP
Get medical advice within 24 hours.

Is your child suffering from either of the following symptoms?

- RED OR HOT JOINTS
- SWOLLEN JOINTS
- NEITHER

If you cannot identify your child's problem from this chart or if the affected joint remains painful for more than 24 hours, talk to your doctor.

Does your child have any of the following symptoms?

- FEVER
- SEEMS UNWELL
- PURPLISH RASH ON LIMBS
- NONE OF THE ABOVE

POSSIBLE CAUSE

HENOCH-SCHÖNLEIN PURPURA (p.147).

ACTION NEEDED

MEDICAL HELP
✚ URGENT! Phone your doctor immediately!

POSSIBLE CAUSES

JUVENILE CHRONIC ARTHRITIS (p.132) or transient arthritis after any acute infection.

ACTION NEEDED

MEDICAL HELP
Get medical advice within 24 hours.

21 FOOT PROBLEMS

The majority of foot problems in childhood are minor. Most common are those resulting from falls and those that affect the skin of one or both feet. Ill-fitting shoes may also cause foot problems. If the foot is very painful or very swollen, or if walking is difficult, you should consult your doctor.

START HERE

Does your child's foot hurt, or does it appear out of shape?
- PAINFUL
- MISSHAPEN

Which of the following describes your child's feet?
- FLAT FEET
- BENT OR CURLY TOES

Might your child's shoes or socks be too small?
- POSSIBLY
- UNLIKELY

Might your child have fallen, or has he or she been injured recently?
- POSSIBLY
- UNLIKELY

How old is your child?
- 3 YEARS OR OVER
- UNDER 3 YEARS

POSSIBLE CAUSE

Shoes or socks that are too small may cause your child's toes to curl.

ACTION NEEDED

SELF-HELP
Replace your child's shoes and socks as soon as they become tight.

If you cannot identify your child's problem from this chart, talk to your doctor within 48 hours.

How has the injury affected your child's walking?
- CHILD CANNOT WALK ON AFFECTED FOOT
- WALKING POSSIBLE BUT PAINFUL

POSSIBLE CAUSES

Bruised or strained muscles or strained ligaments (see STRAINS AND SPRAINS, p.127).

ACTION NEEDED

MEDICAL HELP
If the pain or swelling is severe, consult your doctor.

SELF-HELP
See panel: *Treating strains and sprains* (p.73).

POSSIBLE CAUSE

Undeveloped muscles and ligaments in the soles of the feet, which are not a cause for concern at this age (see MINOR SKELETAL PROBLEMS, p.129).

ACTION NEEDED

MEDICAL HELP
If you feel your child's feet are not developing properly, make an appointment to see your doctor.

POSSIBLE CAUSE

Flat feet (see MINOR SKELETAL PROBLEMS, p.129).

ACTION NEEDED

MEDICAL HELP
If your child's feet are painful or if you are worried about them, make an appointment to see your doctor.

POSSIBLE CAUSE

A bone in your child's foot, toe, or ankle may have been fractured (see FRACTURES AND DISLOCATIONS, p.128).

ACTION NEEDED

MEDICAL HELP
✚ EMERGENCY! Take your child to the nearest hospital accident and emergency department. If you are unable to move your child, you should call an ambulance.

POSSIBLE CAUSE

Your child's shoes may not fit properly, or the lining may be worn.

ACTION NEEDED

SELF-HELP
Replace your child's shoes as soon as they become tight or worn with new shoes that are long and wide enough. Try to buy from shops where the assistants are trained to fit children's shoes.

POSSIBLE CAUSE

Verruca (see WARTS, p.141).

ACTION NEEDED

MEDICAL HELP
Make an appointment to see your doctor.

POSSIBLE CAUSE

Athlete's foot (see FUNGAL INFECTIONS, p.142).

ACTION NEEDED

MEDICAL HELP
If the rash does not clear up within 2 weeks of starting self-help treatment, or if your child's toenails are affected, make an appointment to see your doctor.

SELF-HELP
Apply an antifungal powder, cream, or spray to the rash. Ensure your child's feet are dried properly after bathing.

When does your child feel pain?

> ONLY WHEN WEARING SHOES

> ONLY WHEN WEIGHT IS PUT ON THE FOOT

> AT ALL TIMES

Is there anything abnormal on the sole of your child's foot?

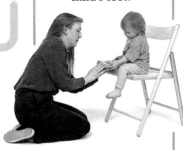

> FLATTENED, HARD LUMP OF SKIN

> ITCHY, PEELING RASH

> NOTHING

Can you see any redness or swelling on one of your child's feet or toes?

> REDNESS OR SWELLING

> NEITHER

> **If you cannot identify your child's problem from this chart, talk to your doctor within 48 hours.**

POSSIBLE CAUSE

Infection from a cut or a foreign body, such as a thorn or a splinter, may cause redness or swelling.

ACTION NEEDED

MEDICAL HELP
Get medical advice within 24 hours.

SELF-HELP
Remove a foreign body with sterilized tweezers. Cover the affected area with a clean, sterile bandage, then elevate and support the foot to reduce swelling.

22 RASH WITH FEVER

The combination of rash and fever – a temperature of 38°C (100°F) or over – is usually caused by an infectious disease. Most of these diseases are caused by viruses and generally clear up quickly without special treatment. You should, however, consult your doctor for a diagnosis.

START HERE

What are the features of your child's rash?

- FLAT SPOTS THAT DO NOT DISAPPEAR WHEN PRESSED
- FINE RED RASH THAT TURNS WHITE WHEN PRESSED
- BLOTCHY, RAISED RED RASH
- CROPS OF ITCHY SPOTS THAT BLISTER AND DRY INTO SCABS
- FLAT, PINK SPOTS STARTING ON THE FACE OR TRUNK
- BRIGHT RED RASH CONFINED TO THE CHEEKS
- NONE OF THE ABOVE

If you cannot identify your child's problem from this chart, talk to your doctor within 48 hours.

DANGER SIGNS
Phone your doctor at once if your child has any of the following symptoms during, or after apparent recovery from, any of the common childhood infectious diseases:
- Abnormal drowsiness or floppiness.
- Seizures.
- Temperature of 40°C (104°F) or above.
- Abnormally fast breathing.
- Noisy or difficult breathing.
- Severe headache.
- Refusing to drink for over 6 hours.

POSSIBLE CAUSE
Blood infection with meningococcus, a bacterium that causes MENINGITIS (p.158).

ACTION NEEDED
MEDICAL HELP
✚ EMERGENCY! Call an ambulance!

POSSIBLE CAUSE
CHICKENPOX (p.120).

ACTION NEEDED
MEDICAL HELP
If the spots become infected, make an appointment to see your doctor.

SELF-HELP
See panel: *Bringing down a high temperature* (p.37).

POSSIBLE CAUSE
ERYTHEMA INFECTIOSUM (p.119).

ACTION NEEDED
MEDICAL HELP
If you are concerned about your child's condition or if your child has SICKLE-CELL ANAEMIA (p.199), make an appointment to see your doctor.

SELF-HELP
See panel: *Bringing down a high temperature* (p.37).

How high was your child's temperature during the 3 to 4 days before the rash appeared?

- 38.5°C (101°F) OR ABOVE
- BELOW 38.5°C (101°F)

POSSIBLE CAUSE
RUBELLA (p.119).

ACTION NEEDED
MEDICAL HELP
Make an appointment to see your doctor.

SELF-HELP
See panel: *Bringing down a high temperature* (p.37).

POSSIBLE CAUSE

MEASLES (p.118).

ACTION NEEDED

MEDICAL HELP
Get medical advice within 24 hours.

SELF-HELP
See panel: *Bringing down a high temperature (p.37).*

Before the rash appeared, did your child also have any of the following symptoms?

RUNNY NOSE

COUGH

RED EYES

SORE THROAT

VOMITING

NONE OF THE ABOVE

POSSIBLE CAUSE

ROSEOLA INFANTUM (p.121).

ACTION NEEDED

MEDICAL HELP
If you are concerned about your child's condition, make an appointment to see your doctor.

SELF-HELP
See panel: *Bringing down a high temperature (p.37).*

COMMON RASHES

This is an identification guide to some of the childhood rashes. However, rashes may differ in appearance depending on how severely your child is affected and the colour of the skin, so a firm diagnosis should always be made by a doctor. Call an ambulance if your child's rash resembles the meningitis rash.

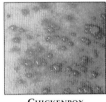
MENINGITIS

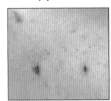
SCARLET FEVER

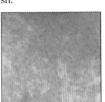
MEASLES

CHICKENPOX

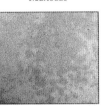
RUBELLA

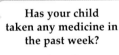
ROSEOLA INFANTUM

POSSIBLE CAUSE

SCARLET FEVER (p.121).

ACTION NEEDED

MEDICAL HELP
Get medical advice within 24 hours.

SELF-HELP
See panels: *Bringing down a high temperature (p.37)* and *Relieving a sore throat (p.91).*

POSSIBLE CAUSE

Drug allergy (see ALLERGIES, p.152).

ACTION NEEDED

MEDICAL HELP
✚ URGENT! Phone your doctor immediately to find out whether the medicine may be causing your child's symptoms and whether you should stop giving it.

Has your child taken any medicine in the past week?

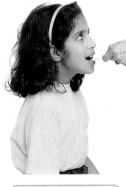

MEDICINE

NO MEDICINE

If you cannot identify your child's problem from this chart, talk to your doctor within 48 hours.

23 SPOTS AND RASHES

For other skin problems in infants, see chart 7

Most spots and rashes are a response to local or general infection or a symptom of an allergic reaction. The spots or rashes are unlikely to be serious if there are no other signs of being unwell. However, if the skin is very itchy or sore or if your child is distressed, you should consult your doctor.

DANGER SIGNS
Call an ambulance at once if your child develops any of the following symptoms:
- Swelling of face or mouth.
- Noisy or difficult breathing.
- Difficulty swallowing.
- Abnormal drowsiness.

START HERE

Does your child have a fever – a temperature of 38°C (100°F) or above?

FEVER

NO FEVER

Is there itchiness?

NO ITCHINESS

ITCHINESS

How far does the itchiness extend?

AFFECTS SOME SKIN THAT DOES NOT HAVE A RASH

CONFINED TO RASH AREA

Where is the rash?

MAINLY ON THE FACE AND AROUND THE JOINTS

ON THE SCALP, TRUNK, OR LIMBS

What is the nature of the rash?

RED, SCALY, OR BLISTER-LIKE PATCHES

SLIGHTLY RAISED, BRIGHT RED, BLOTCHY PATCHES

SMALL, INFLAMED SPOTS IN ONE AREA

NONE OF THE ABOVE

Go to chart **22 RASH WITH FEVER**

POSSIBLE CAUSE

ATOPIC ECZEMA (p.135).

ACTION NEEDED

MEDICAL HELP
If your child's rash is very itchy, extensive, or weeping, make an appointment to see your doctor.

POSSIBLE CAUSE

Ringworm (see FUNGAL INFECTIONS, p.142).

ACTION NEEDED

MEDICAL HELP
Make an appointment to see your doctor.

POSSIBLE CAUSE

Insect bites (see INSECT BITES AND STINGS, p.138), possibly from mosquitoes or cat or dog fleas.

ACTION NEEDED

SELF-HELP
Apply cool compresses or calamine lotion to the spots to relieve the itching.

What does the rash or spot look like?

- GROUPS OF LUMPS, EACH WITH A CENTRAL DEPRESSION
- PUS-FILLED AREAS OR GOLDEN CRUSTS, OFTEN ON THE FACE
- ONE OR MORE FIRM, ROUGH LUMPS
- A PAINFUL, RED LUMP, POSSIBLY WITH A YELLOW TOP
- TINY, RED, ITCHY SPOTS OR FLUID-FILLED BLISTERS
- NONE OF THE ABOVE

POSSIBLE CAUSE

MOLLUSCUM CONTAGIOSUM (p.141).

ACTION NEEDED

MEDICAL HELP
Make an appointment to see your doctor.

POSSIBLE CAUSE

IMPETIGO (p.139).

ACTION NEEDED

MEDICAL HELP
Get medical advice within 24 hours.

continued on p.82, top

POSSIBLE CAUSE

WARTS (p.141).

ACTION NEEDED

MEDICAL HELP
If the warts are troublesome, make an appointment to see your doctor.

POSSIBLE CAUSE

URTICARIA (p.138).

ACTION NEEDED

MEDICAL HELP
If the rash does not disappear within 4 hours, or if your child has repeated attacks, make an appointment to see your doctor.

SELF-HELP
Apply cool compresses or calamine lotion to the spots to relieve the itchiness.

POSSIBLE CAUSE

A BOIL (p.137).

ACTION NEEDED

MEDICAL HELP
If a boil is very painful or if more than one boil forms, make an appointment to see your doctor.

POSSIBLE CAUSE

Prickly heat, a rash caused by unevaporated sweat.

ACTION NEEDED

SELF-HELP
Apply cool compresses as often as needed to relieve the itchiness. Do not use soap on the affected areas.

POSSIBLE CAUSE

SCABIES (p.143).

ACTION NEEDED

MEDICAL HELP
Make an appointment to see your doctor.

Is your child's face or mouth swollen?

- NOT SWOLLEN
- SWOLLEN

POSSIBLE CAUSE

An allergic reaction, which may be caused by insect stings, peanuts, or other factors, and can lead to ANAPHYLACTIC SHOCK (p.154).

ACTION NEEDED

MEDICAL HELP
✚ EMERGENCY! Call an ambulance!

continued on p.82, bottom

23 Spots and rashes (continued)

continued from p.81, top

Has your child reached puberty?

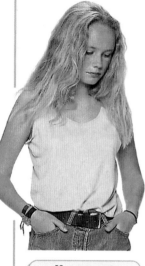

HAS REACHED PUBERTY

HAS NOT REACHED PUBERTY

continued from p.81, bottom

Have you noticed any of the following types of spots?

ROUND, SCALY SPOTS ON THE TRUNK, UPPER ARMS, OR THIGHS

TINY BLACK SPOTS (BLACKHEADS)

WHITE-CENTRED, INFLAMED SPOTS (WHITEHEADS)

SMALL, SOLID, TENDER SWELLINGS UNDER THE SKIN

NONE OF THE ABOVE

Does your child have small, oval pink spots arranged along the lines of the ribs?

YES

NO

Are you giving your child any medicine?

MEDICINE

NO MEDICINE

POSSIBLE CAUSE

PITYRIASIS VERSICOLOR (p.142).

ACTION NEEDED

MEDICAL HELP
Make an appointment to see your doctor.

POSSIBLE CAUSE

ACNE (p.140).

ACTION NEEDED

MEDICAL HELP
If the acne is severe, make an appointment to see your doctor.

POSSIBLE CAUSE

An allergic reaction to certain medicines can cause a rash (see ALLERGIES, p.152).

ACTION NEEDED

MEDICAL HELP
✚ URGENT! Phone your doctor immediately to find out whether the medicine may be causing your child's symptoms and whether you should stop giving it.

POSSIBLE CAUSE

PITYRIASIS ROSEA (p.140).

ACTION NEEDED

MEDICAL HELP
Make an appointment to see your doctor.

SELF-HELP
See panel: *Relieving itchiness* (p.49).

> If you cannot identify your child's problem from this chart, talk to your doctor within 48 hours.

24 ITCHINESS

Itchiness may affect the whole of your child's body or just one area. The causes of itchiness are varied and range from allergic reactions to infestation by parasites. Intense itchiness can be very distressing and scratching may lead to infection, so prompt treatment of any underlying disorder is essential.

START HERE

Is there a rash of itchy spots or patches of inflamed skin?

- ITCHY RASH
- INFLAMED PATCHES
- NEITHER

Has your child been wearing either of the following next to his or her skin?

- WOOL
- SYNTHETIC MATERIAL
- NEITHER

Go to chart
23 SPOTS AND RASHES

Which parts of your child's body are itchy?

- BETWEEN THE TOES, OR THE SOLES OF THE FEET
- ANAL AREA
- SCALP
- GENITAL AREA (IN A GIRL)
- A LARGE AREA OF THE BODY
- NONE OF THE ABOVE

Are there thin grey lines on your child's fingerwebs, wrists, palms, or soles?

- NO
- YES

POSSIBLE CAUSE

Athlete's foot (see FUNGAL INFECTIONS, p.142).

ACTION NEEDED

MEDICAL HELP
If the rash does not clear up within 2 weeks or if it affects your child's toenails, make an appointment to see your doctor.

SELF-HELP
Apply an antifungal powder, cream, or spray to the rash.

POSSIBLE CAUSE

THREADWORMS (p.188).

ACTION NEEDED

MEDICAL HELP
Make an appointment to see your doctor.

Go to chart
25 HAIR AND SCALP PROBLEMS

Go to chart
41 GENITAL PROBLEMS IN GIRLS

If you cannot identify your child's problem from this chart, talk to your doctor within 48 hours.

POSSIBLE CAUSE

Sensitive skin.

ACTION NEEDED

SELF-HELP
Use a washing powder made for people with delicate or sensitive skin. Ensure cotton is worn next to the skin.

POSSIBLE CAUSE

SCABIES (p.143).

ACTION NEEDED

MEDICAL HELP
Make an appointment to see your doctor.

25 HAIR AND SCALP PROBLEMS

Although problems with the hair and scalp are fairly common in children, they are rarely serious. Skin conditions, infections, or infestations by parasites are the most likely causes of scalp problems, while pulling on the hair or having the hair tied back tightly are the most probable reasons for hair loss.

START HERE

Does your child have any of the following symptoms?

- BALD PATCHES
- FLAKY SCALP
- ITCHY SCALP
- HAIR BECOMING GENERALLY THIN
- CRUSTY YELLOW PATCHES ON THE SCALP
- NONE OF THE ABOVE

How old is your child?

- UNDER 1 YEAR
- 1 YEAR OR OVER

POSSIBLE CAUSE

If your infant often rubs his or her head on the cot or baby seat, bald patches may develop as the delicate first hair falls out. This hair loss is normal and the bald patches will soon be replaced by new, stronger hair.

ACTION NEEDED

SELF-HELP
If your baby is bald or has little hair you should always cover his or her head to protect it from the sun and to keep it warm in cold weather.

POSSIBLE CAUSE

Dandruff (see SEBORRHOEIC DERMATITIS, p.134).

ACTION NEEDED

SELF-HELP
Wash your child's hair with an anti-dandruff shampoo. If the symptoms do not improve within 2 weeks, make an appointment to see your doctor.

Does the itchiness get better for a few days after a thorough shampoo?

- IMPROVEMENT
- NO IMPROVEMENT

POSSIBLE CAUSE

HEAD LICE (p.143).

ACTION NEEDED

SELF-HELP
Wash your child's hair with one of the anti-lice shampoos available over the counter. If your child is under 2 years old or has an allergy, consult your doctor before starting any treatment.

POSSIBLE CAUSE

Cradle cap (see SEBORRHOEIC DERMATITIS, p.134).

ACTION NEEDED

MEDICAL HELP
Make an appointment to see your doctor.

If you cannot identify your child's problem from this chart, make an appointment to see your doctor

How old is your child?

- 1 YEAR OR OVER
- UNDER 1 YEAR

How does the skin in the bald areas look?

- NORMAL
- SCALY AND INFLAMED

POSSIBLE CAUSE

A form of localized baldness, which often may have no apparent cause.

ACTION NEEDED

MEDICAL HELP
Make an appointment to see your doctor.

POSSIBLE CAUSE

Ringworm (see FUNGAL INFECTIONS, p.142)

ACTION NEEDED

MEDICAL HELP
Make an appointment to see your doctor.

Do either of the following apply to your child?

- HAS RECENTLY HAD AN ILLNESS
- IS TAKING MEDICINE
- NEITHER

POSSIBLE CAUSE

General thinning of the hair could be a result of a recent illness. The hair will probably return to its normal thickness over the next few months.

ACTION NEEDED

MEDICAL HELP
If you are worried, consult your doctor.

POSSIBLE CAUSE

The thinning of your child's hair could be a side-effect of the medicine that he or she is taking.

ACTION NEEDED

MEDICAL HELP
Phone your doctor to find out whether the medicine may be causing your child's symptoms and whether you should stop giving it.

Does your child play with his or her hair or is it tied back?

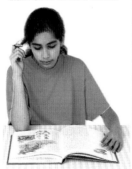

- HABITUALLY PULLS OR TWISTS HAIR
- WEARS HAIR IN TIGHT PLAITS OR BRAIDS
- NEITHER

POSSIBLE CAUSE

As the baby hair falls out, your infant's hair will be noticeably thinner until the new, stronger hair grows in. This process is normal and is not a cause for concern.

ACTION NEEDED

SELF-HELP
Cover your baby's head to protect it from the sun and to keep it warm in cold weather.

POSSIBLE CAUSE

Habitual hair pulling may indicate an underlying psychological problem (see HABITUAL BEHAVIOUR, p.169).

ACTION NEEDED

MEDICAL HELP
If your child is losing a lot of hair or if he or she has other behavioural problems, make an appointment to see your doctor.

POSSIBLE CAUSE

Damage to the hair roots, caused by excessive pulling of the hair, can result in temporary hair loss.

ACTION NEEDED

SELF-HELP
Change your child's hairstyle or have his or her hair cut.

If you cannot identify your child's problem from this chart, make an appointment to see your doctor

26 BREATHING PROBLEMS

Breathing problems range from noisy or fast breathing to difficulty breathing. Many babies and children wheeze slightly when they have a minor respiratory infection. However, breathing problems that are accompanied by danger signs (see right) constitute a medical emergency.

DANGER SIGNS

If your child's breathing problems are accompanied by any of the following symptoms, you should call an ambulance at once:
- Blue-tinged lips or tongue.
- Abnormal drowsiness.
- Inability to talk or produce sounds normally.

START HERE

How long has your child had breathing problems?
- STARTED SUDDENLY A FEW MINUTES AGO
- STARTED MORE THAN A FEW MINUTES AGO

Are any of the following danger signs present?
- BLUE-TINGED LIPS OR TONGUE
- ABNORMAL DROWSINESS
- INABILITY TO TALK OR PRODUCE SOUNDS NORMALLY
- NONE OF THE ABOVE

How old is your child?
- 18 MONTHS OR OVER
- UNDER 18 MONTHS

Could your child be choking on a small object?
- POSSIBLY
- UNLIKELY

Has your child had an asthma attack in the past or is he or she being treated for asthma?

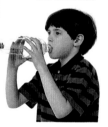

- HAS HAD AN ASTHMA ATTACK
- IS BEING TREATED FOR ASTHMA
- NEITHER

POSSIBLE CAUSE

Severe ASTHMA (p.153) attack.

ACTION NEEDED

MEDICAL HELP
✚ EMERGENCY! Call an ambulance!

SELF-HELP
Administer medications as prescribed. See panel: *Easing breathing in an asthma attack* (opposite) and FIRST AID: *Artificial ventilation* (p.205).

POSSIBLE CAUSES

BRONCHIOLITIS (p.155), PNEUMONIA (p.155), severe CROUP (p.150), or ASTHMA (p.153).

ACTION NEEDED

MEDICAL HELP
✚ EMERGENCY! Call an ambulance!

SELF-HELP
See FIRST AID: *Artificial ventilation* (p.205).

POSSIBLE CAUSE

Inhalation of a foreign body.

ACTION NEEDED

MEDICAL HELP
✚ EMERGENCY! Call an ambulance!

SELF-HELP
See FIRST AID: *Choking* (p.204).

Does your child suffer from repeated episodes of any of these symptoms?

- WHEEZING
- SHORTNESS OF BREATH
- COUGHING AT NIGHT
- NONE OF THE ABOVE

SELF-HELP: EASING BREATHING IN AN ASTHMA ATTACK

If your child is having difficulty breathing, the following measures may help:
- Help your child to sit up, leaning forwards against a table or the back of a chair.
- If medicine has been prescribed, make sure it is used as soon as breathing difficulties start.
- Try to keep other people away as crowds may cause further worry, making breathing harder.

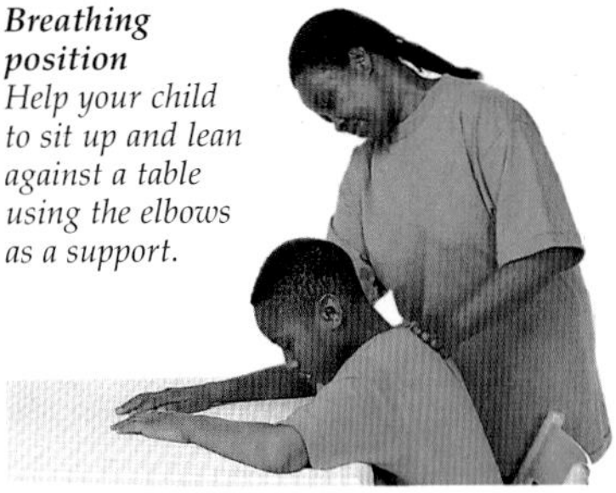

Breathing position
Help your child to sit up and lean against a table using the elbows as a support.

POSSIBLE CAUSE

ASTHMA (p.153).

ACTION NEEDED

MEDICAL HELP
If your child seems very unwell or if breathing difficulties develop, phone your doctor immediately.

SELF-HELP
See panel: *Easing breathing in an asthma attack* (above).

POSSIBLE CAUSES

PNEUMONIA (p.155) or BRONCHIOLITIS (p.155).

ACTION NEEDED

MEDICAL HELP
✚ URGENT! Phone your doctor immediately!

SELF-HELP
See panel: *Easing breathing in an asthma attack* (above).

Has your child had noisy, crowing breathing since birth but otherwise been well?

- NO
- YES

Do either of the following apply to your child?

- FAST BREATHING, FEVER, AND COUGH
- HOARSE VOICE, NOISY BREATHING, AND BARKING COUGH
- NEITHER

POSSIBLE CAUSE

CROUP (p.150).

ACTION NEEDED

MEDICAL HELP
✚ URGENT! Phone your doctor immediately!

Has there been a recent change in your child's breathing?

- CHANGE IN BREATHING
- NO CHANGE IN BREATHING

POSSIBLE CAUSE

Congenital laryngeal stridor, a harmless condition that your child will outgrow.

ACTION NEEDED

MEDICAL HELP
If there is no improvement by the age of 3 months, make an appointment to see your doctor.

POSSIBLE CAUSES

ASTHMA (p.153) or BRONCHITIS (p.154).

ACTION NEEDED

MEDICAL HELP
Get medical advice within 24 hours.

SELF-HELP
See panel: *Easing breathing in an asthma attack* (above).

27 COUGHING

In very young babies, coughing is rare and may indicate a serious lung infection. In older children, however, coughing is usually caused by a minor respiratory infection, such as a cold. A sudden cough in any child who is otherwise well can be serious as it may be caused by an airway obstruction.

DANGER SIGNS
Call an ambulance at once if your child has any of the following symptoms:
- Blue-tinged lips or tongue.
- Abnormal drowsiness.
- Inability to talk or produce sounds.
Phone your doctor at once if your child has the following symptom:
- Areas between ribs appear sunken.

START HERE

How old is your child?
- UNDER 1 YEAR
- 1 YEAR OR OVER

Is your child's breathing abnormally rapid or noisy (see panel, p.90)?
- ABNORMALLY RAPID
- NOISY
- NEITHER

Does your child have a fever – a temperature of 38°C (100°F) or above?
- FEVER
- NO FEVER

POSSIBLE CAUSES
A COMMON COLD (p.148) or, rarely, BRONCHIOLITIS (p.155) or PNEUMONIA (p.155).

ACTION NEEDED
MEDICAL HELP
If your child is very unwell or if breathing difficulties develop, phone your doctor immediately.
SELF-HELP
See panel: *Relieving a cough* (p.90).

Go to chart
26 BREATHING PROBLEMS

POSSIBLE CAUSE
PERTUSSIS (p.123) or ASTHMA (p.153).

ACTION NEEDED
MEDICAL HELP
Get medical advice within 24 hours.
SELF-HELP
See panel: *Relieving a cough* (p.90).

When does your child cough?
- MAINLY AT NIGHT
- AT ANY TIME

When does your child cough?
- AT ANY TIME
- MAINLY AT NIGHT

POSSIBLE CAUSE
PERTUSSIS (p.123) or ASTHMA (p.153).

ACTION NEEDED
MEDICAL HELP
Get medical advice within 24 hours.
SELF-HELP
See panel: *Relieving a cough* (p.90).

Does the cough have either of these characteristics?
- COMES IN FITS ENDING WITH A WHOOP
- IS ACCOMPANIED BY VOMITING
- NEITHER

Do either of the following apply to your child?

- HAS A RASH
- HAS RECENTLY BEEN EXPOSED TO MEASLES
- NEITHER

Does your child have any nasal symptoms?

- STUFFY NOSE
- RUNNY NOSE
- NEITHER

POSSIBLE CAUSE

MEASLES (p.118).

ACTION NEEDED

MEDICAL HELP
Get medical advice within 24 hours.

SELF-HELP
See panel: *Bringing down a high temperature* (p.37).

POSSIBLE CAUSE

A COMMON COLD (p.148).

ACTION NEEDED

MEDICAL HELP
If your child is distressed by the symptoms, consult your doctor.

SELF-HELP
See panel: *Relieving a cough* (p.90).

POSSIBLE CAUSES

A COMMON COLD (p.148) or INFLUENZA (p.151).

ACTION NEEDED

MEDICAL HELP
If breathing difficulties develop, phone your doctor. If a rash appears, get medical advice within 24 hours.

SELF-HELP
See panels: *Relieving a cough* (p.90) and *Bringing down a high temperature* (p.37).

POSSIBLE CAUSE

Inhalation of a foreign body.

ACTION NEEDED

MEDICAL HELP
✚ URGENT! Phone your doctor immediately!

SELF-HELP
See FIRST AID: *Choking* (p.204).

POSSIBLE CAUSE

ENLARGED ADENOIDS (p.149).

ACTION NEEDED

MEDICAL HELP
Make an appointment to see your doctor.

SELF-HELP
If the ear infections are causing pain, see panel: *Relieving earache* (p.101).

How long has your child been coughing?

- LESS THAN 24 HOURS
- 24 HOURS OR MORE

Does your child also have either of the following symptoms?

- FREQUENT EAR INFECTIONS
- NASAL VOICE
- NEITHER

POSSIBLE CAUSE

Recurrent colds (see COMMON COLD, p.148).

ACTION NEEDED

MEDICAL HELP
If your child seems generally unwell or is upset by the cough, consult your doctor.

SELF-HELP
See panel: *Relieving a cough* (p.90).

Is your child's nose persistently runny?

- PERSISTENTLY RUNNY
- NOT RUNNY

continued on p.90, top

27 Coughing (continued)

continued from p.89, bottom

Do either of the following apply to your child?

- HAS HAD PERTUSSIS WITHIN THE LAST FEW MONTHS
- HAS BEEN DIAGNOSED AS HAVING ASTHMA
- NEITHER

POSSIBLE CAUSE

ASTHMA (p.153).

ACTION NEEDED

MEDICAL HELP
If there is no improvement within 24 hours, consult your doctor.

SELF-HELP
Make sure that your child is taking his or her asthma medicine as directed. See panels: *Easing breathing in an asthma attack* (p.87) and *Relieving a cough* (below).

Are there smokers in your home, or might your child have been smoking?

- SMOKERS IN THE HOME
- CHILD MIGHT SMOKE
- NEITHER

ASSESSMENT: CHECKING BREATHING RATES

A child whose breathing rate is unusually rapid may need medical attention. To check your child's breathing, make sure that he or she is resting, then count the number of breaths over one minute.

Normal breathing rates
As a child grows older and the breathing apparatus matures, his or her normal breathing rate (the breathing rate at rest, not when active or crying) decreases. A young baby breathes much faster than a child who is aged 5 years or over.

AGE	NORMAL RATE
Under 2 months	Less than 60 breaths per minute
2 to 11 months	Less than 50 breaths per minute
1 to 5 years	Less than 40 breaths per minute
Over 5 years	Less than 30 breaths per minute

POSSIBLE CAUSE

Cough persisting after PERTUSSIS (p.123).

ACTION NEEDED

MEDICAL HELP
If your child is distressed by the cough or feels unwell, or if the cough persists for more than 3 months, make an appointment to see your doctor.

SELF-HELP
See panel: *Relieving a cough* (below).

POSSIBLE CAUSE

Irritation of the throat and lungs as a result of smoking or of being in a smoky atmosphere.

ACTION NEEDED

SELF-HELP
Make sure no one smokes around your child. If your child smokes, encourage him or her to give it up (see SUBSTANCE ABUSE, p.174).

If you cannot identify your child's problem from this chart, talk to your doctor within 48 hours.

SELF-HELP: RELIEVING A COUGH

The following measures may help to relieve your child's cough:
- Give soothing liquids, such as warm water mixed with honey (do not give honey to children under 1 because it may cause food poisoning), and plenty of other warm or cool drinks.
- Moisten the air by hanging a wet towel in front of a radiator.
- Do not overheat your child's room because this will dry out the air and increase coughing.

Relieving a coughing fit
Sit a young child on your lap, leaning slightly forwards, and pat his or her back to loosen any phlegm.

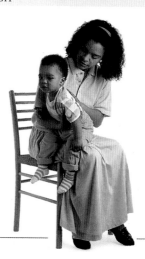

28 SORE THROAT

Most sore throats in children are caused by minor viral
infections that clear up quickly without treatment.
Occasionally, however, a sore throat may indicate a more
serious problem, such as tonsillitis. In very young children,
reluctance to eat or drink may be a sign of a sore throat.

START HERE

Does your child have any of the following symptoms?

- FEVER
- SEEMS UNWELL
- SNEEZING
- RUNNY NOSE
- COUGHING
- NONE OF THE ABOVE

Is your child suffering from any of the following symptoms?

- VOMITING
- RASH
- BRIGHT RED TONGUE AND THROAT
- PAIN ON SWALLOWING OR REFUSAL TO EAT SOLIDS

POSSIBLE CAUSE

SCARLET FEVER (p.121).

ACTION NEEDED

MEDICAL HELP
Get medical advice within 24 hours.

SELF-HELP
See panel: *Bringing down a high temperature* (p.37).

POSSIBLE CAUSE

Tonsillitis (see PHARYNGITIS AND TONSILLITIS, p.151).

ACTION NEEDED

MEDICAL HELP
If your child is no better after 24 hours, consult your doctor.

SELF-HELP
See panel: *Bringing down a high temperature* (p.37).

POSSIBLE CAUSES

A COMMON COLD (p.148) or ALLERGIC RHINITIS (p.152).

ACTION NEEDED

MEDICAL HELP
If the symptoms persist for more than a week, make an appointment to see your doctor.

SELF-HELP
See panel: *Relieving a cough* (opposite).

POSSIBLE CAUSE

Inflammation of the throat caused by a minor infection or irritation.

ACTION NEEDED

MEDICAL HELP
If your child's throat is still sore after 48 hours, make an appointment to see your doctor.

SELF-HELP: RELIEVING A SORE THROAT

The following measures will help
to reduce the discomfort of your
child's sore throat:
- Give your child as many cold,
  non-acidic drinks, and as much
  ice cream and jelly to eat, as he
  or she wants.
- Give regular doses of liquid
  paracetamol.
- Offer throat lozenges if your
  child is old enough to suck
  rather than chew them.
- If your child is over 8 years old,
  he or she can gargle with a
  diluted antiseptic.

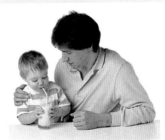

Soothing a sore throat
*Cold, non-acidic drinks, such as milk,
may help to soothe your child's sore
throat. A straw makes drinking easier.*

29 ABNORMAL DROWSINESS OR CONFUSION

Drowsiness may simply be a result of lack of sleep or a minor illness, or it may be a symptom of a serious disease, such as meningitis. Confusion – which includes appearing dazed or agitated, or talking nonsense – is always a serious symptom that requires immediate medical attention.

DANGER SIGNS
Call an ambulance at once if your child has any of the following symptoms:
- Unconscious for 3 minutes.
- Unresponsive or difficult to rouse from sleep.
- Blood or fluid leaking from the nose or ears.
- Irregular or slow breathing.

START HERE

Did your child have a recent accident or fall that involved banging the head?

- **BLOW TO HEAD**
- **NO BLOW TO HEAD**

Might your child have swallowed any poisonous plants or fungi, household cleaners, alcohol, or other substance?

- **UNLIKELY**
- **POSSIBLY**

Does your child have any of the following symptoms?

- **FEVER**
- **DIARRHOEA WITH OR WITHOUT VOMITING**
- **HEADACHE**
- **VOMITING WITHOUT DIARRHOEA**
- **STIFF NECK**
- **FLAT SPOTS THAT DO NOT DISAPPEAR WHEN PRESSED**
- **NONE OF THE ABOVE**

POSSIBLE CAUSE
HEAD INJURY (p.159).

ACTION NEEDED
MEDICAL HELP
✚ **EMERGENCY!** Call an ambulance! While waiting, do not give your child anything to eat or drink.

POSSIBLE CAUSE
Swallowed poisons may make your child unusually drowsy or confused, and may lead to a loss of consciousness.

ACTION NEEDED
MEDICAL HELP
✚ **URGENT!** Phone your doctor immediately!

SELF-HELP
See FIRST AID: *Swallowed poisons* (p.211).

POSSIBLE CAUSE
MENINGITIS (p.158).

ACTION NEEDED
MEDICAL HELP
✚ **EMERGENCY!** Call an ambulance!

POSSIBLE CAUSE
DIABETES MELLITUS (p.190).

ACTION NEEDED
MEDICAL HELP
✚ **URGENT!** Phone your doctor immediately!

POSSIBLE CAUSES

A high fever, resulting from any infection but especially MENINGITIS (p.158) or a kidney or liver infection, may cause delirium, particularly if your child's temperature exceeds 39°C (102°F).

ACTION NEEDED

MEDICAL HELP
✚ URGENT! Phone your doctor immediately!

SELF-HELP
See panel: *Bringing down a high temperature* (p.37).

POSSIBLE CAUSE

Your child may be suffering from dehydration as a result of GASTROENTERITIS (p.180).

ACTION NEEDED

MEDICAL HELP
✚ URGENT! Phone your doctor immediately!

SELF-HELP
See panel: *Preventing dehydration in babies* (p.38) or *Preventing dehydration in children* (p.53).

POSSIBLE CAUSE

DIABETES MELLITUS (p.190).

ACTION NEEDED

MEDICAL HELP
✚ URGENT! Phone your doctor immediately!

Has your child been passing an unusually large quantity of urine?

- LARGE AMOUNT OF URINE
- NORMAL AMOUNT OF URINE

POSSIBLE CAUSE

Certain medicines, such as antihistamines given for ALLERGIES (p.152), can cause confusion or have a sedative effect on some children.

ACTION NEEDED

MEDICAL HELP
Phone your doctor to find out whether the medicine may be causing your child's symptoms and whether you should stop giving it.

POSSIBLE CAUSE

SUBSTANCE ABUSE (p.174).

ACTION NEEDED

MEDICAL HELP
Make an appointment to see your doctor.

Is your child suffering from any of the following symptoms?

- EXCESSIVE THIRST
- LOSS OF WEIGHT
- UNCHARACTERISTIC TIREDNESS DURING THE LAST FEW WEEKS
- NONE OF THE ABOVE

Have you noticed any of the following changes in your child's appearance or behaviour?

- RED EYES
- LOSS OF APPETITE
- MOOD SWINGS
- WITHDRAWAL
- AGGRESSION
- NONE OF THE ABOVE

Have you been giving your child any medicine?

- MEDICINE
- NO MEDICINE

If you cannot identify your child's problem from this chart, talk to your doctor at once.

30 DIZZINESS, FAINTING, AND SEIZURES

Dizziness is a spinning sensation. It may be accompanied by an attack of faintness or lightheadedness. Fainting is a brief loss of consciousness that is caused by a fall in blood pressure. A seizure may also involve a loss of consciousness, but it is a result of abnormal electrical activity in the brain.

DANGER SIGNS
Call an ambulance at once if your child has lost consciousness and any of the following occur:
- Consciousness is not regained within 3 minutes.
- Breathing becomes slower.
- Breathing is irregular or noisy.

START HERE

Does your child have any of the following symptoms?

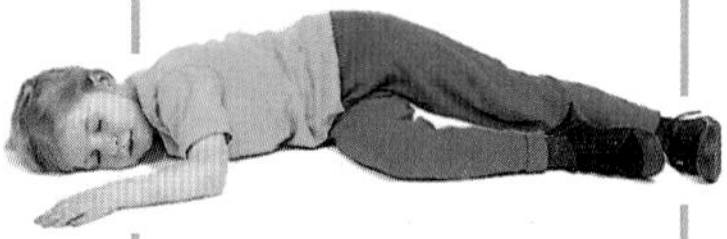

- FELL TO GROUND UNCONSCIOUS
- FEELS SURROUNDINGS ARE GOING ROUND AND ROUND
- SEEMS UNAWARE OF SURROUNDINGS FOR A FEW MOMENTS
- FEELS FAINT OR UNSTEADY
- NONE OF THE ABOVE

POSSIBLE CAUSE
LABYRINTHITIS (p.164).

ACTION NEEDED
MEDICAL HELP
Make an appointment to see your doctor.

POSSIBLE CAUSE
A petit mal seizure (see EPILEPSY, p.157).

ACTION NEEDED
MEDICAL HELP
Make an appointment to see your doctor.
SELF-HELP
Sit your child down quietly until fully recovered.

During your child's loss of consciousness, did any of the following occur?

- TWITCHING OF THE FACE OR LIMBS
- PASSING URINE
- INJURY, SUCH AS BITING THE TONGUE
- NONE OF THE ABOVE

POSSIBLE CAUSE
Low blood sugar level (hypoglycaemia), caused by DIABETES MELLITUS (p.190).

ACTION NEEDED
MEDICAL HELP
If your child often feels faint, make an appointment to see your doctor.
SELF-HELP
As soon as your child feels faint, give glucose tablets or a glucose or sugary drink. See panel: *Dealing with faintness and fainting* (opposite).

Is your child being treated for diabetes mellitus?

- YES
- NO

If you cannot identify your child's problem from this chart, talk to your doctor within 48 hours.

Is your child being treated for diabetes mellitus?

YES

NO

How old is your child?

UNDER 5 YEARS

5 YEARS OR OVER

Does your child have a fever – a temperature of 38°C (100°F) or above?

NO FEVER

FEVER

POSSIBLE CAUSE

Extremely low blood sugar level (severe hypoglycaemia), caused by DIABETES MELLITUS (p.190), may cause your child to lose consciousness and, in some cases, to have a seizure.

ACTION NEEDED

MEDICAL HELP
✚ URGENT! Phone your doctor immediately!

POSSIBLE CAUSE

A grand mal seizure (see EPILEPSY, p.157).

ACTION NEEDED

MEDICAL HELP
✚ URGENT! Phone your doctor immediately!

POSSIBLE CAUSE

FEBRILE CONVULSIONS (p.156).

ACTION NEEDED

MEDICAL HELP
✚ URGENT! Phone your doctor immediately!

SELF-HELP
See panel: *Bringing down a high temperature* (p.37).

POSSIBLE CAUSES

Your child's unconsciousness is probably a fainting attack. Fainting may be due to a fall in blood pressure, possibly caused by emotional stress or anxiety; or a low blood sugar level as a result of not eating for some time; or from being in an overcrowded or stuffy atmosphere for too long.

ACTION NEEDED

MEDICAL HELP
If your child faints regularly, make an appointment to see your doctor.

SELF-HELP
See panel: *Dealing with faintness and fainting* (below).

POSSIBLE CAUSES

Hunger, anxiety, or being in a stuffy atmosphere are all possible causes of faintness. A child who is feeling faint may experience dizziness, nausea, and weakness; the child will also have a very pale face.

ACTION NEEDED

MEDICAL HELP
If your child has not shown any signs of recovery within 30 minutes, phone your doctor immediately.

SELF-HELP
See panel: *Dealing with faintness and fainting* (right).

SELF-HELP: DEALING WITH FAINTNESS AND FAINTING

A child who feels faint should be laid down with legs propped up on several cushions, and the following measures should be carried out:
• Loosen any tight clothing and make sure there is plenty of fresh air.
• Calm and reassure your child.
• Faintness can be caused by low blood sugar, so a sugary drink or small snack may help. Do not offer food or drink if your child is not fully conscious.
• If your child loses consciousness, monitor his or her condition using the ABC of resuscitation (pp.202–203). Place in the recovery position (p.203) if he or she is unconscious but breathing.

First aid for fainting
Lay your child down with feet raised, to increase the supply of blood to the brain.

31 EYE PROBLEMS

Any child with an eye injury, or a foreign body in the eye that cannot be removed by self-help measures (opposite), should receive immediate medical attention. Most other problems, such as itching, redness, watering, and discharge, are caused by infections or irritation and are seldom serious.

START HERE

Does your child have any obvious damage to an eye?

DAMAGE

NO OBVIOUS DAMAGE

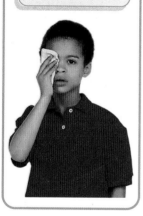

Can you see a foreign body, such as a speck of dirt, in your child's eye?

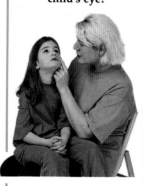

NO FOREIGN BODY

FOREIGN BODY

Does your child have any of the following symptoms?

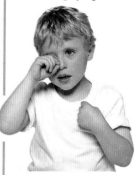

RED LUMP ON EYELID

EYES PRODUCE TEARS EVEN WHEN CHILD IS NOT CRYING

WHITE OF EYE IS RED

RED, ITCHY EYELIDS

NONE OF THE ABOVE

If you cannot identify your child's problem from this chart, talk to your doctor within 48 hours.

POSSIBLE CAUSE

Eye injury.

ACTION NEEDED

MEDICAL HELP
✚ EMERGENCY! Call an ambulance or take your child to the nearest hospital accident and emergency department.
SELF-HELP
See FIRST AID: *Eye wound* (p.209).

POSSIBLE CAUSE

A foreign body often causes redness and watering.

ACTION NEEDED

MEDICAL HELP
If you cannot remove the foreign body or if your child is in pain, phone your doctor immediately.
SELF-HELP
See panel: *Removing a foreign body from the eye* (opposite).

POSSIBLE CAUSES

Blepharitis (see EYELID DISORDERS, p.166) or CONJUNCTIVITIS (p.165).

ACTION NEEDED

MEDICAL HELP
Make an appointment to see your doctor.

SELF-HELP: REMOVING A FOREIGN BODY FROM THE EYE

A foreign body, such as an eyelash or a speck of dirt, can usually be removed as illustrated. If the foreign body is metal, or if it is embedded in your child's eye, do not try to remove it. See FIRST AID: *Eye wound* (p.209) and take your child to hospital at once.

• If you can see the foreign body on your child's lower eyelid or white of the eye, use a corner of a clean, damp handkerchief to lift it off.

• If your child cannot dislodge the object from the upper eyelid as shown, hold the lashes, pull the eyelid outwards, and fold it over a cotton wool bud. Remove the object with a handkerchief.

• If the foreign body is still not visible, seek medical assistance.

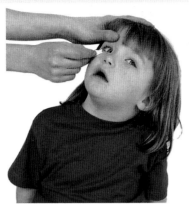

Foreign body on lower eyelid
Lift the foreign body off your child's eyelid with the corner of a clean handkerchief that has been moistened with water.

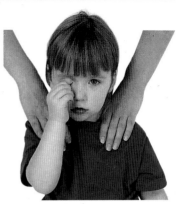

Foreign body on upper eyelid
Tell your child to pull the upper eyelid down over the lower one to dislodge a foreign body caught under it.

POSSIBLE CAUSE

Stye (see EYELID DISORDERS, p.166).

ACTION NEEDED

MEDICAL HELP
If the eye becomes red and painful, if the stye does not heal within 1 week, or if it recurs, make an appointment to see your doctor.

How old is your child?
- UNDER 1 YEAR
- 1 YEAR OR OVER

If you cannot identify your child's problem from this chart, talk to your doctor within 48 hours.

POSSIBLE CAUSE

BLOCKED TEAR DUCT (p.165).

ACTION NEEDED

MEDICAL HELP
Make an appointment to see your doctor.

POSSIBLE CAUSES

Eye irritation may be caused by chemicals, fumes, or viral or allergic CONJUNCTIVITIS (p.165). IRITIS (p.164), a more serious condition, is also a possibility.

ACTION NEEDED

MEDICAL HELP
✚ URGENT! Phone your doctor immediately if your child is in pain. If there is no pain but redness continues for more than 24 hours, make an appointment to see your doctor.

SELF-HELP
See FIRST AID: *Chemical in eye* (p.209).

Does your child's eye have a sticky discharge?
- DISCHARGE
- NO DISCHARGE

POSSIBLE CAUSE

Severe CONJUNCTIVITIS (p.165).

ACTION NEEDED

MEDICAL HELP
Get medical advice within 24 hours.

32 VISION PROBLEMS

Any problem with a child's vision should be investigated promptly. Usually, any defects are picked up in the routine eye tests that most children undergo at school. Alternatively, you or the teacher may notice that your child is having difficulty seeing or that there are other eye problems.

START HERE

How is your child's vision affected?

- DOUBLE OR BLURRED VISION
- ALL OR PART OF VISION IS LOST
- HAS DIFFICULTY SEEING DISTANT OR NEAR OBJECTS
- NONE OF THE ABOVE

POSSIBLE CAUSE

Injury to the eye or part of the brain is possible.

ACTION NEEDED

MEDICAL HELP
✚ EMERGENCY! Take your child to the nearest hospital accident and emergency department!
SELF-HELP
See FIRST AID: *Eye wound* (p.209).

POSSIBLE CAUSES

A REFRACTIVE ERROR (p.167), such as shortsightedness or longsightedness.

ACTION NEEDED

MEDICAL HELP
Make an appointment to see your doctor or optician.

Do your child's eyes seem out of alignment?

- RARELY
- OFTEN

POSSIBLE CAUSE

SQUINT (p.166).

ACTION NEEDED

MEDICAL HELP
If your child is over 4 months old, make an appointment to see your doctor.

Do either of the following apply to your child?

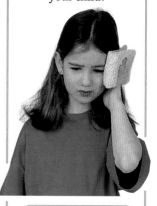

- HAD A RECENT HEAD INJURY
- VISION PROBLEMS ASSOCIATED WITH HEADACHES
- NEITHER

Does your child have recurrent attacks of seeing flashing lights or floating spots, with a severe headache afterwards?

- YES
- NO

POSSIBLE CAUSE

Bleeding inside skull (see HEAD INJURY, p.159).

ACTION NEEDED

MEDICAL HELP
✚ URGENT! Phone your doctor immediately!

Is your child taking any medicine, or might he or she have taken someone else's medicine?

> TAKING MEDICINE

> POSSIBLY TOOK SOMEONE ELSE'S MEDICINE

> NEITHER

POSSIBLE CAUSE

Some drugs may cause blurred vision.

ACTION NEEDED

MEDICAL HELP
Phone your doctor to find out whether the medicine may be causing your child's symptoms and whether you should stop giving it.

POSSIBLE CAUSE

Accidental poisoning by drugs, particularly certain antidepressants, may cause blurred vision.

ACTION NEEDED

MEDICAL HELP
✚ URGENT! Phone your doctor immediately!

SELF-HELP
See FIRST AID: *Swallowed poisons* (p.211).

Is one or both of your child's eyes red and painful?

> NOT RED OR PAINFUL

> RED AND PAINFUL

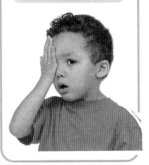

POSSIBLE CAUSES

A REFRACTIVE ERROR (p.167), such as shortsightedness or longsightedness, or a SQUINT (p.166) is possible.

ACTION NEEDED

MEDICAL HELP
Make an appointment to see your doctor or optician.

POSSIBLE CAUSE

IRITIS (p.164).

ACTION NEEDED

MEDICAL HELP
✚ URGENT! Phone your doctor immediately!

POSSIBLE CAUSE

Migraine (see RECURRENT HEADACHES, p.161).

ACTION NEEDED

MEDICAL HELP
If this is your child's first attack, phone your doctor. If the attacks are frequent, make an appointment to see your doctor.

SELF-HELP
See panel: *Relieving a headache* (p.65).

> If you cannot identify your child's problem from this chart, talk to your doctor within 48 hours.

ASSESSMENT: CHECKING YOUR BABY'S VISION

You can use the following method to check developing vision in a baby who is at least 6 weeks old.

- Your baby should sit on another adult's lap, preferably someone with whom your baby is familiar.
- Crouch down so that your face is level with your baby's face, and at arm's length away. Your baby should fixate on your face.
- Move your head from side to side. Your baby should hold your gaze.

An alternative method
Ask another adult to sit your baby on his or her lap and hold a toy at arm's length. Note whether your baby fixates on the toy.

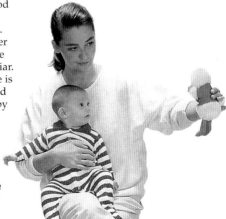

33 PAINFUL OR ITCHY EAR

Earache is usually caused by infection. Young children are particularly prone to middle ear infections because the tubes connecting the ears and nose are short and easily blocked by infected material. The outer ear can be affected by disorders that cause symptoms such as itchiness or discharge.

START HERE

How would you describe your child's earache?

- NOT SEVERE
- SEVERE

Might there be something in your child's ear?

- POSSIBLY
- UNLIKELY

POSSIBLE CAUSE

A foreign body, such as an insect or bead, in the ear.

ACTION NEEDED

MEDICAL HELP
Get medical advice within 24 hours.

SELF-HELP
If you can see the foreign body in your child's ear and it is not stuck, you should remove it but should take care not to push the object further into the ear canal. An insect may be floated out by pouring tepid water into your child's ear.

Does your child seem unwell in any other way?

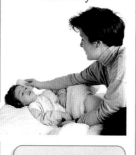

- HAS A FEVER
- HAS A COLD
- SEEMS GENERALLY UNWELL
- SEEMS WELL

Can you see a red lump inside your child's ear?

- RED LUMP
- NO RED LUMP

POSSIBLE CAUSE

OTITIS MEDIA (p.162).

ACTION NEEDED

MEDICAL HELP
✚ URGENT! Phone your doctor immediately!

SELF-HELP
See panels: *Relieving earache* (opposite) and *Bringing down a high temperature* (p.37).

POSSIBLE CAUSE

A BOIL (p.137) in the outer ear canal.

ACTION NEEDED

MEDICAL HELP
Get medical advice within 24 hours.

SELF-HELP
See panel: *Relieving earache* (opposite).

POSSIBLE CAUSE

OTITIS EXTERNA (p.163).

ACTION NEEDED

MEDICAL HELP
Get medical advice within 24 hours.

SELF-HELP
See panel: *Relieving earache* (opposite).

What are your child's other symptoms?

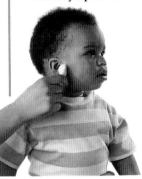

DISCHARGE FROM EAR

ITCHY EAR

NEITHER

What is the effect of gently tugging on your child's earlobe?

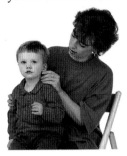

MAKES PAIN WORSE

NO EFFECT

POSSIBLE CAUSES

ATOPIC ECZEMA (p.135) or OTITIS EXTERNA (p.163).

ACTION NEEDED

MEDICAL HELP
Get medical advice within 24 hours.

SELF-HELP
See panel: *Relieving earache* (below).

POSSIBLE CAUSE

OTITIS MEDIA (p.162).

ACTION NEEDED

MEDICAL HELP
Get medical advice within 24 hours.

SELF-HELP
See panel: *Relieving earache* (below).

POSSIBLE CAUSES

ATOPIC ECZEMA (p.135) or OTITIS EXTERNA (p.163).

ACTION NEEDED

MEDICAL HELP
Get medical advice within 24 hours.

SELF-HELP
See panel: *Relieving earache* (below).

Did the pain start during or soon after a journey by air?

STARTED DURING OR AFTER A FLIGHT

DID NOT START DURING OR AFTER A FLIGHT

POSSIBLE CAUSE

BAROTRAUMA (p.164).

ACTION NEEDED

MEDICAL HELP
If the earache persists or if your child seems unwell, make an appointment to see your doctor.

SELF-HELP
See panel: *Relieving earache* (right).

SELF-HELP: RELIEVING EARACHE

The following measures may reduce the pain of an earache:
- Give liquid paracetamol.
- Provide a hot water bottle covered with a towel to hold against the ear. For a baby, use a warmed soft cloth.
- Tell your child to lie down or sit up, with his or her head propped up with pillows.
- Do not insert either ear drops or oil into your child's ear.

Easing the pain of earache
If lying flat makes the earache worse, prop up your child, supported by a couple of pillows or cushions.

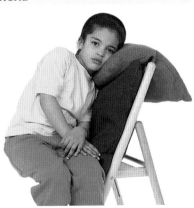

34 HEARING PROBLEMS

Hearing defects are often first noticed by the child's parents. In babies, the first sign of deafness is a failure to respond to sounds. In older children, the onset of hearing problems may cause school work to deteriorate. Although hearing loss may be only temporary, it should be checked by your doctor.

START HERE

Has your child had hearing problems for long?

- STARTED RECENTLY
- DID NOT START RECENTLY

Did your child have earache before the hearing loss started?

- HAD EARACHE
- DID NOT HAVE EARACHE

Might your child's hearing difficulties have been present since birth?

- POSSIBLY
- UNLIKELY

Has your child had any of the following infectious diseases recently?

- MUMPS
- MEASLES
- MENINGITIS
- ENCEPHALITIS
- NONE OF THE ABOVE

POSSIBLE CAUSES

Rarely, infectious diseases, such as MUMPS (p.122), MEASLES (p.118), MENINGITIS (p.158), and ENCEPHALITIS (p.159), may damage parts of the nervous system that are involved with hearing, and may result in permanent hearing loss.

ACTION NEEDED

MEDICAL HELP
If your child experiences difficulty hearing following any of these illnesses, make an appointment to see your doctor.

POSSIBLE CAUSE

GLUE EAR (p.163).

ACTION NEEDED

MEDICAL HELP
Make an appointment to see your doctor.

POSSIBLE CAUSE

A congenital defect is possible, although unlikely unless there is a family history of deafness or your child was exposed to RUBELLA (p.119) before he or she was born.

ACTION NEEDED

MEDICAL HELP
Make an appointment to see your doctor. He or she may arrange for your child to have a hearing test.

> If you cannot identify your child's problem from this chart, talk to your doctor within 48 hours.

Is your child suffering from earache or has he or she had earache recently?

- HAS EARACHE NOW
- HAD EARACHE RECENTLY
- NEITHER

Did the hearing problems start during or shortly after a journey by air?

- STARTED DURING OR AFTER A FLIGHT
- DID NOT START DURING OR AFTER A FLIGHT

POSSIBLE CAUSE

BAROTRAUMA (p.164).

ACTION NEEDED

MEDICAL HELP
If hearing problems persist, make an appointment to see your doctor.

SELF-HELP
See panel: *Relieving earache* (p.101).

Which of the following apply to your child?

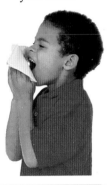

- HAS BEEN SNEEZING
- RECENTLY HAD A COLD
- NEITHER

POSSIBLE CAUSE

OTITIS MEDIA (p.162).

ACTION NEEDED

MEDICAL HELP
Get medical advice within 24 hours.

SELF-HELP
See panel: *Relieving earache* (p.101).

POSSIBLE CAUSES

A COMMON COLD (p.148) or ALLERGIC RHINITIS (p.152) may have caused the tubes connecting the ears and throat to become blocked.

ACTION NEEDED

MEDICAL HELP
Make an appointment to see your doctor.

POSSIBLE CAUSE

Earwax blockage (see OTITIS EXTERNA, p.163).

ACTION NEEDED

MEDICAL HELP
Make an appointment to see your doctor.

ASSESSMENT: CHECKING YOUR BABY'S HEARING

While only a professional can test your child's hearing accurately, you can easily make the following observations of your baby's hearing. A negative response at any age may indicate a problem.

- Shortly after birth, your baby should respond to a sudden loud noise, such as clapped hands, by blinking or opening the eyes.
- By the age of 1 month, your baby should respond to a prolonged sound that starts suddenly, such as the noise of a vacuum cleaner.
- By the age of 4 months, your baby should react to the sound of your voice, even if you are out of sight.
- By the age of 12 months, your baby should respond to his or her own name as well as familiar words such as "mama" and "no".

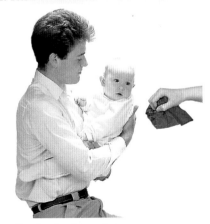

Hearing development
By the age of 7 months, your baby should turn towards a soft sound made behind him or her, such as paper being crackled.

35 MOUTH PROBLEMS

Most problems affecting the lips, tongue, gums, and inside of the mouth are minor. However, a sore mouth may make your child miserable and eating and drinking painful. In an infant, the most likely cause of mouth pain is teething, which may be relieved by chewing on a hard or cold object.

START HERE

Does your child have any of the following symptoms?

- SORE AREAS ON OR AROUND THE LIPS
- SORENESS AFFECTING THE TONGUE ONLY
- PAINFUL, RED, SWOLLEN GUMS
- PAINFUL, DISCOLOURED AREAS INSIDE MOUTH
- PAINFUL, DISCOLOURED AREAS ON TONGUE
- NONE OF THE ABOVE

Might your child be teething?
- POSSIBLY
- UNLIKELY

What is the nature of the discoloured areas?
- LIGHT YELLOW SPOTS
- CREAMY-YELLOW AND EASILY SCRAPED OFF
- NEITHER

POSSIBLE CAUSE
Irritation of the tongue caused by a rough tooth.

ACTION NEEDED
DENTAL HELP
Make an appointment to see your dentist.

POSSIBLE CAUSE
TEETHING (p.33).

ACTION NEEDED
SELF-HELP
You can help your baby by providing a hard object, such as a teething ring, for him or her to chew on. A variety of gels, drops, and powders, available over the counter, may also ease the pain.

POSSIBLE CAUSE
GINGIVITIS (p.176).

ACTION NEEDED
DENTAL HELP
Make an appointment to see your dentist.
SELF-HELP
Your child should continue to brush his or her teeth with care. Your child can also use an antibacterial mouthwash to relieve the inflammation. See How can I prevent dental caries? (p.177).

POSSIBLE CAUSE
ORAL THRUSH (p.176).

ACTION NEEDED
MEDICAL HELP
Make an appointment to see your doctor.

If you cannot identify your child's problem from this chart, talk to your doctor within 48 hours.

If you cannot identify your child's problem from this chart, talk to your doctor within 48 hours.

What is the appearance of the affected area?

- TINY BLISTERS ON OR AROUND THE LIPS
- REDNESS AROUND MOUTH
- CRACKS AT CORNERS OF LIPS
- NONE OF THE ABOVE

POSSIBLE CAUSE
COLD SORES (p.139).

ACTION NEEDED
MEDICAL HELP
If the blisters are severe, have lasted for more than 2 weeks, or are causing your child embarrassment, make an appointment to see your doctor.

SELF-HELP
Apply a cream or gel, available over the counter, to the sores several times daily until they disappear.

POSSIBLE CAUSE
LICK ECZEMA (p.136).

ACTION NEEDED
SELF-HELP
Apply petroleum jelly to the affected area every few hours. Use a lip salve to moisturize and protect the lips themselves.

> If you cannot identify your child's problem from this chart, talk to your doctor within 48 hours.

Does your child have any of the following symptoms?

- FEELS GENERALLY UNWELL
- HAS A FEVER
- HAS SPOTS ON THE HANDS AND FEET
- NONE OF THE ABOVE

POSSIBLE CAUSE
GINGIVOSTOMATITIS (p.176).

ACTION NEEDED
MEDICAL HELP
Make an appointment to see your doctor.

SELF-HELP
See panels: *Relieving a sore mouth* (below) and *Bringing down a high temperature* (p.37).

POSSIBLE CAUSE
HAND, FOOT, AND MOUTH DISEASE (p.120).

ACTION NEEDED
SELF-HELP
See panel: *Relieving a sore mouth* (below).

POSSIBLE CAUSE
MOUTH ULCERS (p.175).

ACTION NEEDED
MEDICAL HELP
If the mouth ulcers have failed to heal within 10 days, make an appointment to see your doctor.

SELF-HELP
See panel: *Relieving a sore mouth* (right).

SELF-HELP: RELIEVING A SORE MOUTH

The following measures may help to relieve your child's discomfort:
- A sore mouth should be rinsed out every hour with ¼ teaspoon bicarbonate of soda dissolved in 100 ml (3.5 fl.oz) of warm water.
- If your child's symptoms are causing pain, you can give the appropriate dose of paracetamol.
- Your child may prefer a diet of soft foods, such as soup and ice cream, while the soreness lasts.
- Avoid giving acidic drinks, such as fruit juices. Drinking through a straw may stop irritating liquids bathing the ulcers.

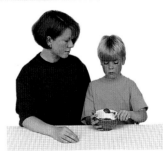

Foods for a sore mouth
Give your child plenty of fluids and soft foods, including yoghurt and soup, until his or her mouth heals.

36 ABDOMINAL PAIN

Every child suffers from abdominal pain from time to time and some children have recurrent bouts of pain. Usually the cause is minor and the pain disappears within a few hours without any treatment. Rarely, however, there may be a serious underlying disorder that requires medical attention.

DANGER SIGNS
Call an ambulance at once if your child has any of the following symptoms:
- Abdominal pain for 6 hours.
- Pain or swelling in the groin or testes.
- Greenish-yellow vomit.

START HERE

What are the features of your child's abdominal pain?

- PAINFUL SWELLING IN GROIN OR SCROTUM
- CONTINUOUS PAIN FOR 6 HOURS
- PAIN AGGRAVATED WHEN ABDOMEN IS GENTLY PRESSED
- NONE OF THE ABOVE

POSSIBLE CAUSES
Strangulated inguinal hernia (see HERNIA, p.187) or testicular torsion (see PENIS AND TESTIS DISORDERS, p.197).

ACTION NEEDED

MEDICAL HELP
✚ EMERGENCY! Call an ambulance! While waiting, do not give your child anything to eat or drink.

POSSIBLE CAUSE
APPENDICITIS (p.179).

ACTION NEEDED

MEDICAL HELP
✚ EMERGENCY! Call an ambulance! While waiting, do not give your child anything to eat or drink.

POSSIBLE CAUSE
APPENDICITIS (p.179).

ACTION NEEDED

MEDICAL HELP
If the pain continues for more than 3 hours, phone your doctor immediately.

SELF-HELP
See panel: *Relieving abdominal pain* (opposite).

Does your child have any of the following symptoms?

- VOMITING
- PAIN RELIEVED BY PASSAGE OF FAECES OR VOMITING
- DIARRHOEA WITH OR WITHOUT VOMITING
- NONE OF THE ABOVE

POSSIBLE CAUSE
APPENDICITIS (p.179).

ACTION NEEDED

MEDICAL HELP
✚ URGENT! Phone your doctor immediately!

SELF-HELP
See panel: *Relieving abdominal pain* (opposite).

Does your child have either of the following symptoms?

- CONTINUOUS PAIN FOR 3 HOURS
- GREENISH-YELLOW VOMIT
- NEITHER

POSSIBLE CAUSE
GASTROENTERITIS (p.180).

ACTION NEEDED

MEDICAL HELP
Get medical advice within 24 hours.

SELF-HELP
See panel: *Preventing dehydration in children* (p.53).

POSSIBLE CAUSE

INTESTINAL OBSTRUCTION (p.185).

ACTION NEEDED

MEDICAL HELP
✚ **EMERGENCY!** Call an ambulance! While waiting, do not give your child anything to eat or drink.

POSSIBLE CAUSE

An upper respiratory tract infection, such as a COMMON COLD (p.148).

ACTION NEEDED

MEDICAL HELP
If your child is distressed by his or her symptoms, consult your doctor.

SELF-HELP
See panels: *Relieving a cough* (p.90), *Relieving a sore throat* (p.91), and *Relieving abdominal pain* (above).

SELF-HELP: RELIEVING ABDOMINAL PAIN

The following measures may help to relieve your child's pain:
- Give your child a hot water bottle, filled with warm water and wrapped in a towel, to hold against his or her abdomen.
- Your child should not have anything to eat, and only plain water to drink, while in pain. If there is any possibility of appendicitis or another serious disorder for which your child might require surgery, do not give anything to eat or drink until you have a doctor's advice.

Easing abdominal pain
A well-wrapped hot water bottle held against your child's abdomen, while lying on a bed or sofa or sitting in a chair, may soothe the pain.

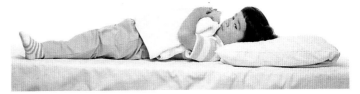

Does your child have any of the following symptoms?

| FEVER |
| PAIN ON PASSING URINE |
| BED-WETTING (AFTER BEING DRY AT NIGHT) |

TWO OR MORE

ONE OR NONE

POSSIBLE CAUSE

URINARY TRACT INFECTION (p.193).

ACTION NEEDED

MEDICAL HELP
Get medical advice within 24 hours.

SELF-HELP
If your child has a fever, see panel: *Bringing down a high temperature* (p.37).

POSSIBLE CAUSE

Anxiety (see ANXIETY AND FEARS, p.170) may be the cause of recurrent abdominal pain, but in many cases there is no obvious explanation.

ACTION NEEDED

MEDICAL HELP
Make an appointment to see your doctor.

SELF-HELP
Try to determine the reason for your child's anxiety, if you feel this is causing your child's pain, and alleviate it. See panel: *Relieving abdominal pain* (above).

Does your child have any of the following symptoms?

SORE THROAT

COUGH

STUFFY OR RUNNY NOSE

NONE OF THE ABOVE

Does your child often have abdominal pain without seeming unwell?

HAS RECURRENT BOUTS

NOT USUALLY

If you cannot identify your child's problem from this chart, talk to your doctor within 48 hours.

37 CONSTIPATION

Children pass faeces from as often as four times a day to once every 4 days; anything within this range is normal as long as the faeces are not runny, hard, or painful to pass. Changes in your child's diet, minor illness, or emotional stress may temporarily affect the frequency of defecation.

START HERE

Has your child passed any faeces in the last 24 hours?

- FAECES
- NO FAECES

Does your child have any of the following problems?

- PAINFUL DEFECATION
- BLOOD ON FAECES
- HARD, PELLET-LIKE FAECES

POSSIBLE CAUSE

Anal fissure (see CONSTIPATION, p.181).

ACTION NEEDED

MEDICAL HELP
Make an appointment to see your doctor.

SELF-HELP
See panel: *Preventing constipation* (opposite).

POSSIBLE CAUSE

Your child's diet may not contain enough fibre or fluid.

ACTION NEEDED

SELF-HELP
See panel: *Preventing constipation* (opposite).

Does your child have abdominal pain?

- ABDOMINAL PAIN
- NO ABDOMINAL PAIN

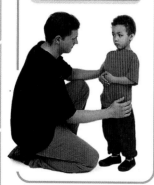

Go to chart
36 ABDOMINAL PAIN

How often does your child usually defecate?

- DAILY
- ONCE EVERY 2 TO 4 DAYS
- LESS THAN ONCE EVERY 4 DAYS

Has your child had a fever – a temperature of 38°C (100°F) or above – or has he or she been vomiting?

- FEVER
- VOMITING
- NEITHER

POSSIBLE CAUSE

CONSTIPATION (p.181).

ACTION NEEDED

MEDICAL HELP
Make an appointment to see your doctor.

SELF-HELP
See panel: *Preventing constipation* (opposite).

POSSIBLE CAUSE

For many children, defecating only once every few days is quite normal.

ACTION NEEDED

MEDICAL HELP
If your child is uncomfortable, make an appointment to see your doctor.

POSSIBLE CAUSE

Loss of fluid as a result of fever or vomiting can disrupt bowel movements, which will return to normal once your child has recovered.

ACTION NEEDED

SELF-HELP
Encourage your child to drink plenty of fluids.
See also panels: *Bringing down a high temperature* (p.37), and *Preventing dehydration in babies* (p.38) or *Preventing dehydration in children* (p.53).

POSSIBLE CAUSE

Anal fissure (see CONSTIPATION, p.181).

ACTION NEEDED

MEDICAL HELP
Make an appointment to see your doctor.

SELF-HELP
See panel: *Preventing constipation* (below).

POSSIBLE CAUSE

Your child's diet may not contain enough fibre or fluid, resulting in hard faeces.

ACTION NEEDED

SELF-HELP
See panel: *Preventing constipation* (below).

Has your child had either of the following symptoms in the past few days?

- PAINFUL DEFECATION
- BLOOD ON FAECES
- NEITHER

When was your child toilet-trained?

- HAS NOT STARTED YET
- SOME TIME AGO
- LEARNING NOW
- RECENTLY

Have you changed your child's diet recently?

- DIET CHANGED
- DIET UNCHANGED

If you cannot identify your child's problem from this chart, talk to your doctor within 48 hours.

SELF-HELP: PREVENTING CONSTIPATION

The following measures may help to relieve or prevent constipation:

- Increase the amount of fluids (except milk, which can cause constipation), fruit, vegetables, and other fibre-rich foods, such as wholegrain cereals and bread, in your child's diet.
- Your child should be encouraged to sit on the potty or toilet at the same time every day, to establish a regular bowel habit.
- Laxatives should never be used for children unless specifically recommended or prescribed by your doctor.

A fibre-rich meal
Give your child fibre-rich foods, such as wholemeal bread and salad or fruit, at all meals if possible.

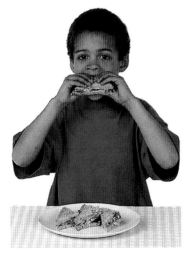

POSSIBLE CAUSE

Children who are nervous about toilet-training may resist the urge to defecate.

ACTION NEEDED

MEDICAL HELP
If no faeces are passed for 4 days, make an appointment to see your doctor.

SELF-HELP
You should adopt a more relaxed attitude towards your child's toilet-training.
See also chart 14, TOILET-TRAINING PROBLEMS.

38 ABNORMAL-LOOKING FAECES

Sudden differences in colour, smell, consistency, or content of faeces are almost always due to changes in diet. It is very rare for any such change to last for more than a few days. However, if there are other symptoms or if the altered faeces persist, you should take your child to see a doctor.

POSSIBLE CAUSE

Intussusception (see INTESTINAL OBSTRUCTION, p.185).

ACTION NEEDED

MEDICAL HELP
✚ **EMERGENCY!** Call an ambulance! While waiting, do not give your child anything to eat or drink.

START HERE

How old is your child?

- **UNDER 1 YEAR**
- **1 YEAR OR OVER**

What are your child's faeces like?

- **RED AND JELLY-LIKE**
- **GREEN; MAY BE RUNNY**
- **NEITHER**

How is your baby fed?

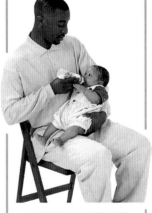

- **BREAST- AND BOTTLE-FED**
- **BOTTLE-FED ONLY**
- **BREAST-FED ONLY**

Is your child taking any medicines?

- **MEDICINE**
- **NO MEDICINE**

POSSIBLE CAUSES

Some types of cow's milk formula may result in green faeces. If the faeces are also runny, your baby may have GASTROENTERITIS (p.180).

ACTION NEEDED

MEDICAL HELP
If you think your baby may have gastroenteritis, get medical advice within 24 hours.

SELF-HELP
If you think the milk formula is responsible, you can try another brand. If you think your baby has gastroenteritis, see panel: *Preventing dehydration in babies* (p.38).

POSSIBLE CAUSE

Many medicines can affect the appearance of faeces.

ACTION NEEDED

MEDICAL HELP
Phone your doctor to find out whether the medicine may be causing your child's symptoms and whether you should stop giving it.

POSSIBLE CAUSE

Green, runny faeces are normal in breast-fed babies and are not a cause for concern.

ACTION NEEDED

MEDICAL HELP
If your baby seems unwell or has other symptoms, make an appointment to see your doctor.

Has your child recently recovered from a bout of diarrhoea or vomiting?

- DIARRHOEA
- VOMITING
- NEITHER

POSSIBLE CAUSE

GASTROENTERITIS (p.180) may sometimes cause faeces to be pale for several days.

ACTION NEEDED

MEDICAL HELP
If your child seems unwell or if the faeces do not return to their normal colour in a few days, make an appointment to see your doctor.

SELF-HELP
See panel: *Preventing dehydration in babies* (p.38) or *Preventing dehydration in children* (p.53).

What are the characteristics of your child's faeces?

- VERY PALE
- VERY PALE, FLOATING, AND FOUL-SMELLING
- BLOOD ON FAECES
- RUNNY

POSSIBLE CAUSE

MALABSORPTION (p.183), often caused by an underlying disorder, such as FOOD INTOLERANCE (p.182).

ACTION NEEDED

MEDICAL HELP
Make an appointment to see your doctor.

Does your child have any of the following symptoms?

- YELLOWISH SKIN
- YELLOWISH WHITES OF THE EYES
- DARK URINE
- NONE OF THE ABOVE

POSSIBLE CAUSES

GASTROENTERITIS (p.180) or anal fissure (see CONSTIPATION, p.181).

ACTION NEEDED

MEDICAL HELP
Get medical advice within 24 hours.

Go to chart
9 DIARRHOEA IN CHILDREN

POSSIBLE CAUSE

HEPATITIS (p.188), which may cause jaundice.

ACTION NEEDED

MEDICAL HELP
Get medical advice within 24 hours.

If you cannot identify your child's problem from this chart, talk to your doctor within 48 hours.

39 URINARY PROBLEMS

For toilet-training problems, see chart 14

Urinary problems may be caused by various conditions, ranging from minor infections to serious disorders, such as diabetes mellitus. Pain on passing urine usually indicates a disorder but variations in frequency of passing urine or in the colour of urine are not necessarily symptoms of disease.

START HERE

Does your child have either of the following symptoms?

> FREQUENT PASSING OF URINE

> PAIN ON PASSING URINE

> NEITHER

Has there been an increase in the quantity of urine your child passes?

> PASSES INCREASED AMOUNTS

> NO INCREASE

Does your child seem generally unwell or does he or she have a fever – a temperature of 38°C (100°F) or above?

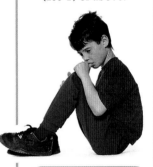

> SEEMS UNWELL

> HAS A FEVER

> NEITHER

Does your child have either of the following symptoms?

> LOSS OF WEIGHT

> ABNORMAL TIREDNESS

> NEITHER

POSSIBLE CAUSE

URINARY TRACT INFECTION (p.193).

ACTION NEEDED

MEDICAL HELP
Get medical advice within 24 hours.

POSSIBLE CAUSE

DIABETES MELLITUS (p.190).

ACTION NEEDED

MEDICAL HELP
✚ URGENT! Phone your doctor immediately!

POSSIBLE CAUSE

URINARY TRACT INFECTION (p.193).

ACTION NEEDED

MEDICAL HELP
Get medical advice within 24 hours.

SELF-HELP
See panel: *Bringing down a high temperature* (p.37).

Has your child been taking any medicines recently?

MEDICINE

NO MEDICINE

Is there any reason why your child might be feeling insecure?

SCHOOL DIFFICULTIES

FAMILY UPHEAVAL, SUCH AS A NEW BABY

CHANGE OF ROUTINE

NONE OF THE ABOVE

POSSIBLE CAUSES

Anxiety (see ANXIETY AND FEARS, p.170) or stress may result in your child going to the toilet more often than usual.

ACTION NEEDED

MEDICAL HELP
If the problem does not clear up within a few days, phone your doctor.

SELF-HELP
Try to establish the reason for your child's anxiety or stress, and alleviate it, if possible.

POSSIBLE CAUSE

Some drugs may cause frequent passing of urine.

ACTION NEEDED

MEDICAL HELP
Phone your doctor to find out whether the medicine may be causing your child's symptoms and whether you should stop giving it.

POSSIBLE CAUSES

GLOMERULONEPHRITIS (p.194) or URINARY TRACT INFECTION (p.193).

ACTION NEEDED

MEDICAL HELP
✚ URGENT! Phone your doctor immediately!

If you cannot identify your child's problem from this chart, talk to your doctor within 48 hours.

POSSIBLE CAUSE

HEPATITIS (p.188).

ACTION NEEDED

MEDICAL HELP
Get medical advice within 24 hours.

What colour is your child's urine?

PINK, RED, OR SMOKY

DARK BROWN AND CLEAR

DARK YELLOW OR ORANGE

GREEN OR BLUE

NONE OF THE ABOVE

What colour are your child's faeces?

PALE

NORMAL

POSSIBLE CAUSES

The urine has probably darkened because it has become concentrated as a result of low fluid intake, fever, vomiting, or diarrhoea.

ACTION NEEDED

SELF-HELP
Make sure that your child has plenty to drink and the urine should soon return to its normal colour. If your child has had been ill with a fever or diarrhoea, or has been vomiting, see panel: *Preventing dehydration in babies* (p.38) or *Preventing dehydration in children* (p.53).

POSSIBLE CAUSE

Artificial colouring in food, drink, or medicine is almost always the cause of such discoloration.

ACTION NEEDED

No action is required. The artificial colouring will soon pass out of your child's system without causing any problems.

If you cannot identify your child's problem from this chart, talk to your doctor within 48 hours.

40 GENITAL PROBLEMS IN BOYS

Pain or swelling in the penis or scrotum, discharge from the penis, or pain on passing urine can affect boys of any age. Injuries to the genitals tend to be most common in school-age boys. Any boy who has severe or persistent genital pain needs urgent medical help.

START HERE

Does your son have any of the following symptoms?

- PAINLESS SWELLING IN GROIN OR SCROTUM
- PAINFUL SWELLING IN GROIN OR SCROTUM
- PAIN OR BURNING SENSATION ON PASSING URINE
- SWELLING OF PENIS TIP OR DISCHARGE FROM FORESKIN
- GREYISH-YELLOW DISCHARGE FROM PENIS
- NONE OF THE ABOVE

POSSIBLE CAUSES

Inguinal hernia (see HERNIA, p.187) or hydrocele (see PENIS AND TESTIS DISORDERS, p.197).

ACTION NEEDED

MEDICAL HELP
Get medical advice within 24 hours.

POSSIBLE CAUSE

URINARY TRACT INFECTION (p.193).

ACTION NEEDED

MEDICAL HELP
Get medical advice within 24 hours.

POSSIBLE CAUSE

Balanitis (see PENIS AND TESTIS DISORDERS, p.196).

ACTION NEEDED

MEDICAL HELP
Get medical advice within 24 hours.

POSSIBLE CAUSE

A foreign body in your son's urethra.

ACTION NEEDED

MEDICAL HELP
Make an appointment to see your doctor.

If you cannot identify your son's problem from this chart, talk to your doctor within 48 hours.

POSSIBLE CAUSE

Orchitis (see PENIS AND TESTIS DISORDERS, p.197).

ACTION NEEDED

MEDICAL HELP
Get medical advice within 24 hours.

POSSIBLE CAUSE

Pain that does not subside following an injury may indicate damage to the testes.

ACTION NEEDED

MEDICAL HELP
⊕ URGENT! Phone your doctor immediately!

Might your son have suffered an injury to his genitals?

- POSSIBLY
- UNLIKELY

Has your son had mumps in the past 2 weeks?

- HAS HAD MUMPS
- HAS NOT HAD MUMPS

POSSIBLE CAUSES

Testicular torsion (see PENIS AND TESTIS DISORDERS, p.197) or strangulated inguinal hernia (see HERNIA, p.187).

ACTION NEEDED

MEDICAL HELP
⊕ EMERGENCY! Call an ambulance! While waiting, do not give your son anything to eat or drink.

41 GENITAL PROBLEMS IN GIRLS

The most common genital symptoms in girls are itching and inflammation of the genital area, which may cause pain on passing urine or an unusual vaginal discharge. An infection or irritation by scented soaps, bubble baths, or deodorants may be the underlying cause of these symptoms.

START HERE

Is your daughter's genital area itchy or uncomfortable?
- ITCHY
- SORE
- NEITHER

Is there a thin white vaginal discharge?
- DISCHARGE
- NO DISCHARGE

How old is your daughter?
- 10 YEARS OR UNDER
- OVER 10 YEARS

Does your daughter have a vaginal discharge?
- GREYISH-YELLOW OR GREENISH DISCHARGE
- THICK WHITE DISCHARGE
- NO DISCHARGE

If you cannot identify your daughter's problem from this chart, talk to your doctor within 48 hours.

POSSIBLE CAUSE

Infection of the vagina (see VULVOVAGINITIS, p.195), which, in young girls, may be caused by a foreign object or, in older girls, a forgotten tampon.

ACTION NEEDED

MEDICAL HELP
Get medical advice within 24 hours.

POSSIBLE CAUSE

Inflammation of the vulva and vagina (see VULVOVAGINITIS, p.195), which may be due to poor hygiene, external irritants, such as soap or bubble baths, or sometimes, infection.

ACTION NEEDED

MEDICAL HELP
Make an appointment to see your doctor.

SELF-HELP
Make sure your daughter changes her underwear daily, washes her vaginal area carefully, and avoids irritants, such as bubble baths.

POSSIBLE CAUSE

Poor hygiene or VULVOVAGINITIS (p.195).

ACTION NEEDED

MEDICAL HELP
Get medical advice within 24 hours.

SELF-HELP
Make sure your daughter changes her underwear daily, washes her vaginal area carefully, and avoids irritants, such as bubble baths.

POSSIBLE CAUSE

Increased production of sex hormones at puberty.

ACTION NEEDED

MEDICAL HELP
If irritation accompanies the discharge, make an appointment to see your doctor.

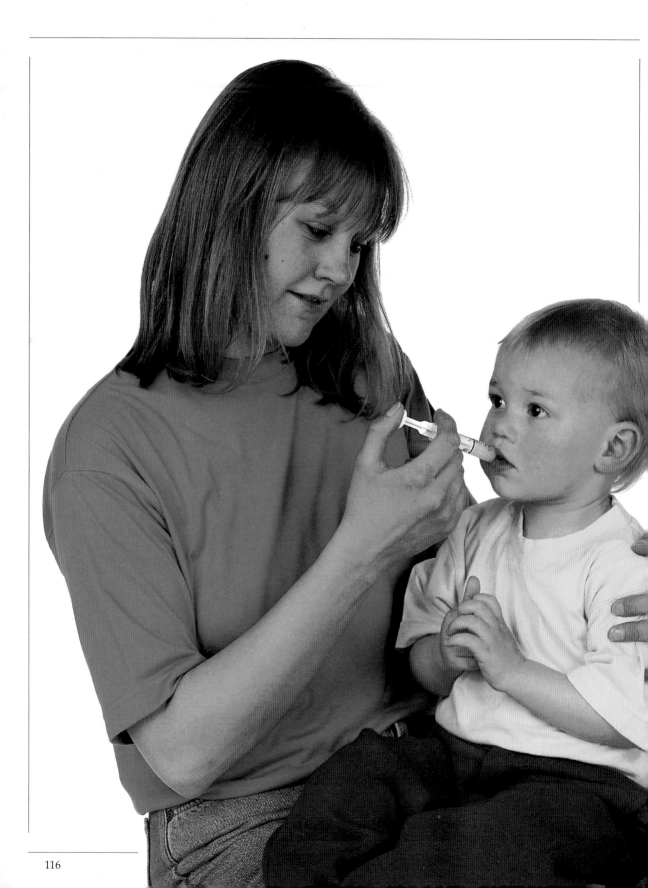

DISEASES & DISORDERS

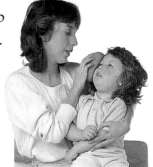

CHILDREN TEND TO SUFFER from a variety of illnesses and problems that do not affect adults or that affect them differently. In this section all the most common childhood diseases and disorders are described, including all possible causes that are pinpointed on the symptom charts. Each article gives detailed information about a particular disease, including a list of the symptoms, causes, if and when a doctor should be consulted, medical and self-help treatment, and the outlook. Photographs and artworks show aspects of the disease or demonstrate self-help techniques that can be used at home. Turn to these pages for information that your doctor has provided but which you may have forgotten or not taken in during the consultation.

ELECTRON MICROGRAPH OF A COLD VIRUS

BRINGING DOWN A HIGH TEMPERATURE

INFECTIOUS DISEASES

CHILDREN ARE MORE SUSCEPTIBLE to infectious diseases than adults because their immune systems have not yet built up resistance. Most childhood infections are not serious. A few can be dangerous. However, because of routine immunization, the main serious viral infections, such as measles, mumps, and rubella, are less common than they once were. Bacterial infections can usually be cured rapidly and completely by antibiotics.

MEASLES

A once common disease of childhood, measles is a viral infection that causes fever and a characteristic rash. The disease itself is not usually serious, but a child with measles typically feels very unwell. There is also a slight possibility of serious complications, especially in children with chronic heart or lung disease or in those who have a depressed immune system. Measles is highly infectious, but widespread IMMUNIZATION (p.30) has now made it a rare disease in the UK and other developed countries.

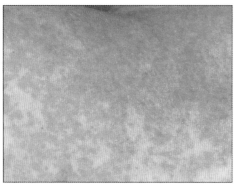

Measles rash
The rash of measles appears 3 to 4 days after the first signs of illness. Initially, the rash consists of separate spots. The spots then merge to give the skin a blotchy appearance.

What are the symptoms?
The measles virus produces the initial symptoms after an incubation period of 10 to 14 days. These symptoms are:
- Fever.
- Red, watering eyes.
- Runny nose.
- Dry cough.

The following characteristic features then appear:
- Tiny white spots with a red base (Koplik's spots), which can sometimes be seen on the insides of the cheeks a couple of days after the first symptoms appear.
- A flat, blotchy, red rash, which develops 3 to 4 days after the start of the illness. The rash appears first on the face and behind the ears, and then spreads down to cover the whole body.

The rash starts to fade after 3 or 4 days. Also at this time, the child's fever subsides and he or she begins to feel better. In the majority of cases, the rash disappears within a week.

What are the complications?
Infection of the middle ear (see OTITIS MEDIA, p.162) and PNEUMONIA (p.155) are the most common complications. In about 1 in 1,000 cases of measles, a serious complication called ENCEPHALITIS (p.159) occurs; this inflammation of the brain is caused by spread of infection to the brain or by an abnormal immune response to the measles virus.

Should I consult a doctor?
Your child should be seen by a doctor within 24 hours if you suspect measles. You should phone a doctor at once if your child has any of the following symptoms: earache, abnormally rapid breathing, drowsiness, seizures, severe headache, or vomiting.

What might the doctor do?
The doctor will examine your child to confirm the diagnosis. He or she will prescribe antibiotics for otitis media or pneumonia. If the doctor suspects encephalitis, he or she will arrange for your child to be admitted to hospital.

What can I do to help?
Let your child choose whether or not to stay in bed. Give him or her paracetamol to reduce fever and plenty of fluids.

The infectious period lasts for about 5 days after the onset of the rash. Try to keep your child away from anyone who might be at risk of infection. However, attempts to isolate siblings from a child with measles may be futile; very often brothers and sisters have been infected before the disease is diagnosed.

What is the outlook?
Most children recover completely from measles within about 10 days of the onset of symptoms. A single attack of measles should give lifelong immunity.

RUBELLA

Formerly known as German measles, rubella is a mild viral infection that may cause a rash and swelling of the lymph nodes. In about a quarter of cases, there is no rash and the infection often passes unnoticed, although blood tests can show that it has occurred. If rubella is contracted early in pregnancy, it can cause serious damage to the developing baby. A once common disease, rubella has become rare because of routine IMMUNIZATION (p.30).

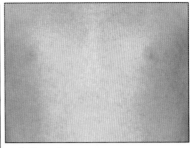

Rubella rash
The rash of rubella consists of tiny, flat pink spots. It first appears on the face and then spreads rapidly to the trunk and limbs. The spots merge as the rubella rash spreads.

What are the symptoms?
After an incubation period of between 2 and 3 weeks, the rubella virus may cause the following symptoms:
- Slight fever.
- Swollen lymph nodes at the back of the neck and behind the ears. In some cases, there is enlargement of lymph nodes throughout the body, including those in the armpits and groin.
- A non-itchy rash (see illustration right) that develops on the second or third day of illness. The rash usually disappears within about 3 days.
- In some children, joint pain.
Rare complications are inflammation of the brain (see ENCEPHALITIS, p.159) and THROMBOCYTOPENIA (p.147), a disorder in which the number of platelets (clotting agents) in the blood is abnormally low.

Should I consult a doctor?
You should phone a doctor if you think your child may have rubella. Do not take the child to the surgery because of the risk of infecting a pregnant woman.

You should phone a doctor at once if your child develops joint pain or if a complication is signalled by any of the following symptoms: a rash of flat, dark-red spots that do not fade when they are pressed, severe headache, vomiting, lack of energy, or abnormal drowsiness.

What might the doctor do?
The doctor will examine your child. To confirm the diagnosis of rubella, a sample of your child's blood may be sent to the laboratory, to be examined for antibodies to the virus. There is no specific medical treatment for rubella.

What can I do to help?
Give your child paracetamol to reduce fever, and provide plenty of fluids. Try to prevent your child from having any contact with pregnant women. Rubella is infectious from 1 week before until 4 days after the rash appears.

What is the outlook?
Children usually recover completely from rubella within about 10 days of the onset of symptoms. A single attack usually gives lifelong immunity.

ERYTHEMA INFECTIOSUM

Also known as fifth disease, erythema infectiosum is a mildly contagious viral illness. It usually occurs in small outbreaks in the spring among children over the age of 2 years. The most distinctive symptom of the disease is a red rash on both cheeks.

What are the symptoms?
After a typical incubation period of between 4 and 14 days, the following symptoms appear:
- Bright red cheeks, contrasting with a pale area around the mouth.
- Fever.
- A rash that usually develops 1 to 4 days after the cheeks become red. The rash appears on the arms and legs, and occasionally on the trunk. It is blotchy or lace-like, especially on the limbs, and may be more pronounced after a warm bath. The rash usually lasts for 7 to 10 days.
- Rarely, joint pain.

What are the complications?
Erythema infectiosum sometimes leads to severe illness in children who have certain uncommon blood disorders, including anaemias such as SICKLE-CELL ANAEMIA (p.199) or THALASSAEMIA (p.200). If erythema infectiosum is contracted during pregnancy, the condition can, in rare cases, lead to miscarriage.

Distinctive red cheeks
Erythema infectiosum is sometimes referred to as "slapped cheek" disease because the first symptom is a bright red rash that suddenly appears on the cheeks. In this child, the rash has also spread to the arms.

Should I consult a doctor?
Phone a doctor if you are concerned about your child's condition, or if he or she has a blood disorder. In some cases, the doctor will arrange for a blood test to confirm the diagnosis. There is no specific treatment for the disease.

What can I do to help?
Give your child paracetamol to reduce a fever, and provide plenty of fluids. Sufferers are unlikely to be infectious after the rash appears; nevertheless, for as long as the rash persists, it may be safest to keep your child away from anyone who might be pregnant.

What is the outlook?
The rash may recur over a period of several weeks or months, and it may vary in intensity in response to changes in temperature or exposure to sunlight. Once your child has had erythema infectiosum, he or she is not likely to have a recurrence of the disease.

CHICKENPOX

Sometimes called varicella, chickenpox is typically a mild viral infection that is characterized by a distinctive, itchy rash and a slight fever. Chickenpox is one of the common childhood infections, mainly affecting children under the age of 10 years. The number of cases is highest in the late winter and spring.

What are the symptoms?
After an incubation period of usually between 2 and 3 weeks, the following symptoms of chickenpox appear:
- Mild fever or headache that develops a few hours before the rash.
- Rash, mainly on the trunk, made up of crops of spots that rapidly turn into itchy blisters. After a few days, the blisters dry up to form scabs. Spots at different stages of development are usually present at the same time.
- Sometimes, discomfort during eating caused by spots in the mouth that have developed into ulcers.
- In some cases, a severe cough.

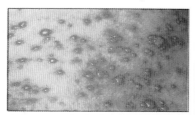

Appearance of a chickenpox rash
A chickenpox rash initially consists of raised pimples. The pimples rapidly turn into small, fluid-filled blisters that have red bases.

What are the complications?
The most common complication is a secondary infection with streptococcal bacteria, which are introduced into the body by scratching. Two other possible complications are PNEUMONIA (p.155) and, rarely, inflammation of the brain (see ENCEPHALITIS, p.159). Those most at risk of complications are children who have a depressed immune system (due to chemotherapy or taking oral cortico-steroids, for example) and newborn babies, who can develop chickenpox if the mother contracted the illness late in pregnancy. The illness in early pregnancy may, rarely, cause fetal birth defects.

Should I consult a doctor?
Phone a doctor at once if your child is a young baby, or has reduced immunity and has been exposed to chickenpox or has symptoms. You should also phone a doctor at once if any of the following symptoms develop: coughing, seizures, rapid breathing, abnormal drowsiness, or unsteadiness when walking.
Your child should be seen by a doctor if there is a discharge of pus from spots or if the skin around the spots is red.

What might the doctor do?
If your child has a secondary bacterial infection, the doctor may prescribe an oral antibiotic. A child at high risk of complications may be given injections of immune globulin, which will give some protection. Alternatively, your child may be admitted to hospital and given injections of the antiviral drug acyclovir over about 5 days.

What can I do to help?
Itchiness may be relieved by applying calamine lotion to the rash; by giving oral antihistamines (available over the counter); and by bathing your child in warm water containing a handful of bicarbonate of soda. Give paracetamol to reduce a fever, and plenty of fluids.
To avoid infection, you should keep your child's fingernails short and tell him or her not to scratch the spots.
Chickenpox is infectious from 1 day before the rash has appeared until all the blisters have formed scabs. During this period, keep your child away from anyone at high risk of complications.

What is the outlook?
Children usually recover completely from chickenpox within 7 to 10 days of the onset of symptoms. An attack of chickenpox leads to lifelong immunity from this disease, but the virus remains dormant in the body and may become active later in life to cause shingles.

HAND, FOOT, AND MOUTH DISEASE

This mild viral infection causes blisters to appear in the mouth, on the hands, and on the feet. Hand, foot, and mouth disease is common in children up to the age of 4 years, and usually occurs in epidemics during the summer and early autumn.

What are the symptoms?
After an incubation period of usually between 3 and 5 days, hand, foot, and mouth disease causes:
- Mild fever.
- Blisters on the inside of the mouth, which sometimes develop into sore, shallow ulcers.
- Reluctance to eat.
- Blisters on the hands and feet, which typically develop 1 or 2 days after the symptoms in the mouth. The blisters are not usually itchy or painful.

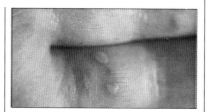

Blisters on the fingers
A child with hand, foot, and mouth disease develops blisters on the hands and feet. They commonly appear on the fingers, the backs of the hands, or the top surfaces of the feet.

What is the treatment?
No specific treatment exists, apart from measures to relieve the symptoms. Give liquid paracetamol for painful mouth ulcers. Rinsing the mouth out with salty water may also help to soothe the pain (see panel: *Relieving a sore mouth,* p.105). Give plenty of bland fluids, such as water or milk. Do not give fruit juices, which are acidic and may make the pain worse. There is no need for your child to eat solid foods.

What is the outlook?
Blisters on the hands and feet usually disappear within 3 or 4 days, as does the fever. However, mouth ulcers may persist for as long as 4 weeks. A single attack provides lifelong immunity.

ROSEOLA INFANTUM

Caused by a virus, roseola infantum is a common infection of early childhood. Most children have had the illness by the time they are 2 years old. Roseola infantum characteristically causes the abrupt onset of a high fever, which lasts for about 4 days, followed by the appearance of a rash of tiny pink spots.

What are the symptoms?
Roseola occurs in two stages. After an incubation period of 5 to 15 days, the first symptoms appear, which are:
- A raised temperature of 39–40°C (102–104°F), although your child may otherwise appear well.
- Sometimes, one or more FEBRILE CONVULSIONS (p.156).

Some children also have:
- Mild diarrhoea.
- Cough.
- Enlargement of the lymph nodes in the neck.
- Earache.

After about 4 days, the illness enters its second stage, characterized by:
- Sudden return of the temperature to its normal level.
- Appearance of a rash, which is made up of tiny, distinct pink spots, usually distributed over the head and trunk. The rash lasts for about 4 days.

What are the complications?
A child who has a suppressed immune system may develop HEPATITIS (p.188) or PNEUMONIA (p.155). Complications are rare in otherwise healthy children.

Should I consult a doctor?
Phone a doctor at once if your child has a temperature of 39°C (102°F) or above, or he or she has a febrile convulsion or is drowsy or irritable. While waiting for the doctor, try to reduce the fever (see photograph right and panel: *Bringing down a high temperature*, p.37).

What might the doctor do?
The doctor will decide whether your child can be looked after at home, or whether he or she should be admitted to hospital for tests to confirm that the illness is not due to bacterial MENINGITIS (p.158), which can produce symptoms similar to those of roseola. No specific treatment is needed for roseola.

What is the outlook?
Recovery from roseola is rapid. Your child should feel completely better by the time the rash has gone.

Reducing a fever
Sponging your child with lukewarm water helps to bring down a high fever. Another way of reducing a fever is to place your child in a lukewarm bath.

SCARLET FEVER

Once fairly common, this illness has become rare in developed countries since the introduction of antibiotics. Scarlet fever is caused by toxins produced by bacteria. A prominent feature is a widespread rash, which gives the child a scarlet appearance.

What are the symptoms?
After an incubation period, typically lasting for 2 to 4 days, the following symptoms of scarlet fever appear:
- Vomiting.
- Fever.
- Sore throat and headache.
- Rash (see photograph right), which develops within 12 hours of the first symptoms appearing. The rash affects the neck and chest first and spreads rapidly, but does not affect the face. It is most dense on the neck and in the armpits and groin. The rash lasts for up to 6 days; the skin then peels.
- Flushed cheeks and an obvious pale area around the mouth.
- The tongue in the early stages has a thick white coating through which red spots project. The coating peels on the third or fourth day to reveal a bright red "strawberry tongue", still with the projecting spots.

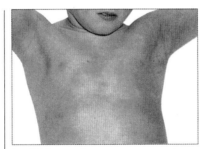

Scarlet fever rash
The rash of scarlet fever consists of a mass of tiny red spots, which may be slightly raised. The spots usually disappear when pressed.

What are the complications?
Possible complications of scarlet fever are rheumatic fever, a disorder that can lead to permanent heart damage, and the kidney disorder GLOMERULONEPHRITIS (p.194). Antibiotic treatment has now made these complications rare.

Should I consult a doctor?
Consult a doctor within 24 hours of the onset of your child's symptoms. Phone a doctor at once if your child's urine is red, pink, or smoky, because this is a symptom of glomerulonephritis.

What might the doctor do?
The doctor will probably confirm the diagnosis from the child's symptoms. He or she may also take a throat swab to be examined for bacteria. Scarlet fever is usually treated with a 10-day course of an antibiotic medicine.

What can I do to help?
Give your child liquid paracetamol to reduce fever and relieve pain. Ensure that your child finishes the course of medication, and keep him or her away from other children until this time.

What is the outlook?
Your child should feel better within about a week of the onset of symptoms. If normal vigour has not returned, you should consult the doctor; rheumatic fever is a possibility. A single attack of scarlet fever confers lifelong immunity.

MUMPS

A mild viral infection, mumps was common among children until routine IMMUNIZATION (p.30) was introduced. Mumps causes a fever and characteristic swelling of one or both of the parotid (salivary) glands, which are situated just in front of and below the ears, inside the angle of the jaw.

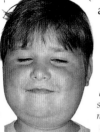

Swollen glands
The most obvious feature of mumps is the swelling of the parotid (salivary) glands, which obscures the angle of the jaw. If both sides are affected, the child may have a hamster-like appearance. The swollen glands may be painful.

What are the symptoms?
The following symptoms develop after an incubation period of 14 to 24 days:
• Fever.
• Tenderness and swelling of one or both sides of the face, which occurs 1 or 2 days after the onset of fever and typically lasts from 4 to 8 days.

What are the complications?
Occasionally, adolescent boys develop inflamed testes, a condition called orchitis (see PENIS AND TESTIS DISORDERS, p.197). It develops about a week after mumps has started. Rarely, ENCEPHALITIS (p.159) or MENINGITIS (p.158), both of which affect the brain, or pancreatitis (inflammation of the pancreas) may occur, either before or after the parotid glands have become swollen.

Should I consult a doctor?
Your child should be seen by a doctor if you think he or she has mumps. Phone a doctor immediately if your child has a severe headache (with or without vomiting) or has pain in the abdomen.

What might the doctor do?
The doctor will usually confirm the diagnosis by examining your child. A child who has a severe headache will be admitted to hospital for tests to rule out encephalitis or bacterial meningitis.

What can I do to help?
You may give your child paracetamol to reduce fever and relieve pain. You should make sure that your child drinks plenty of fluids but do not give fruit juices: they stimulate the flow of saliva and may increase gland pain.

What is the outlook?
In most cases, a child recovers in about 10 days. Problems affecting the testes and pancreas do not usually have long-term ill effects. Contrary to popular belief, infertility following orchitis is extremely rare. However, encephalitis or meningitis can result in permanent hearing loss. A single attack of mumps usually provides lifelong immunity.

TETANUS

A serious illness affecting the central nervous system, tetanus is due to infection by bacterial spores, which enter the body through a wound. A deep wound contaminated by garden soil or animal manure is most likely to result in tetanus. The disease is now rare in developed countries because of IMMUNIZATION (p.30).

What are the symptoms?
After an incubation period of between 3 and 21 days, the following symptoms of tetanus develop:
• Inability to open the mouth (lockjaw).
• Difficulty in swallowing.
• Contraction of facial muscles, giving the appearance of a fixed smile.
• Spasms of muscles in the neck, back, abdomen, and limbs, which typically occur over a period of 10 to 14 days, and may make breathing difficult.

Should I consult a doctor?
Tetanus is a medical emergency. You should consult a doctor at once if symptoms suggesting tetanus develop.

What is the treatment?
Your child will be admitted to hospital if the doctor suspects tetanus. Mild cases may require only a light diet and sedative drugs. The treatment for more severe cases of tetanus may include a tracheostomy (insertion of a tube into the windpipe) to aid breathing, muscle-relaxant and sedative drugs to relieve muscle contractions, and mechanical ventilation to maintain breathing.

What is the outlook?
Tetanus is still a rare cause of death, but with prompt hospital treatment most children recover completely. The time it takes to recover depends on the severity of the illness, but is usually within 3 weeks.

How is tetanus prevented?
Routine immunization against tetanus is usually given in early childhood (see illustration right). If your child has a deep wound, you should take him or her immediately to the nearest accident and emergency department, even if he or she has been immunized against tetanus. Do not wait to see if any symptoms develop. To prevent the disease developing, the hospital doctor may operate on the wound to make sure that all foreign bodies and dead tissue are removed. Your child may be given injections of tetanus vaccine.

Prevention of tetanus
Babies receive a course of three injections of vaccine. Boosters are given before school entry and again when schooling has finished; they are needed every 10 years subsequently.

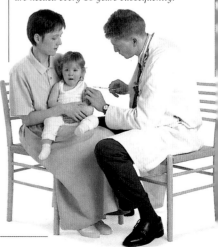

PERTUSSIS

Also known as whooping cough, pertussis is a childhood illness caused by bacterial infection. The major symptom is a cough, sometimes followed by a whoop. Infants under 6 months of age are most severely affected. Pertussis has become uncommon in developed countries because of IMMUNIZATION (p.30).

What are the symptoms?
Symptoms develop after an incubation period of about 7 days. Pertussis occurs in two stages. For the first 7 to 10 days, the main symptoms are:
- A short, dry cough that typically occurs only at night.
- Runny nose.
- Slight fever.

During the next stage of the illness, which may last 8 to 12 weeks, the symptoms are easier to recognize:
- Bouts of 10 to 20 short, dry coughs that occur day and night.
- Long attacks of coughing followed by a sharp indrawing of breath, which may produce a crowing or whooping sound. (Babies may not whoop.)
- Vomiting caused by coughing.
- Sometimes, seizures.

In rare cases, blockage of a bronchus (air passage) by thick mucus causes collapse of a segment of the lung.

Should I consult a doctor?
Consult a doctor within 24 hours if a child with a cough is under 6 months; coughing causes vomiting; or a cough does not improve after a week. Phone a doctor at once if your child's tongue or lips turn blue during a coughing attack or if he or she has a seizure.

To confirm the diagnosis, the doctor may collect a sample from your child's throat for laboratory testing. A 10-day course of antibiotics may be prescribed for the child and for any brothers and sisters. Antibiotics can shorten the duration of pertussis, but are effective only if given in the early stages.

A child who has turned blue or had a seizure may be admitted to hospital, especially if he or she is under 6 months old. If a child is generally ill or the cough has not improved after 6 weeks, a chest X-ray may be arranged.

What can I do to help?
Give your child soft food (but avoid crumbly food, which could trigger vomiting) and plenty of fluids.

You may halt a coughing attack by slapping your child gently on the back. If necessary, you will be shown how to give your child simple physiotherapy to help clear lung secretions.

To avoid becoming exhausted from lack of sleep while caring for your sick child, ask other family members to take turns sleeping in his or her room.

What is the outlook?
Coughing may continue for several months. In some children, the cough recurs if they catch a viral infection in the following year. Permanent lung damage is extremely rare.

MALARIA

A serious health problem in the tropics and subtropics, malaria is increasingly occurring in other areas as a result of travel to malarial regions. It is caused by malarial parasites, which enter a human's bloodstream via a bite from an infected mosquito. The most serious form of the illness is falciparum malaria.

What are the symptoms?
Symptoms of malaria usually appear 6 to 30 days after infection. Sometimes, however, they may not appear for as long as a year if antimalarial drugs have been taken and been only partly effective. The main symptoms are:
- High fever alternating with shivering.
- Headache.

There may also be:
- Nausea and vomiting.
- Pain in the abdomen and back.
- Joint pain.

Falciparum malaria can result in very serious complications affecting the kidneys, liver, brain, and blood.

Should I consult a doctor?
Phone a doctor at once if your child has any symptoms of malaria. You should take your child to the nearest hospital

accident and emergency department if he or she has any of the following symptoms of complications: seizures, drowsiness, yellowing of the skin, or extreme paleness of the skin.

What might the doctor do?
Your child will be admitted to hospital, and a blood test will be performed to look for malarial parasites. Treatment is by means of antimalarial drugs. If there are complications, your child may need treatment in an intensive care unit

How can malaria be prevented?
If you plan to visit a malarial region, you and your family will need to take antimalarial drugs. By taking measures such as wearing protective clothing and sleeping under mosquito nets, you may be able to prevent mosquito bites.

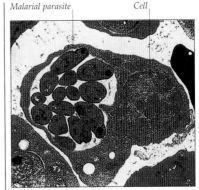

Malarial parasite   *Cell*

An infected cell
Malarial parasites mature and multiply inside cells. The infected cells eventually burst, releasing parasites to infect more cells. Liver and red blood cells are most often affected.

What is the outlook?
With prompt treatment, recovery may take only a few days or up to 2 weeks, depending on how severe the illness is. However, falciparum malaria may be life threatening if complications affect the brain or the kidneys.

TYPHOID FEVER

Also known as enteric fever, typhoid fever is caused by bacteria called *Salmonella typhi*. The infection is usually acquired from food or water contaminated with bacteria from the faeces of an infected person. Typhoid fever occurs when the bacteria pass into the bloodstream, resulting in fever and other symptoms of blood poisoning. Immunization is advisable for people travelling to developing countries, where the disease is common.

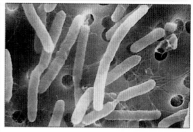

Salmonella typhi *bacteria*
After ingestion, the bacteria responsible for typhoid fever invade the wall of the small intestine and enter the bloodstream.

What are the symptoms?
After an incubation period lasting for 7 to 14 days, the following may appear:
• Fever that rises gradually to 39–40°C (102–104°F) and then stays at this level without daily fluctuations for up to 4 weeks.
• Headache.
• Lack of energy.
• Abdominal pain.
• Constipation or diarrhoea.
• Rash, consisting of raised pink spots, on the abdomen and chest. The rash develops during the second week of illness and lasts for about a day.

Intestinal bleeding or perforation or other complications may develop in the second or third week of illness if typhoid fever is not treated.

Should I consult a doctor?
Your child should be seen by a doctor within 24 hours of the appearance of possible typhoid symptoms.
　If the doctor suspects that your child might have typhoid fever, he or she will probably arrange for your child to be admitted to hospital. The diagnosis is confirmed by culturing a sample of faeces or urine or by a blood test.

The doctor may treat your child with antibiotics, which are sometimes given intravenously if symptoms are severe.

What is the outlook?
The symptoms usually start to subside several days after the start of treatment. Most children are completely recovered within 2 or 3 weeks. Complications are unlikely to occur if treatment is prompt.

INFECTIOUS MONONUCLEOSIS

Commonly known as glandular fever, infectious mononucleosis is a viral infection that typically causes a high fever, lack of energy, and swollen lymph nodes (glands). It is caused by the Epstein-Barr virus. Infectious mononucleosis can occur at any age, but is most common in adolescents and young adults.

What are the symptoms?
Infectious mononucleosis causes the following typical symptoms after an incubation period of about 10 days:
• High fever (39–40°C/102–104°F), which may last for a few days or for several weeks.
• Poor appetite and loss of weight.
• Lack of energy.
• Sore throat, which may be severe.
• Swollen lymph nodes in the neck and/or elsewhere in the body.
• Headache.
• Sometimes, muscle pain.
• Occasionally, a rash of raised pimples or flat spots.

What are the complications?
The liver condition HEPATITIS (p.188) is the most common complication. Rare complications include PNEUMONIA (p.155); rupture of the spleen; and nervous system, blood, and respiratory problems.

Should I consult a doctor?
Your child should be seen by a doctor if you suspect that he or she may have infectious mononucleosis.

A typical symptom
Children with infectious mononucleosis usually have swollen lymph nodes in the neck. The nodes can be felt just under the jaw.

The doctor may diagnose the disease solely from your child's symptoms. Alternatively, he or she may arrange for a blood test to confirm the diagnosis or to make sure that your child does not have one of several other infections that produce similar symptoms. There is no specific medical treatment for infectious mononucleosis; antibiotic drugs do not help and may actually bring on the rash.

What can I do to help?
Give paracetamol to reduce the fever and make sure your child drinks plenty of fluids. Your child may stay in bed during the day if he or she wishes. However, he or she may be more comfortable sitting in a chair.

What is the outlook?
Most children feel well enough to return to school after a couple of weeks. However, your child may require extra rest for a few more weeks. Strenuous sports should be avoided for a month after your child has recovered because they may result in extreme tiredness. A small minority of children develop CHRONIC FATIGUE SYNDROME (p.161).

KAWASAKI DISEASE

First observed in Japan in the 1960s, Kawasaki disease is being diagnosed increasingly in Western countries. It occurs mainly in children under the age of 5 years and is believed to be due to an infection, although no causative organism has been found. The disease causes fever, swollen lymph nodes, and symptoms that affect the skin and mucous membranes. In a few cases, children who have Kawasaki disease develop heart disease.

What are the symptoms?
Typical symptoms of the disease are:
- Fever, lasting more than 5 days.
- CONJUNCTIVITIS (p.165).
- Dry, cracked, swollen lips.
- Sore throat.
- Swelling of one or more lymph nodes in the neck.
- Swelling of the hands and feet.
- Blotchy, red rash over the entire body.
- Reddening of the palms and soles.
- Skin peeling from the tips of fingers and toes (in second week of illness).

What are the complications?
Possible complications of Kawasaki disease include arthritis, myocarditis (inflammation of the heart muscle), myocardial infarction (heart attack), and coronary artery disease.

Should I consult a doctor?
Your child should be seen by a doctor within 24 hours if you think he or she may have Kawasaki disease.

The doctor may admit your child to hospital, where his or her condition can be monitored and treatment may be given promptly for any complications. Your child may be given aspirin and injections of gammaglobulin to reduce the risk of heart complications.

What is the outlook?
Most children make a full recovery from the disease after about 3 weeks. Myocarditis or arthritis may last for 6 to 8 weeks. Coronary artery disease improves gradually over about a year. In perhaps 1 or 2 per cent of cases, serious heart complications may occur.

HIV INFECTION AND AIDS

Most of the children affected by HIV (human immunodeficiency virus) contracted the virus from their infected mother either before or around the time of birth. HIV infection produces few symptoms, but it progressively damages the immune system, leading to AIDS (acquired immune deficiency syndrome). In AIDS, the immune system is so weakened that it allows illnesses, such as PNEUMONIA (p.155), to develop unhindered.

What are the symptoms?
Most infants infected before or around the time of birth will have symptoms before they are 2 years old. However, some may not develop symptoms until they are over 5 years old, and a few cases have been diagnosed as late as 11 years. Typical among the wide range of possible symptoms in children are:
- Failure to thrive.
- Recurrent diarrhoea.
- Enlarged lymph nodes.
- Frequent infections.
- Attacks of pneumonia.
- Developmental delay.

Should I consult a doctor?
Children who are infected with HIV or who have developed AIDS require careful medical supervision.

What might the doctor do?
If the doctor suspects that a baby has HIV, counselling is arranged for the parents. If both parents give their consent after counselling, a blood test is performed. Diagnosis is difficult in babies who do not have symptoms, because the mother's HIV antibodies may remain in the baby's blood for a year or more.

The doctor may prescribe drugs, such as zidovudine, to attack the virus and to slow the development and progress of the disease. He or she might give your child regular injections of gamma globulin and prescribe antibacterial drugs, such as cotrimoxazole, which will help to prevent or fight opportunistic infections, such as pneumonia.

What can I do to help?
If you are HIV-positive and the mother of a baby, you are advised not to breast-feed, because there is a small but definite risk that you might transmit the virus in your milk to your baby, who might otherwise escape infection.

If your child has HIV infection or AIDS you will be given counselling and advice on how to manage the illness.

What is the outlook?
It has been found that children who are infected with HIV may survive into young adulthood. However, the progressive nature of HIV infection is such that all infected people eventually succumb to it.

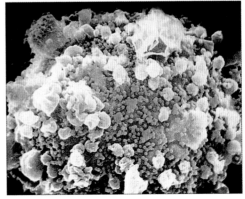

An infected white blood cell
HIV particles (green spheres) are seen here on the surface a white blood cell. White blood cells play a crucial role in the body's immune system. The HIV virus destroys these cells, thus reducing the efficiency of the immune system.

MUSCLE, BONE, AND JOINT DISORDERS

CHILDREN HAVE A HIGH RISK of problems with their muscles, bones, and joints for two main reasons: they are very active, and the bones and joints are still growing and are immature. Some disorders result from genetic abnormalities or birth defects. For all these reasons, musculoskeletal disorders are common. Orthopaedics is the science of correcting these problems. The outlook is generally good because children have great potential for rapid and complete recovery.

LIMPING

A child with a limp may have a minor injury that will get better on its own. However, the child may have an underlying disorder that requires prompt treatment to prevent permanent disability. Therefore, you should never ignore a limp in a child.

How is it caused?
The most common cause of a limp or a reluctance to walk is pain. Some causes of the pain are shown on the right.

Unequal leg length may also cause a limp. A bone may be short from birth or may fail to grow because of a spinal cord abnormality or CEREBRAL PALSY (p.160) involving muscular weakness of one side of the body. A limp may also be due to apparent shortening of a leg, as a result of CONGENITAL HIP DISLOCATION (p.130) that was detected late or of spinal curvature (see SCOLIOSIS, p.128).

Children who have a disorder of the muscles and/or the nervous system, such as MUSCULAR DYSTROPHY (p.133) or cerebral palsy, may have muscle weakness or incoordination, causing walking problems that resemble a limp.

Rarely, a limp develops as part of a behavioural problem in a child with emotional or psychological difficulties.

Should I consult a doctor?
A doctor should see your child if he or she has a limp, or is old enough to walk but refuses to do so, and you are unable to find an obvious cause, such as a splinter in the foot. You should phone a doctor at once if your child also has a fever, rash, or hot, swollen joints; these symptoms could indicate bone or joint infection, conditions that require immediate medical treatment.

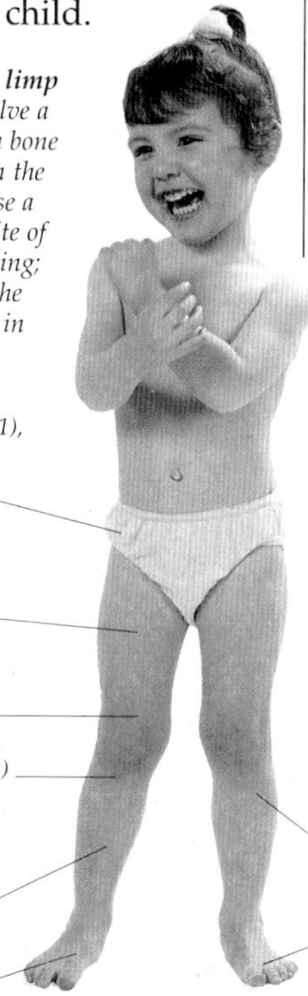

What might the doctor do?
Your child will be examined and blood tests, X-rays, and/or scanning may be carried out in order to help diagnose the cause of the problem. The child may be referred to a paediatrician or orthopaedic surgeon and admission to hospital may be required for tests or observation. The treatment will depend on the underlying cause.

What is the outlook?
A limp due to a minor injury should disappear in a few days. A limp due to most other causes should disappear once the underlying problem has been treated. In a few cases, the underlying cause, such as unequal leg length or muscular weakness, cannot be cured, and walking problems may be lifelong.

Causes of painful limp
Disorders that involve a joint, a muscle, or a bone around the hip or in the leg or foot may cause a painful limp. The site of pain can be misleading; an abnormality in the hip may cause pain in the thigh or knee.

IRRITABLE HIP (p.130), PERTHES' DISEASE (p.131), SLIPPED FEMORAL EPIPHYSIS (p.131)

Muscle strain (see STRAINS AND SPRAINS, *opposite)*

Bone infection (see BONE AND JOINT INFECTION, p.133)

KNEE DISORDERS (p.132)

Fractured bone (see FRACTURES AND DISLOCATIONS, p.128)

JUVENILE CHRONIC ARTHRITIS (p.132)

Joint infection (see BONE AND JOINT INFECTION, *p.133).*

A verruca (see WARTS, *p.141) or a sharp object in the sole of the foot*

STRAINS AND SPRAINS

A strain, which is also known as a pulled muscle, occurs when a muscle is overstretched and some of the muscle fibres are damaged. A joint is sprained when one or more of its ligaments (the fibrous bands that connect bones at joints) is overstretched or torn. Strains and sprains often result from falls or vigorous physical activity. Treatment for the injuries can usually be given at home; medical attention is needed only if they are severe.

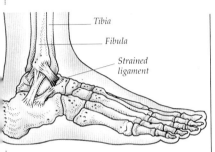

Tibia
Fibula
Strained ligament

Sprained ankle
The ankle is the most commonly sprained joint. The injury may occur during a fall when the foot is twisted onto its outside edge.

What are the symptoms?
The severity of symptoms depends on how badly the muscle or ligaments are damaged. The symptoms may include:
• Pain and tenderness, which increase with movement of the affected area.
• Swelling at the site of injury.
• Muscle spasm (tightness of a muscle produced by involuntary contractions).
• A limp, if a leg is affected.
• Bruising, which may appear a few days after the injury.

What can I do to help?
For about the first 48 hours after injury, a strain or a sprain is best treated by means of RICE – rest, ice, compression, and elevation (see panel: *Treating strains and sprains*, p.73). You should not apply heat to the injury for the first 48 hours. You may give your child paracetamol in order to help relieve the pain.

After 1 or 2 days of rest, the pain and swelling should begin to subside, and your child may begin gently to exercise the sprained or strained limb.

Should I consult a doctor?
Your child should be seen by a doctor if pain and swelling are severe just after the injury (for example, if a child cannot walk on an injured ankle) or if milder symptoms have not shown any improvement within a few days.

What might the doctor do?
The doctor will examine the injured area and may arrange for an X-ray to be taken in hospital to make sure that no bones have been fractured. The injured part may be strapped or wrapped in a compression bandage. Your child may have to use crutches for a leg injury or wear a sling if the arm is affected.

If the strain or sprain is very severe, non-steroidal anti-inflammatory drugs (NSAIDs) may be prescribed to reduce pain and swelling and speed healing. Your child may have to wear a splint or plaster cast for a severe sprain.

Once the pain has disappeared, the doctor may suggest exercises that will strengthen the affected part, or may refer your child to a physiotherapist.

How can I prevent strains and sprains?
Try to make sure that your child warms up before taking part in any sport or strenuous physical activity. A warm-up routine should include movements that mobilize the joints and warm up the muscles, followed by gentle stretches.

What is the outlook?
A strain or a sprain should heal within 2 weeks. If the affected ligament or muscle is allowed to heal properly and is exercised, it will regain full mobility and will not be permanently weakened.

CRAMP

The onset of cramp, a strong, painful contraction (spasm) of a muscle, is usually sudden and severe. However, cramp usually lasts only a few minutes. As well as being painful, the muscle feels hard and tight, and a lump or distortion may be visible in the affected area. Cramp frequently affects the calf muscle.

How is it caused?
Cramp may be triggered by vigorous exercise, by repetitive movement, or by lying or sitting awkwardly. Exercise-related cramp may be partly caused by loss of salt from sweating. Rarely, a recurrent or prolonged cramp may be caused by lack of calcium in the blood.

What can I do to help?
Your child's cramp can be relieved by gently massaging and stretching the affected muscle. You can teach your child to stretch the calf muscle by using the method shown in the illustration (right). The exercise may be repeated until the pain starts to subside. If there is still some pain, apply a hot water bottle wrapped in a towel to the affected area; or your child may take a hot bath or shower. Paracetamol or ibuprofen may also be given. Cramp can be frightening; reassure your child that cramp is common and temporary. To help prevent cramp, make sure that your child drinks plenty of fluids during exercise, particularly in hot weather.

If the cramps continue and there is no obvious cause, you should consult a doctor to exclude the possibility of an underlying disorder.

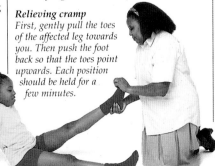

Relieving cramp
First, gently pull the toes of the affected leg towards you. Then push the foot back so that the toes point upwards. Each position should be held for a few minutes.

FRACTURES AND DISLOCATIONS

Bones commonly fractured (broken) in children are those of the leg and arm, and the clavicle (collarbone). A dislocation occurs when the ligaments that hold the bones of a joint are stretched or torn, so that the bones are displaced. The elbow is the joint most often dislocated in children. When a joint is dislocated, bones may also be fractured. Fractures and dislocations usually result from falls, sports activities, or traffic accidents.

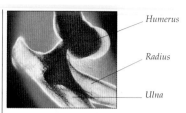

Dislocated elbow joint
This X-ray shows severe displacement of the ball-like end of the humerus from its normal position in the socket of the ulna.

What are the symptoms?
A minor fracture may cause only mild symptoms and may be mistaken for a STRAIN OR SPRAIN (p.127). More severe fractures and dislocations may cause:
• Severe pain; the child will not want to move the injured part.
• Extreme tenderness if pressure is put on the area directly over the site of the injury.
• Swelling and skin discoloration at the site of the injury.
• Visible deformity (in the case of a dislocated joint and some serious fractures).
A fracture or a dislocation may damage surrounding tissues, nerves, and blood vessels. If fractured bone breaks the skin, infection is a risk.

Should I consult a doctor?
Do not move your child if his or her neck or back may be injured; call an ambulance. If you suspect a fracture or dislocation of another part of the body, take your child to a hospital accident and emergency department immediately or call an ambulance. While waiting for an ambulance, you may immobilize an affected arm or leg (see BROKEN ARM, p.211; BROKEN COLLARBONE, p.210; BROKEN LEG, p.210).

What might the doctor do?
An X-ray will be taken of the injured area to confirm whether a bone is fractured and/or dislocated, and to pinpoint the site of the injury and its severity. The doctor may give your child a local or a general anaesthetic and manipulate any displaced bones back into position. In some cases, surgery is required to reposition bones and repair damage to surrounding tissues. The affected limb may be immobilized to hold the bones in the correct position as they heal. Plaster casts or splints are used to immobilize some fractures; traction

Greenstick fracture
Because children's bones are supple, the long bones of the arms and legs tend to bend and to crack on only one side.

may also be used. In some cases, metal screws, rods, pins, or plates may be inserted to hold bones in position.

Fractures in children heal much more quickly than they do in adults. A small bone that does not bear weight, such as a finger bone, may take only a week or two to heal; large, weight-bearing bones such as the femur (thighbone) may take several months. Dislocations usually heal within a week or two.

As soon as it is safe for your child to use the affected part, physiotherapy will be given to prevent muscles and joints from becoming stiff and weak.

What is the outlook?
As long as bones have been properly repositioned and immobilized, your child should recover completely from a fracture or dislocation, but stiffness may not disappear for several weeks or months. Joint fractures slightly increase the risk of arthritis in later life.

SCOLIOSIS

Abnormal sideways curvature of the spine is called scoliosis. Usually, scoliosis has no known cause. Rarely, it is due to a structural abnormality of one or more vertebrae or to a local muscle weakness. Scoliosis most often affects girls, starting around the time of the adolescent growth spurt.

What are the symptoms?
The main symptoms are:
• Sideways curve of the spine.
• Shoulders are not level.
• Chest is more prominent on one side than the other.

Appearance of scoliosis
In scoliosis, the spine curves to one side, usually the right, and one shoulder is higher than the other.

The curve of the spine will probably be accentuated when your child bends forwards to touch his or her toes with the knees kept straight.

What is the treatment?
A doctor should be consulted if you think your child has scoliosis. After examining your child, the doctor will refer him or her to an orthopaedic surgeon, who will monitor your child to see whether the curvature is getting worse. A mild curvature that is not progressive does not usually need any treatment. In progressive cases, a child may be fitted with a plastic body cast or brace to prevent the curvature of the spine from becoming worse.

What is the outlook?
As long as scoliosis is treated promptly, it should not become any worse and your child is unlikely to have any long-term ill effects. If progressive scoliosis is not treated, it may, in some children, eventually cause severe deformity of the spine and ribcage. The deformity may lead to breathing difficulties and recurrent chest infections.

MINOR SKELETAL PROBLEMS

When a child first starts to stand and walk, parents often worry that the position of his or her legs or feet may be abnormal. The most common sources of concern are in-toeing or out-toeing (walking pigeon-toed or splay-footed), bowlegs, knock-knees, and flat feet. In most cases, these conditions result from the position of the baby in the uterus or are a normal variation. In a very few cases, they may indicate an underlying disorder.

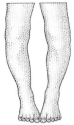 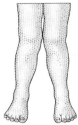

Bowlegs
Outward-curved legs prevent the knees from touching; the shinbone is rotated inwards.

Knock-knees
The legs are curved inwards so that the knees touch and the feet lie apart.

IN-TOEING; OUT-TOEING

Both of these conditions are common. Inward rotation of the whole leg from the hip is the most frequent cause of in-toeing. Other causes are curving of the front part of the foot (see illustration below) and bowlegs (see right). Out-toeing is caused by outward rotation of the whole leg at the hip.

In-toeing
Inward curving of the front part of the foot (known as hooked forefoot) is a common cause of in-toeing. The web space between the big toe and the second toe is also often increased.

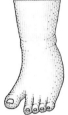

Should I consult a doctor?
Consult a doctor if you are worried about the position of your child's legs or feet. Inward-curving feet usually get better on their own by the age of 3 or 4 years. If they persist, they can be treated by gentle manipulation of the feet and immobilization in casts.

Rarely, surgery is needed. Hip rotation usually corrects itself by the age of 8 years. An operation is rarely required for a persistent problem.

Out-toeing almost always corrects itself within a year of the child starting to walk. Even if out-toeing does persist, it does not cause problems.

BOWLEGS; KNOCK-KNEES

Slight outward curving of the leg bones is normal in toddlers; in bowlegs, the outward curve is exaggerated and the tibia (shinbone) is rotated inwards. In knock-knees, the legs curve inwards. Bowlegs usually correct themselves by the age of 3 or 4 years; knock-knees are usually outgrown by the age of 11 years.

Should I consult a doctor?
If you are worried, you should consult a doctor, who will probably reassure you that nothing is wrong with your child. Very rarely, an operation is required to correct a severe or persistent deformity, which can be the result of a disorder of bone growth, such as rickets.

FLAT FEET

It is normal for children to have flat feet (meaning that the soles of the feet rest on the ground) up to the age of about 2 or 3 years. In some children, they persist but are not associated with any problems. Rarely, flat feet are due to an underlying abnormality of the bones or joints that makes the feet painful, stiff, and weak.

Should I consult a doctor?
Consult a doctor if you are worried about your child's feet. The doctor will check the appearance, mobility, and strength of the feet. If all these features are normal, the feet are normal and no treatment is needed.

If there is an underlying disorder, treatment may include immobilizing the feet in casts and, rarely, surgery.

CLUBFOOT

In this congenital deformity, the foot is twisted out of shape or position. Clubfoot affects three times more male babies than female babies, and in half of all cases, both feet are affected. Clubfoot is detected during the routine examination at birth.

How is it caused?
Clubfoot may be due to the position of the baby's foot in the uterus (postural clubfoot) or to an abnormality of the bones in the foot (structural clubfoot).

What might the doctor do?
The doctor will check the mobility of the foot. If it is normal, your child has postural clubfoot, and no treatment is required. Restricted mobility indicates structural clubfoot. Treatment consists

of manipulation of the foot followed by adhesive strapping and splinting to hold the foot in position. If the foot has not straightened by the age of 3 to 6 months, an operation to straighten it may be performed. The foot is then put in a plaster cast for at least 3 months.

What is the outlook?
Postural clubfoot corrects itself within a few weeks of birth. In about half of all cases of structural clubfoot, the

Features of clubfoot
The heel of the foot is turned inwards and the rest of the foot is bent downwards and inwards. In some cases, the tibia (shinbone) is turned inwards and the leg muscles are underdeveloped.

baby's foot is corrected after 2 to 3 months of manipulation and strapping. An operation successfully corrects the deformity in most of the remaining cases. In a small number of children, a series of operations may be performed over a 5-year period to improve the function and appearance of the foot, but it may never be completely normal.

CONGENITAL HIP DISLOCATION

One newborn baby in about 250 has congenital hip dislocation. In this condition, the head of the femur (thighbone) lies outside the socket of the pelvis or is unstable and likely to slip out of position. Babies are screened for congenital hip dislocation soon after birth, and tests for the condition are included in routine check-ups during the first year of life. Congenital hip dislocation runs in families and is more common in girls than in boys.

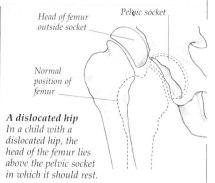

A dislocated hip
In a child with a dislocated hip, the head of the femur lies above the pelvic socket in which it should rest.

How is it caused?
Although the underlying cause is not known, one or both of a baby's hips may be dislocated or unstable because the fibrous capsule surrounding the hip joint is weak or because the pelvic socket is abnormally shallow.

What are the symptoms?
Congenital hip dislocation is usually detected soon after birth. The technique shown below or, in some hospitals, ultrasound scanning may be used

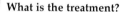

Examining a baby's hips
The doctor manipulates a newborn baby's thighs and hips to check for congenital hip dislocation. If a hip is dislocated, the doctor may feel a jolting or jerking sensation as the head of the femur moves into the socket.

to diagnose the condition. The problem may be found later, during one of the routine checkups in the first year of life. Occasionally, the disorder may not be discovered until your child begins to walk, when you may notice:
• A limp.
• The back of the affected leg has more skin folds below the buttock than the unaffected leg.
Your child should be seen by a doctor if you suspect that he or she may have congenital hip dislocation.

What is the treatment?
An unstable hip often corrects itself soon after birth. If your baby's hip abnormality has not corrected itself by about 2 weeks of age, a splint may be applied to move the head of the femur into the socket and keep it there. The splint is usually worn for 2 to 4 months. You will be advised about how to care for your baby while he or she is wearing the splint. When the splint is removed, the hip joint should be normal. However, if your baby's congenital hip dislocation is not

discovered until his or her next routine examination (which is carried out at 6 weeks or more) the head of the femur may have to be moved into the socket and held in place by traction for several weeks. Following traction, your child will probably have to wear a splint or plaster cast for several months.

If your child begins to walk before the condition is discovered, a series of operations will probably be necessary to correct the disorder.

What is the outlook?
The earlier that treatment is given, the better the outlook. If a child is treated in early infancy, he or she should be able to walk normally and is not likely to suffer from any ill effects later in life. However, if treatment is delayed or if no treatment is given, there may be a risk of a permanent limp and the early onset of arthritis in the affected hip.

IRRITABLE HIP

This condition occurs when the lining of the hip joint becomes inflamed and fluid accumulates inside the joint. The cause is unknown, but irritable hip often develops within about 2 weeks of a mild upper respiratory tract infection, such as a cold. Children aged 2 to 12 years are most susceptible to irritable hip.

What are the symptoms?
The symptoms of irritable hip start suddenly and may include:
• A limp.
• Pain in the hip, groin, thigh, or knee.
• Sometimes, mild fever.
Your child should be seen by a doctor within 24 hours if he or she has pain in the hip, groin, thigh, or knee, and/or a limp without an obvious cause.

What is the treatment?
The doctor will probably advise you to give painkillers, such as paracetamol, and to make sure that your child rests in bed until the pain improves, which usually takes 1 to 7 days.

Occasionally, if the pain is severe, a child may be admitted to hospital, where blood tests may be carried out to exclude an infection. The child may

also have X-rays and ultrasound scans of the hip to rule out conditions such as PERTHES' DISEASE (opposite) or joint infection (see BONE AND JOINT INFECTION, p.133). Traction may be applied to the hip to relieve muscle spasm and pain.

What is the outlook?
Once the pain has subsided, a child can usually return to normal activities. If a child becomes active too early, there is a risk that symptoms may return and non-steroidal anti-inflammatory drugs (NSAIDs) may be required. If pain recurs in the hip despite treatment, the problem may be due to Perthes' disease or JUVENILE CHRONIC ARTHRITIS (p.132).

SLIPPED FEMORAL EPIPHYSIS

The growth of a long bone occurs near the ends at growth plates, which separate regions called the epiphyses from the main shaft. A slipped femoral epiphysis occurs when the upper epiphysis of the femur (thighbone), which forms part of the hip joint, slips into an abnormal position. This rare disorder affects adolescents during the growth spurt (about 10 to 14 years of age in girls and 12 to 16 years of age in boys). Children who are overweight or growing very rapidly are most susceptible to the condition.

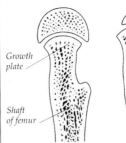 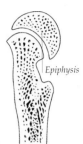

NORMAL POSITION   SLIPPED EPIPHYSIS

Slipped femoral epiphysis
In this condition, the growth plate shears and the upper epiphysis (end) of the femur slips and comes to lie below and behind its normal position, causing the leg to rotate outwards.

How is it caused?
In growing children, the femur grows mainly at the upper end. The growth plate, where new bone is formed, is made of cartilage and so is an area of relative weakness in the bone; as a result, the upper epiphysis is vulnerable to displacement (see illustration right). A femoral epiphysis may slip suddenly out of position as a result of an injury that shears the growth plate; or it may slip gradually, for unknown reasons.

What are the symptoms?
The symptoms may include:
• Pain in the hip, knee, or thigh.
• Inability to bear weight on affected leg.
• A limp or a splay-footed walk, because the leg is rotated outwards.
• Restricted movement of the hip.

If your child has a painful hip, thigh, or knee and/or a limp, he or she should be seen by a doctor within 24 hours.

What is the treatment?
The doctor will examine your child, and will probably send him or her to hospital for a hip X-ray. If the X-ray shows a slipped femoral epiphysis, an operation will be performed. If the slip is mild, your child's epiphysis may be left where it is and fixed with screws to prevent further slipping. During the same operation, the epiphysis of the other hip joint may be strengthened in a similar way. For a more severe slip, a wedge of bone may be removed from below the upper epiphysis, so that the epiphysis is returned to its normal position within the pelvic socket.

What is the outlook?
Provided the hip is treated promptly, the long-term outlook is good, and after recovering from the operation, your child will probably be able to lead a normal, active life. A subsequent slipped femoral epiphysis is unlikely to occur, especially once the pubertal growth spurt is over. In a few cases, however, the affected hip may become stiff and painful, and there may be vulnerability to arthritis in later life.

PERTHES' DISEASE

Progressive softening, followed by re-forming and hardening, of the head of the femur (thighbone) is known as Perthes' disease. It is caused by poor blood supply to the head of the femur. The condition affects children, particularly boys, aged 4 to 8 years. Although Perthes' disease gets better spontaneously within 2 to 4 years, treatment should be carried out as early as possible in order to prevent the hip joint from becoming deformed.

What are the symptoms?
The main symptoms of the disease are:
• A limp.
• Pain in the hip or knee.
• Restricted movement at the hip.
If your child has pain in the hip or knee and/or a limp, he or she should be seen by a doctor within 24 hours.

What is the treatment?
The doctor will examine your child and may send him or her to hospital for an X-ray of the hip joint to help establish the cause of the symptoms. The type of

Flattened head   Pelvic socket
of femur

Femur

Femoral deformity
If the hip joint continues to bear a child's weight while he or she has Perthes' disease, the head and neck of the femur may become deformed.

Shortened neck of femur

treatment depends on the severity of the disease. In less severe cases, bed rest for 1 to 2 weeks until the joint pain subsides, with regular monitoring by X-ray, may be all that is required. If the joint is at risk of becoming deformed, your child may have to wear calipers, splints, or a plaster cast. In very severe cases, an operation may be performed to fix the head of the femur more firmly within the pelvic socket, which reduces the risk of hip joint deformity.

What is the outlook?
The younger a child is when Perthes' disease is discovered and treatment is given, and the less severe the disease, the better the outcome is likely to be. Usually, deformity of the hip joint can be prevented and the joint will function normally. In some very severe cases, it is impossible to prevent joint deformity, even with treatment, and there is a risk of arthritis of the hip later in life.

KNEE DISORDERS

The most common knee disorders that affect children are chondromalacia patellae and Osgood-Schlatter disease. They occur mainly in adolescents. Both conditions may be brought on by overuse of the joint, usually as a result of strenuous physical activity. One or both knees may be affected.

Tendon from quadriceps muscle

Patella

Tibia

Point of attachment

Osgood-Schlatter disease
The large tendon from the quadriceps muscle of the thigh extends to the patella and then to the tibia, where it is attached. Exercise can cause inflammation of the tendon at its point of attachment.

CHONDROMALACIA PATELLAE

In this condition, the cartilage at the back of the patella (kneecap) becomes soft, swollen, and roughened. Girls aged 15 to 18 years are the group most susceptible to chondromalacia patellae.

The main symptom is aching pain behind the patella. The pain is made worse by exercise (especially climbing stairs) and gets better with rest.

What is the treatment?

The treatment is rest. Your child should avoid any activities that make the pain worse or that involve repetitive knee-bending, such as cycling. You may give paracetamol to relieve the pain. If pain is severe or is no better after 24 hours, your child should be seen by a doctor to exclude a more serious disorder.

What is the outlook?

Bouts of pain behind the patella may recur throughout adolescence. Most children are symptom-free within a year of growth ceasing. In a few cases, early arthritis may develop.

OSGOOD-SCHLATTER DISEASE

In this disorder, there is inflammation of the tibia (shinbone) just below the knee at the point where a large tendon is attached (see illustration above right). Osgood-Schlatter disease mainly affects boys aged between 10 and 14 years.

The main symptoms are tenderness, pain, and swelling just below the knee, which usually worsens with exercise. Your child should be seen by a doctor, who will probably refer him or her to an orthopaedic surgeon.

What is the treatment?

The surgeon may ask your child to avoid strenuous physical activities, such as football, for several months. If the pain is severe or persists for more than a few months, despite avoiding strenuous activities, the knee may have to be immobilized in a plaster cast for 6 to 8 weeks. This treatment almost always cures the problem.

The problem is unlikely to recur, as long as only moderate exercise is taken until the child is over about 14 years.

JUVENILE CHRONIC ARTHRITIS

Three types of chronic arthritis (inflammation of the joints) affect children. Pauciarticular arthritis affects four or fewer large joints (such as the knee). The polyarticular type affects small joints, such as those of the hands and feet. Systemic juvenile arthritis also affects small joints and produces symptoms of general illness.

How is it caused?

Although the underlying cause is not known, the disorder may be inherited. The initial joint inflammation may be triggered by a viral infection, but no specific virus has been identified.

What are the symptoms?

The main symptoms are:
• Pain, redness, swelling, and stiffness of affected joints.
• A limp, if the feet or legs are affected.
• In polyarticular arthritis, a mild fever.
In systemic arthritis, the following symptoms may appear several weeks or months before the joints are affected:
• A temperature above 39°C (102°F).
• Swollen glands throughout the body.
• A blotchy, non-itchy rash.
A rare complication is IRITIS (p.164).

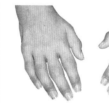

Arthritis affecting the hands
The joints of the fingers are red and swollen because of arthritis. Other small joints that may be affected are those of the neck and jaw.

Should I consult a doctor?

Your child should be seen by a doctor within 24 hours of the onset of joint pain or stiffness, a limp, or a rash with a fever. The doctor will examine your child and arrange for blood tests in order to exclude other disorders.

What is the treatment?

An important part of treatment consists of physiotherapy to maintain muscle strength and joint mobility. Splints may need to be worn at night to prevent joint deformity and sometimes during the day in order to rest the joints.

The doctor may prescribe aspirin and non-steroidal anti-inflammatory drugs (NSAIDs), such as ibuprofen, to relieve pain and swelling. If these drugs are ineffective, more powerful drugs, such as corticosteroids, may be prescribed. In very severe cases, an operation may be performed to replace joints that are damaged and painful or to lengthen muscles that are causing deformity.

Until your child has recovered from arthritis, his or her eyes will probably be examined regularly for signs of iritis.

What is the outlook?

One third of children recover from juvenile arthritis completely; another third continues to have symptoms for many years. In the remaining cases, the condition worsens.

BONE AND JOINT INFECTION

Infection of a bone or joint most commonly occurs when bacteria are carried through the bloodstream from an infected site, such as a wound or a BOIL (p.137), elsewhere in the body. In some cases, infection spreads directly from nearby infected tissue.

BONE INFECTION

Children aged 3 to 14 years, especially boys, are susceptible to bone infection. The long bones of the arms and legs are most often affected. Without prompt treatment, bone infection may become chronic and difficult to eradicate.

What are the symptoms?
The symptoms may include:
- Severe pain in the affected arm or leg, which the child is reluctant to move or allow to be touched.
- Fever.
- If treatment is delayed, swelling and inflammation of the skin overlying the infected bone.

Phone a doctor at once if you think that your child might have a bone infection.

What might the doctor do?
The doctor will examine your child and admit him or her to hospital for tests, including a blood culture and a bone scan. Treatment is with antibiotics. In a few cases, an operation may be carried out to remove infected bone. Your child should make a complete recovery if he or she is treated promptly.

JOINT INFECTION

Infection of a joint is most common in children up to the age of 2 years and in adolescents. The joint becomes inflamed and fluid collects within it. If treatment is delayed, the cartilage that covers bones inside the joint may be damaged, causing stiffness and deformity of the joint.

What are the symptoms?
The symptoms are similar to those of bone infection, but the joint is usually also swollen and hot. Phone a doctor at once if you think that your child might have a joint infection.

What might the doctor do?
The doctor will examine your child and may send him or her to hospital for an ultrasound scan of the joint. To confirm the diagnosis, fluid is taken from the joint for analysis (see illustration below). Blood tests may also be carried out. Treatment is with antibiotic drugs. An operation may be performed to drain the infected fluid from the infected joint. Once the infection has cleared up, your child may receive physiotherapy, which will keep the joint flexible. As long as the infected joint is treated promptly, your child should make a complete recovery.

Femur

Patella

Fluid

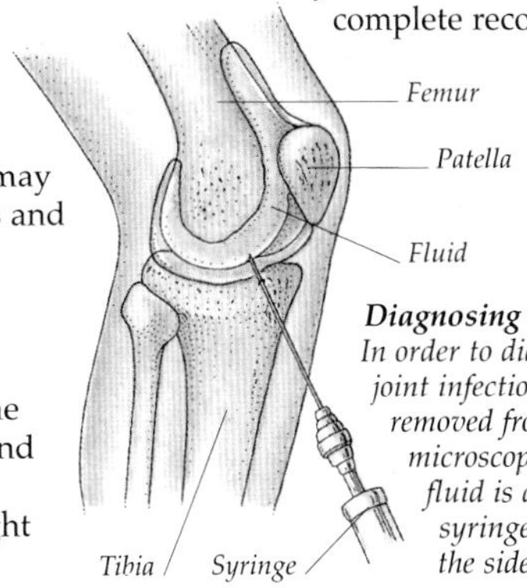

Diagnosing joint infection
In order to diagnose bacterial joint infection, fluid may be removed from the joint for microscopic analysis. The fluid is drawn off using a syringe inserted through the side of the knee.

Tibia / *Syringe*

MUSCULAR DYSTROPHY

The main features of this disorder are progressive weakness and wasting of muscle. There are several types of muscular dystrophy. The most common and most serious type is Duchenne muscular dystrophy; it affects only boys and appears before 5 years of age.

How is it caused?
Duchenne muscular dystrophy is due to an abnormal gene. A boy born to a woman who is a carrier has a 50 per cent chance of having the disorder; his sisters have a 50 per cent chance of being carriers.

What are the symptoms?
The first symptom is weakness in the leg muscles, which may cause your child to:
- Walk late (at over the age of 18 months) and waddle.
- Climb stairs with difficulty.
- Fall easily and roll on to his front, and climb or "hand walk" up his own legs.

Other symptoms may include:
- Enlarged calf muscles.
- Inward curvature of the lower spine.

Your child should be seen by a doctor if you think that muscular dystrophy might be a possibility.

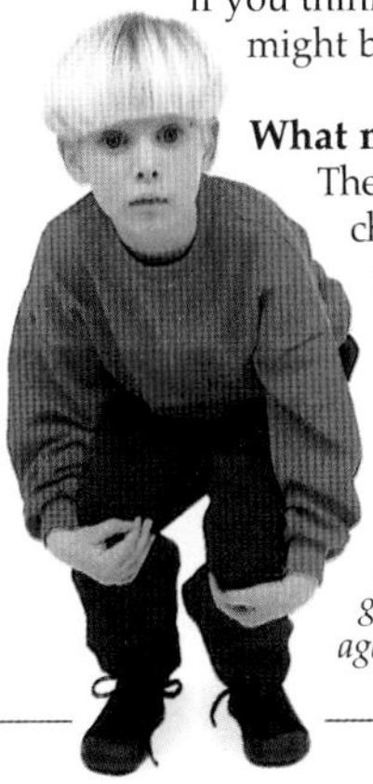

What might the doctor do?
The doctor will examine your child and may send him to a neurologist. Tests in hospital may be arranged in order to confirm the diagnosis. At present, there is no cure for

Weak leg muscles
A child with weak leg muscles gets up from the floor by pushing against his ankles, knees, and thighs.

Duchenne muscular dystrophy. Instead, physiotherapy will be given to maintain mobility, and you will be shown how to help your child exercise.

How can Duchenne muscular dystrophy be prevented?
A woman who has a family history of Duchenne dystrophy and who plans to have a baby may be tested to see if she is a carrier. If she is a carrier, she will be offered genetic counselling to explain the risks of a baby being affected. Tests can also be done during pregnancy to see if the fetus of a woman is affected; if it is, termination can be considered.

What is the outlook?
The child's muscle weakness increases and gradually spreads to affect more and more muscles until the child needs a wheelchair, usually by 8 to 11 years of age. The boy becomes increasingly vulnerable to chest infections and may not survive past his early 20s.

SKIN DISORDERS

YOUNG SKIN IS SENSITIVE, and skin reactions are common in childhood. A rash or other change in the skin may be due to irritation (for example, by chemicals in detergents), infection, or allergy. Skin reactions may also be part of a generalized illness, such as measles. Disorders that are confined to the skin are usually minor and, in most cases, get better rapidly. The first step in dealing with a skin disorder is to identify its cause, and a doctor is the best person to do this.

SEBORRHOEIC DERMATITIS

This common inflammation of the skin has no known cause. It may affect the body and face and/or the scalp. Seborrhoeic dermatitis may appear initially in the first few months of a baby's life. The symptoms vary in severity over a number of months, but generally clear up by the age of about 2 years. However, seborrhoeic dermatitis may reappear after puberty and then recur periodically throughout life.

What are the symptoms?

The main symptoms of the infant form of seborrhoeic dermatitis are:

- A scaly, blotchy rash, most commonly in the skin creases of the nappy area but also sometimes in other areas of the body (see illustration below).
- Occasionally, slight itchiness.
- Thick yellowish scales on the scalp (cradle cap). Scaly areas on the forehead, behind the ears, and in the eyebrows may accompany cradle cap.

Scalp

Sites of seborrhoeic dermatitis in infants
Babies may be affected by seborrhoeic dermatitis at one or more of the sites shown here.

Face

Neck

Armpits

Chest (occasionally)

Nappy area

The main symptoms of the adolescent form of seborrhoeic dermatitis are:

- A scaly, blotchy rash, which may appear on the face, behind the ears, on the neck, chest, and back, and in the armpits and groin.
- Occasionally, itchiness.
- Dandruff, if the scalp is affected. White flakes of dead skin can be seen in the hair, usually near the scalp.

Scratching the affected area sometimes leads to a bacterial infection, such as IMPETIGO (p.139), causing the rash to become raw and weepy.

What can I do to help?

Affected areas of skin should be kept clean with emulsifying ointment, rather than soap, which may irritate the rash. After cleaning the affected areas of skin, apply a corticosteroid cream. This treatment is most effective if started as soon as symptoms appear.

Cradle cap often disappears on its own within a few weeks or months. However, you can remove unsightly cradle cap scales by gently massaging baby oil or olive oil into your baby's scalp and leaving it overnight. The next day, comb your baby's hair in order to dislodge the softened scales, and then wash them away. Over-the-counter salicylic acid ointment and special shampoos are also available for treating cradle cap.

Regular use of a special shampoo or combing your baby's hair daily may stop the scaly patches from forming.

Dandruff can usually be effectively controlled by frequent use of an over-the-counter antidandruff shampoo.

Should I consult a doctor?

Your child should be seen by a doctor if the rash is extensive or looks infected, the scalp is inflamed, other symptoms develop, or the condition does not improve within a few weeks. The doctor may prescribe a corticosteroid cream or ointment containing either an antibiotic or an antiseptic. With treatment, the rash should clear up within a few weeks.

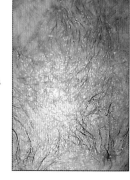

Cradle cap
Scaly yellowish patches of skin on the scalp are the main feature of cradle cap. Although the patches are unsightly, cradle cap is harmless.

ATOPIC ECZEMA

About 1 child in 30 develops the itchy rash of atopic eczema. The rash usually first appears before a child is 18 months old, and may vary in severity over a number of years. The cause of atopic eczema is unknown. Most affected children have a close relative with eczema or an allergic disorder, such as ASTHMA (p.153) or hay fever (see ALLERGIC RHINITIS, p.152). Rarely, intolerance to certain foods may be responsible (see FOOD INTOLERANCE, p.182).

What are the symptoms?
The symptoms of atopic eczema vary, depending on the age of the child. In children less than 4 years old:
- The rash consists of itchy, inflamed pimples, which may be mildly weepy.
- The scalp, cheeks, forearms, fronts of the legs, and trunk are most often affected, although the rash may appear anywhere on the body.

The rash often disappears before a child reaches the age of 4 years and, in some individuals, never returns. The rash may reappear (or appear for the

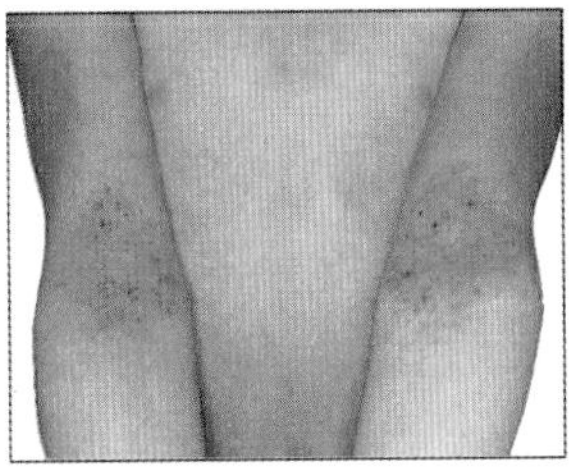

Appearance of eczema
The insides of the elbows are often affected by atopic eczema. The rash seen here has the typical appearance of atopic eczema in children aged 4 years or over: it is scaly, red, and dry, with a rough surface.

first time) in some children between the ages of 4 and 10 years. At this age:
- The rash consists of itchy, dry, scaly patches, and the skin may be cracked.
- The face, neck, insides of the elbows, wrists, backs of the knees, and ankles are most commonly affected (see illustration above right).
- Skin in affected areas may become thickened over time.

Regardless of your child's age, the first sign of an impending flare-up of atopic eczema is generally a small, slightly inflamed area on the skin.

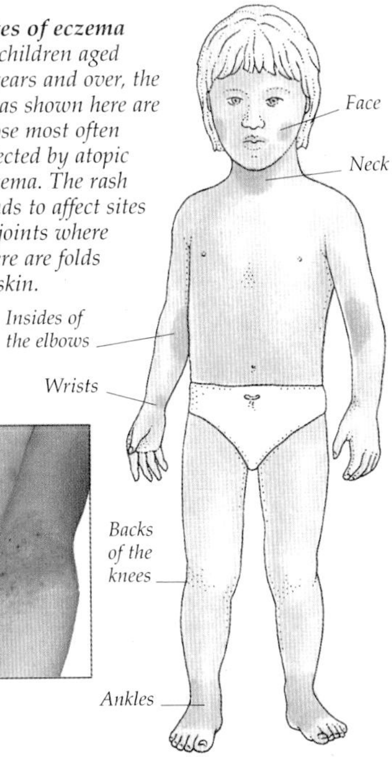

What are the complications?
If your child scratches the rash, the skin may become infected with bacteria, resulting in weeping blisters. A much rarer, but more serious, complication is an illness called eczema herpeticum, which can occur if a child with eczema is infected by the herpes simplex virus (which causes COLD SORES, p.139). This disorder causes a widespread rash

Sites of eczema
In children aged 4 years and over, the areas shown here are those most often affected by atopic eczema. The rash tends to affect sites at joints where there are folds of skin.

Face
Neck
Insides of the elbows
Wrists
Backs of the knees
Ankles

consisting of blisters and open sores, which is often accompanied by a high fever of 40–41°C (104–106°F). The lymph nodes may also be enlarged.

Should I consult a doctor?
Your child should be seen by a doctor within 24 hours if he or she has not had the rash before. If your child has already been diagnosed as having atopic eczema and the rash does not respond to treatment or gets worse, he or she should be seen by a doctor because the rash may be infected.

What might the doctor do?
A corticosteroid cream or ointment may be prescribed by the doctor to reduce inflammation and itchiness during flare-ups of atopic eczema. You should continue to apply the cream to affected areas of skin, according to the doctor's instructions, until the normal

texture of the skin has returned. When slight inflammation indicates that a flare-up of eczema is imminent, apply the prescribed cream to affected areas to prevent the rash from developing. If the itchiness is keeping your child awake at night, an antihistamine may be prescribed. The doctor may suggest that you exclude certain foods from your child's diet if the eczema is persistent, severe, or widespread.

For a bacterial infection, the doctor may prescribe a cream or ointment containing a corticosteroid and an antibiotic or antiseptic. He or she may also prescribe an oral antibiotic.

Your child may be sent to hospital if he or she develops eczema herpeticum; in hospital, the antiviral drug acyclovir may be administered intravenously.

What can I do to help?
Apart from applying any creams or ointments as directed by the doctor, you may be able to keep symptoms to a minimum by preventing your child's skin from becoming too dry. When you bathe your child, use a mild cleanser such as a baby soap or aqueous cream. You may make the bath water less irritating by adding a bath oil that is specially formulated for eczema.

Keep your child's skin soft and well moisturized by regularly applying an emollient, such as aqueous cream or emulsifying ointment. The emollient should be used several times a day on the affected areas. It may be especially effective if it is applied to the skin when it is still warm and wet after your child's daily bath.

In some children, eczema is worse in cold weather, while in others hot weather prompts a flare-up. Bathing and moisturizing the skin more often during hot or cold weather may help to minimize symptoms. Make sure that your child wears cotton clothing next to the skin to help reduce irritation.

Your child should avoid close contact with anyone who has cold sores.

What is the outlook?
As your child grows older, the rash will probably become less extensive, and by adolescence most children no longer have atopic eczema. However, up to 50 per cent of children who are affected by atopic eczema develop other allergic conditions, such as asthma.

Nappy rash

A baby's skin may become irritated if a wet or soiled nappy is worn for too long. Nappy rash affects most babies at some time, but illness and diarrhoea may increase a child's susceptibility. Some children seem to be more prone to nappy rash than others.

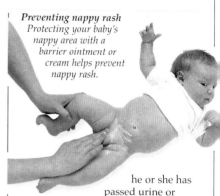

Preventing nappy rash
Protecting your baby's nappy area with a barrier ointment or cream helps prevent nappy rash.

What are the symptoms?
The main symptoms of nappy rash are:
• A sore nappy area.
• Red, raw spots in the nappy area.
An infection by bacteria (see IMPETIGO, p.139) or by the yeast *Candida albicans* (see ORAL THRUSH, p.176) may cause the area to become blistery and weepy.

What is the treatment?
Leave the nappy off and expose your baby's bottom to warm, dry air as much as you can. You should make an appointment to see a doctor if the rash does not improve after a few days. The doctor may prescribe a corticosteroid cream to reduce inflammation. If the rash is infected, a corticosteroid cream combined with an anti-infective drug may be prescribed. With treatment, an infected rash should take between a few days and a week to clear up.

How can nappy rash be prevented?
To help prevent a rash, change your baby's nappy as soon as possible after he or she has passed urine or defecated. After washing and drying the nappy area, protect your baby's skin by applying water-repellent zinc cream or petroleum jelly.

Contact dermatitis

Dermatitis (inflammation of the skin) resulting from contact with irritating substances does not often occur in children aged under about 12 years. Common irritants include nickel (found in jewellery), rubber, fabric dyes, plasters, plants, bubble baths, detergents, medicinal creams, and cosmetics.

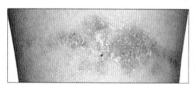

Contact dermatitis
This red, dry, scaly rash on a child's wrist was probably caused by a reaction to the nickel in a metal watchstrap or bracelet.

What are the symptoms?
The rash may be confined to one area, if due to jewellery for example; or it may be widespread, if due to products such as bubble bath or scented soaps. The main symptoms are:
• An inflamed, scaly rash.
• Intense itchiness.
• Sometimes, blistering and weeping (often caused by contact with plants).

The symptoms may take several days to appear after contact; the length of time they last depends on the irritant.

What is the treatment?
If you know what the cause of the dermatitis is, remove it or encourage your child to avoid contact with it. You may apply calamine lotion or a corticosteroid cream to the rash to help relieve the symptoms.

If you cannot identify the cause, consult a doctor, who may arrange for your child to have patch tests. These tests involve applying suspected irritants to small areas of your child's skin and watching for a reaction.

Lick eczema

A child with lick eczema has a rash around his or her mouth. The rash is caused by saliva irritating the lips and surrounding skin as a result of excessive lip-licking or thumb-sucking. Lick eczema clears up when the habit that causes it disappears.

What are the symptoms?
The main symptoms of lick eczema are:
• Inflamed, scaly skin around the lips.
• Dry, chapped lips, which are sore.

What can I do to help?
Apply a corticosteroid cream (available over the counter) to the skin around the lips for a few days to reduce the inflammation, then use petroleum jelly often to protect the skin from saliva. Applying lip salve to the lips will help to moisturize and protect them.

Children usually grow out of lip-licking or thumb-sucking before they reach school age. The habit may be given up more quickly if you gently draw your child's attention to it whenever it occurs. However, nagging your child about the habit may make it worse.

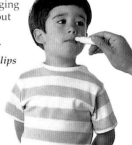

Protecting dry lips
Lip salve helps to protect your child's lips from irritating saliva and also relieves discomfort.

PSORIASIS

In this chronic skin condition, red, scaly, thickened patches develop on the limbs, trunk, or scalp. Children over the age of 10 years are most likely to be affected. The rash does not usually itch, but psoriasis can be uncomfortable and your child may be distressed by its appearance. Psoriasis tends to fluctuate in severity; it often becomes worse during periods of illness or emotional stress, such as impending school examinations.

How is it caused?
The cause of psoriasis is unknown, but it tends to run in families and may be inherited. The psoriasis rash sometimes first appears after an acute infection such as tonsillitis (see PHARYNGITIS AND TONSILLITIS, p.150) or an infection of the middle ear (see OTITIS MEDIA, p.162).

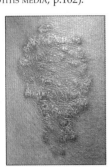

Psoriasis rash
This rash is characteristic of psoriasis. The affected area is a sharply defined, raised red patch covered by silvery white scales of dead skin. A large patch such as this may appear on the elbows or knees.

A psoriasis rash forms when new skin cells are produced at a faster rate than old skin cells are shed. The excess new cells build up to produce the thickened areas, which may be covered with dead, flaking skin.

What are the symptoms?
The psoriasis rash tends to vary in appearance. However, the most common symptoms are:
- Patches of thickened red skin that are covered with silvery scales. The patches are most often located on the elbows, knees, or scalp.
- Numerous small, red, slightly scaly patches, which tend to be scattered over the trunk and face.
- Pitted and thickened nails.
- Pain or discomfort if cracks appear in the affected skin.

What can I do to help?
If your child's psoriasis is mild, you may be able to prevent flare-ups by keeping the skin well moisturized with an emollient cream. Exposing affected areas to the sun sometimes helps clear up the rash, but take care not to let your child get sunburned.

Should I consult a doctor?
Your child should be seen by a doctor if the rash is severe, widespread, or distressing. The doctor will probably refer your child to a dermatologist. For psoriasis limited to a few small areas, such as the scalp, knees, or elbows, the dermatologist may prescribe a cream or ointment containing coal tar, salicylic acid, or a corticosteroid. If the psoriasis is widespread, an ointment containing dithranol may be prescribed. Other treatments, such as bathing in water containing a coal tar preparation and moderate exposure to ultraviolet light, may also be recommended.

What is the outlook?
Psoriasis cannot be cured, and is likely to recur throughout life. However, individual attacks can be controlled if they are treated promptly.

BOIL

A boil is a painful, pus-filled swelling in the skin. It occurs when a hair follicle becomes infected by bacteria. The source of the infection is not usually known, although the bacteria are carried in some people's noses. Boils most commonly occur in damp areas, such as the armpit and groin, and at the back of the neck.

What are the symptoms?
A boil usually starts as a small red lump that becomes larger as it fills with pus. The main symptoms are:
- Pain and tenderness around the boil.
- A white or yellow "head" of pus at the centre of the boil.

Most boils burst, releasing their pus, although occasionally pus drains away into surrounding tissues. In most cases, healing occurs within 2 weeks.

What can I do to help?
If a boil is coming to a head, apply over-the-counter magnesium sulphate paste and cover the boil with a plaster. This treatment may make it burst more

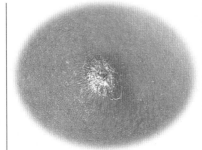

Appearance of a boil
The lump covered by white flakes of dead skin is a boil. Pus has escaped from the boil to form a greenish scab at its centre. The surrounding skin is red because the infection has spread.

quickly and hasten healing. When the boil bursts, carefully wipe away the pus with cotton wool soaked in antiseptic solution and cover the affected skin with an adhesive plaster. You should avoid poking or squeezing the boil to make it burst because you may cause the infection to spread.

Your child should be seen by a doctor if a boil lasts longer than 2 weeks or is very large or painful, or if your child suffers from recurrent boils.

What might the doctor do?
Oral antibiotics may be prescribed to clear up the infection. In some cases, the doctor may make a small cut in the boil in order to release pus. If boils keep recurring, the doctor may prescribe an antibiotic cream to apply inside your child's nose. He or she may suggest that your child washes with antiseptic soap and that an antiseptic solution is added to your child's bath water.

INSECT BITES AND STINGS

Most children experience only localized itchiness or pain when they are bitten or stung by an insect. However, some children, particularly those with allergies, may have a severe, possibly life-threatening, reaction called ANAPHYLACTIC SHOCK (p.154). The most common insect bites in children are those of mosquitoes. Insect stings are most likely to be from bees or wasps. The risk of being stung or bitten increases with warm weather.

INSECT BITES

The reaction to an insect bite causes:
• A small red pimple.
• Local itchiness.
• In some cases, a weal (a smooth, raised red area) or a firm swelling.
The symptoms of an insect bite may last from a few hours to several days.
   Insect bites in some children, most commonly those aged 2 to 7 years, result in groups of itchy, raised spots. The spots last for 2 to 10 days.

What can I do to help?

Apply cool compresses or calamine lotion to relieve itching. Discourage your child from scratching the affected area to prevent possible infection.
   When your child goes outside during times when insects are active, you can apply an insect repellent to exposed areas of his or her skin in order to help protect against insect bites.

INSECT STINGS

The reaction to an insect sting most commonly results in:
• Local irritation or pain.
• Redness and swelling.
The symptoms of an insect sting usually disappear within 48 hours.
   Some children are allergic to insect venom and develop URTICARIA (below) and/or anaphylactic shock, a severe generalized allergic reaction.

Should I consult a doctor?

You should call an ambulance or take your child to the nearest hospital accident and emergency department at once if he or she develops any of the following symptoms of anaphylactic shock: swelling of the face or mouth; noisy or difficult breathing; difficulty swallowing; or abnormal drowsiness. You should make an appointment to see your doctor if your child has had a

severe reaction to a sting. The doctor may give you a kit that contains a syringe filled with adrenaline to use for preventing anaphylactic shock if your child is stung by an insect again.

What can I do to help?

If a bee has left its sting in the skin, you should remove it (see illustration below). Applying a cool compress to the affected area may help relieve the pain and swelling. Oral antihistamines (available over the counter) may also help to relieve inflammation.

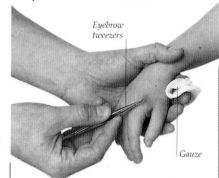
Eyebrow tweezers

Gauze

Removing a sting
Use eyebrow tweezers to remove an insect sting and its attached venom sac. Clean the area with gauze soaked in antiseptic.

URTICARIA

Also known as nettle rash or hives, urticaria is an intensely itchy, raised rash. In many cases, the cause of urticaria is not known. The most common known cause is an allergic reaction, possibly to a specific food (for instance, milk or citrus fruit), a drug (such as penicillin), an insect sting (above), or a plant.

What are the symptoms?

There are two forms of urticaria. Acute urticaria lasts between 30 minutes and several days; chronic urticaria may persist for up to several months. Both types may recur. The symptoms of chronic and acute urticaria are:
• Smooth, raised white or yellow lumps surrounded by an inflamed area of skin.
• Extreme itchiness.
The rash may affect a small area or it may be

widespread. Very rarely, urticaria is part of ANAPHYLACTIC SHOCK (p.154), a severe, generalized allergic reaction. The symptoms of anaphylactic shock include: swelling of the face or mouth; noisy or difficult breathing; difficulty

Urticarial rash
The patches of affected skin in urticaria vary in size and shape. The patches are raised, pale, and have red edges, which distinguish them from the surrounding normal skin.

swallowing; and abnormal drowsiness. Call an ambulance or take your child to the nearest hospital accident and emergency department at once if he or she has any of these symptoms.

What is the treatment?

If your child has recurrent attacks of urticaria, try to identify the cause so that your child can avoid it, if possible. During attacks, an over-the-counter oral antihistamine may relieve the symptoms. It should be continued for several weeks after the rash disappears.
   If severe urticaria is not helped by antihistamines, your child should be seen by a doctor. An oral corticosteroid may be prescribed and/or your child may be sent to a dermatologist for tests to establish the cause of the problem. As your child gets older, attacks of urticaria will probably diminish.

COLD SORES

Caused by a strain of the herpes simplex virus, cold sores are small blisters that develop on and around the lips. The initial infection by herpes simplex often goes unnoticed, but may cause GINGIVOSTOMATITIS (p.176). After this first infection, the virus lies dormant in nerve cells but may be reactivated later to cause cold sores. Cold sores may be triggered by an acute infection, anxiety or emotional stress, or exposure to the sun or cold winds.

What are the symptoms?
Cold sores may appear singly or in clusters. The main symptoms are:
• A tingling sensation around the mouth, which occurs 4 to 12 hours before any blisters appear.
• Small blisters, which may be itchy or sore, surrounded by a slightly inflamed area. The blisters burst within a few days to form a crust and heal on their own within 2 weeks.

What can I do to help?
For most children, cold sores are a minor inconvenience for which no treatment is necessary.

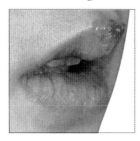

However, if the sores are causing any discomfort, a cold drink or an ice lolly may relieve the soreness. If the blisters recur frequently, are severe, or cause your child embarrassment, a cream containing the antiviral drug acyclovir

Cold sore cluster
Often appearing in clusters, cold sore blisters are clear at first; they become cloudy and then form crusts. Cold sores are smaller and more regular in shape than impetigo sores (below).

may be used. The cream, which can be bought over the counter, reduces the severity and duration of an attack. It is most effective if it is applied as soon as your child feels the initial tingling sensation around the mouth, before any blisters have appeared.

If you are able to identify a particular trigger factor for your child, you can take appropriate preventive action. For example, if cold sores tend to develop after exposure to the sun, you may be able to prevent them by applying a sunscreen or sunblock to your child's lips before he or she goes outside.

To reduce the chance of spreading the virus, both to other people and to other parts of your child's body, try to prevent your child from touching the blisters or sucking his or her fingers, and encourage frequent handwashing.

What is the outlook?
There is no cure for cold sores and your child will probably have recurrences throughout life. However, outbreaks usually become less frequent with time.

IMPETIGO

This common, highly contagious bacterial skin infection occurs mainly in young children, especially babies. Impetigo most often affects the mouth and nose area in children, and the nappy area in babies, although it may appear anywhere on the body. The bacteria that cause impetigo are able to enter and infect the skin when it is broken by a cut, an insect bite, or a skin condition such as ATOPIC ECZEMA (p.135) or SCABIES (p.143).

What are the symptoms?
The symptoms of impetigo change as the infection develops:
• Initially, the skin reddens and crops of small blisters appear.
• The blisters burst, leaving raw, moist sores that gradually enlarge.
• Straw-coloured crusts form as the surface of the sores dries.
Impetigo sores do not hurt, although they may be slightly itchy. Without treatment, the condition may last for weeks, or even months.

Should I consult a doctor?
Your child should be seen by a doctor within 24 hours if you think he or she has impetigo. The doctor may prescribe

an antibiotic ointment, which should be applied to the sores several times a day. If the infection is widespread, an oral antibiotic may also be prescribed.

What can I do to help?
Before you apply the ointment, you should remove the crusts by gently dabbing them with gauze soaked in salt solution and then dry the area. To prevent the infection from spreading, your child should not touch the sores. Keep your child's bedding, washcloth, and towels separate. Your child should stay away from other children until the infection has cleared up completely. With treatment, impetigo usually gets better within about 5 days.

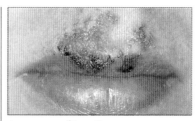

Appearance of impetigo
Impetigo starts as small blisters. Here, the blisters have burst to form large, irregular sores covered in straw-coloured crusts.

How can I prevent impetigo?
Your child should shower or bathe daily. Keeping your baby's nappy area clean and protected from moisture helps to prevent NAPPY RASH (p.136), thus reducing the chance of infection. Making sure that your child's nails are kept short and clean makes infection less likely to be introduced through scratching. When your child has a cold or a runny nose, applying a little petroleum jelly to the nose and upper lip should help to protect the skin from being broken by constant wiping.

ACNE

The most common skin disorder in adolescents, acne consists of inflamed spots on the face and other parts of the body. Acne tends to appear at the onset of puberty, usually between the ages of 12 and 14 years. It may be at its worst in the late teens, after which it begins to subside. The condition often runs in families and is usually more common and severe in boys than in girls. Although acne cannot be prevented, it can be controlled.

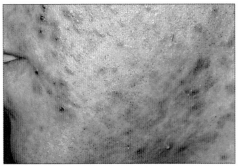

Acne affecting the face
The spots on this boy's face are typical of acne. The slightly indented purplish marks are the result of spots that have healed.

How is it caused?
At puberty, there is an increase in the production of sebum (an oily substance produced by sebaceous glands in hair follicles), which is probably triggered by increased levels of sex hormones. Acne spots occur when excess sebum and, sometimes, dead skin cells form a plug that blocks a hair follicle; trapped bacteria multiply, causing the skin surrounding the follicle to become inflamed.

Oily substances on the skin, such as cosmetics or hair oil, may make the problem worse. However, diet has no effect.

What are the symptoms?
Acne principally affects the face (see illustration left), neck, shoulders, chest, upper arms, and back. The main symptoms are:
- Pimples (small, raised red spots).
- Blackheads (tiny black spots).
- Whiteheads (tender, inflamed lumps with a white centre).
- Cysts (fluid-filled swellings).
- Purplish marks left by healed spots, which gradually fade.

If it is very severe, acne may leave scars and pits in the skin. The condition may also make your child feel considerably embarrassed by his or her appearance, because it coincides with the increased self-consciousness of adolescence.

What is the treatment?
Your child should wash his or her face twice daily with ordinary soap and water. An over-the-counter acne cream or lotion may then be applied to the affected areas. These preparations promote skin peeling, which helps to unblock the pores, and also control bacteria. They are available in different strengths; your child should try the mildest first. Exposure to sunlight may help to clear up acne spots. Your child should avoid picking, squeezing, or scrubbing the spots, all of which may cause the bacteria to spread.

If the acne has not improved after your child has been using an acne preparation for 2 to 3 months, consult a doctor. Treatment with several courses of oral antibiotics may be suggested. Each course the doctor prescribes will last for between 3 and 6 months.

If antibiotics do not help, the doctor may prescribe a retinoid drug, which reduces sebum production. Retinoid drugs are usually effective but may cause side effects, such as dryness of the lips, eyes, and nose.

What is the outlook?
Acne cannot be cured. However, its severity can be reduced and scarring prevented with treatment. Because of the availability of effective remedies, few children should have severe acne. The condition gradually improves and often disappears in the early twenties.

PITYRIASIS ROSEA

A rash of flat, scaly spots, pityriasis rosea most frequently affects the trunk, arms, and legs. It is believed to be caused by a viral infection, although no specific virus has been isolated. Pityriasis rosea most frequently affects adolescents.

What are the symptoms?
The main symptoms are:
- An initial spot, called the herald patch, which is oval or round, flat, scaly, and 1–2 cm (⅜–¾ in) in diameter.
- Flat, oval, copper-coloured or dark-pink spots, which appear 3 to 10 days after the herald patch. After a week, each spot develops a scaly margin.
- Occasionally, itchiness.

The rash appears initially on the trunk, running along the lines of the ribs. It may then spread up towards the neck and down along the arms and legs, fading below the elbows and knees. The rash seldom appears on the face.

Should I consult a doctor?
Although pityriasis rosea is not serious and gets better without treatment, your child should be seen by a doctor within a few days. The doctor will examine your child to make sure he or she does not have a more serious skin disease.

What is the treatment?
The doctor treats the symptoms rather than the condition itself. He or she may prescribe a mild corticosteroid cream to alleviate the itchiness. If the itchiness is severe, the doctor may prescribe an oral antihistamine. Keeping the skin cool, for example by avoiding exertion in hot weather, and moisturizing the affected areas may also relieve the symptoms. Exposure to sunlight may help the rash to clear up more rapidly.

What is the outlook?
Pityriasis rosea generally takes between 3 and 8 weeks to clear up. Once your child has had the condition, he or she is very unlikely to have it again.

WARTS

Caused by a virus, warts are harmless growths on the surface of the skin. They most commonly appear on the hands and feet. Warts are contagious, but some people are more susceptible to them than others. Most warts disappear naturally within a few months, but some last for years if they are not treated.

What are the symptoms?
There are several different types of wart, any of which may occur singly or in clusters. The ones that most often affect children are:
• Common warts. These are firm, raised growths, usually with a hard, rough surface. They generally occur on the hands, feet, knees, and face.
• Plane warts. These smooth growths are level with the skin or slightly raised. They occur on the hands or face and may cause slight itchiness.
• Plantar warts (verrucas). These hard, horny warts occur on the sole of the foot. They appear flat and are often painful because the child's weight has pushed them into the skin.

What can I do to help?
Warts often disappear if left untreated. However, if your child would like to have a wart removed, home treatment is safe for warts on the hands and feet. Never attempt to remove a wart on your child's mouth or face.

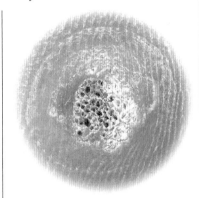

Plantar wart
This wart on the sole of the foot has a hard, rough, calloused surface and is dotted with tiny blood clots (black spots).

The simplest technique for treating common and plane warts is to cover the wart with a plaster, which should be changed daily. If the wart does not respond to this treatment in about 3 weeks, you could try using wart paint (available over the counter). The directions must be followed carefully. To protect normal skin surrounding the wart, cover it with a little petroleum jelly before you apply the paint.

If your child has a plantar wart, rub the wart's surface with a pumice stone to remove as much of the overlying skin as possible. Cut a piece of salicylic acid plaster to the exact size of the wart and tape it in place. Replace the plaster every day until the wart disappears, which may take up to 3 months.

Tell your child not to touch the warts because picking or scratching them may cause them to spread.

Should I consult a doctor?
Consult a doctor if home treatment has not been successful or if a wart on the face or mouth is causing your child discomfort or embarrassment.

The doctor may send your child to a dermatologist. Most warts are removed by freezing (cryotherapy). A plantar wart may be scraped off (curettage).

What is the outlook?
Most warts eventually disappear, even without treatment. However, warts sometimes recur, even if treated, and may require several treatments before they finally disappear for good.

MOLLUSCUM CONTAGIOSUM

This mild viral infection causes small, shiny pimples to appear on the skin. Molluscum contagiosum is common in children between 2 and 5 years of age. It is easily spread, either by direct contact or indirectly, for example in a public swimming pool or by touching infected clothing or towels.

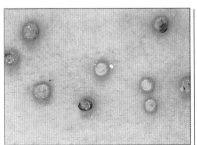

Molluscum contagiosum pimples
The pimples, which are between 2 and 5 mm (⅛ and ¼ in) in diameter, usually appear in groups although they sometimes occur singly.

What are the symptoms?
The pimples appear 2 to 7 weeks after infection. They occur mainly on the trunk, face, hands, and (rarely) on the palms or soles. The pimples are:
• Dome shaped with a central dimple.
• Pearly white or flesh coloured.

Should I consult a doctor?
Your child should be seen by a doctor within 24 hours if you think he or she might have molluscum contagiosum. If it is untreated, the condition will probably disappear within a few weeks to a few months. However, molluscum contagiosum should be treated by a doctor. If it is left alone, the condition may spread to other parts of the body and may become unsightly. It can also spread to other children, with the result that your child could be excluded from his or her school or playgroup for the duration of the condition.

What might the doctor do?
If molluscum contagiosum affects only a small area of the body, the doctor may decide to treat the condition by piercing the pimples with an instrument dipped in podophyllin paint. This treatment releases the white cheesy substance in the pimples and destroys them. If there are many pimples, the doctor may send your child to a dermatologist. The dermatologist will remove the pimples by scraping them off (curettage) or by freezing them (cryotherapy).

FUNGAL INFECTIONS

The skin, hair, and nails may all be affected by fungal infections. Of these infections, the most familiar are ringworm and athlete's foot. Ringworm appears in schoolchildren and may affect the scalp or the skin of the body or face. Adolescents are susceptible to athlete's foot, which usually affects the skin between the toes.

RINGWORM

Children can catch ringworm directly from another person, from an animal, or from soil; or indirectly from hats, combs, clothing, or household items, such as carpets or chairs.

What are the symptoms?
Ringworm of the body or face causes:
• Oval or circular, flaky patches with raised, mildly inflamed borders.
• Itchiness.
Ringworm affecting the scalp causes:
• Flakes resembling severe dandruff.
• Hair loss, with hair tending to break just above the scalp.
• Occasionally, the development of an inflamed, pus-filled area (a kerion).
• Usually, itchiness.
Your child should be seen by a doctor if you think he or she has ringworm.

What is the treatment?
For body or face infections, the doctor may recommend an antifungal lotion or cream. If your child's body or face infection is widespread, or if the scalp is affected, the doctor may prescribe antifungal medicine. Oral antibiotics may be prescribed to treat a kerion.

To help prevent ringworm, keep your child away from any person or animal known to be infected, and encourage him or her not to share personal items, such as combs, with school friends.

ATHLETE'S FOOT

This condition is particularly common during the summer months, especially among adolescents who wear trainers. Athlete's foot is commonly caught from the floors of changing rooms and showers at communal places, such as swimming pools and gymnasiums.

What are the symptoms?
The main symptoms are:
• Cracked, sore skin between the toes, often the fourth and fifth toes.
• Usually, itchiness.
• Occasionally, thick, discoloured, and easily broken toenails.

What is the treatment?
Various powders, creams, and sprays are available over the counter for treating athlete's foot (see illustration right). With treatment, the condition usually begins to clear up in about 1 to 2 weeks. If athlete's foot persists

for longer than 2 weeks, or the toenails are infected, make an appointment for your child to be seen by a doctor. The doctor may prescribe antifungal tablets.

Athlete's foot is less likely to occur if your child thoroughly dries his or her feet after washing and puts on clean cotton socks every day. Wearing open-toed sandals and going barefoot when practical may also help.

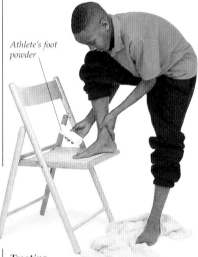

Athlete's foot powder

Treating athlete's foot
Your child should wash and dry his or her feet thoroughly and sprinkle athlete's foot powder (or apply a cream or spray) between the toes twice a day. Socks and shoes should be dusted with athlete's foot powder.

PITYRIASIS VERSICOLOR

This common skin condition results in discoloured patches of skin. It is caused by overgrowth of a yeast normally present on the skin, possibly triggered by exposure to sunlight or a hot, humid environment. The condition usually occurs after puberty.

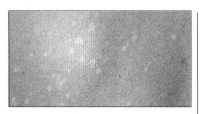

Appearance of pityriasis versicolor
Areas of dark or tanned skin that are affected by pityriasis versicolor appear as round, flat, pale patches with clearly defined borders.

What are the symptoms?
Discoloured patches of skin are the main symptom. The patches typically have the following characteristics:
• On pale skin, they are usually darker than surrounding skin; on dark skin, they are usually lighter.
• Slight flakiness.
• Well-defined borders.
• Sometimes, mild itchiness.
Your child should be seen by a doctor if he or she has symptoms of pityriasis

versicolor. Although it is not harmful or contagious, the condition may persist indefinitely if it is not treated.

What is the treatment?
The doctor will prescribe an antifungal cream or lotion. You should apply the preparation once a day to the affected areas. This treatment reduces the yeast to its normal levels in about a week. However, the antifungal preparation should be used for 3 weeks in order to reduce the chance of the condition recurring. Exposing the affected areas to the air as much as possible also helps to discourage regrowth. The skin may take weeks or months to regain its normal appearance.

SCABIES

This extremely itchy, contagious condition is due to infestation of the skin by parasitic mites. The female mites burrow into the skin to lay their eggs, causing intense itching. Scabies is passed from person to person by close bodily contact. Anyone can catch scabies; it has nothing to do with lack of personal hygiene.

What are the symptoms?
Following infestation, the symptoms of scabies may take up to 6 weeks to appear. They may include:
• Intense itchiness, especially at night.
• Thin grey lines (the mites' burrows) between the fingers, on the wrists, in the armpits, between the buttocks, or around the genitals. In infants, the palms and soles may be affected.
• Sores, blisters, and scabs, resulting from scratching.
• Inflamed lumps on the body.

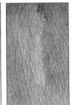

Scabies mite burrow
Thin, grey lines on the skin are the burrows made by female mites. Burrows may be obscured by sores and scabs caused by scratching.

Your child should be seen by a doctor within 24 hours if he or she is scratching intensely or has any other signs of scabies. Scabies will not clear up without treatment and scratching may result in IMPETIGO (p.139).

What is the treatment?
The doctor will prescribe a lotion that kills scabies mites. It should be applied to all areas of your child's body except for the head and neck, and should be washed off after 24 hours. You need to treat all members of your household at the same time, even if they to do not have any obvious signs of scabies. After treatment, you should wash and iron all clothing and bed linen.

The mites usually die within 3 days of treatment. However, itchiness may persist for up to 2 weeks afterwards. The doctor may prescribe an ointment to relieve the itchiness.

People with whom you and your child have had contact should be told about the scabies, so that they can be examined, and treated if necessary.

HEAD LICE

Head lice are very small, flat, wingless insects that live on the scalp and suck blood. Schoolchildren can catch these insects easily through direct contact or by sharing hats or combs. If your child has head lice, you need not worry that he or she is not washing properly: the insects actually prefer clean hair and skin.

What are the symptoms?
The main symptoms of head lice are:
• Intense itchiness of the scalp.
• Tiny red spots (bites) on the scalp.
Adult head lice are very small, almost transparent, and therefore hard to see. The eggs (nits) are more easily seen, particularly after the insects have hatched. The empty nit shells can be seen as small white bumps near the bases of the hairs.

What can I do to help?
If you suspect that your child has lice, examine his or her hair for nits. You can also see if lice are present by wetting your child's hair and combing it with a fine-tooth comb over a white piece of paper. Any lice will be visible as they crawl on the paper.

If your child is infested, check all other members of the family for head lice and tell your child's school so that other parents can be alerted.

Head lice and eggs
The tiny, white ovals are louse eggs. They are firmly attached to the hair shafts. Several head lice are also visible clinging to hairs.

Should I consult a doctor?
You can treat head lice at home without consulting a doctor first. However, if your child is less than 2 years old or has allergies or asthma, you should talk to a doctor before starting treatment.

What is the treatment?
Special lotions and shampoos are available over the counter for the treatment of head lice. Some preparations can be applied just once; others must be applied repeatedly over a number of days. All family members and contacts should be treated at the same time (even if they have no symptoms) to eradicate the head lice completely and to prevent the possibility of your child becoming reinfested. You should wash all combs and brushes in boiling water in order to kill any lice or eggs that might be attached to them.

As long as all close contacts are treated simultaneously, one course of treatment is usually all that is necessary to rid your child of head lice.

How can head lice be avoided?
To reduce your child's chances of catching lice, you should discourage him or her from sharing hats, combs, and brushes with family members or with school friends. If you know that there is an outbreak of lice at your child's school, you can use a head lice repellent to prevent your child from becoming infested. Head lice repellent is available over the counter.

Eradicating head lice
Head lice can be eradicated by washing the hair with a special shampoo or lotion. Follow the directions on the package, and comb your child's hair carefully afterwards with a fine-tooth comb to remove the dead lice and nits.

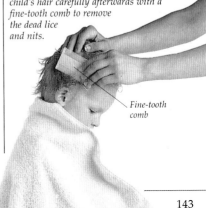

Fine-tooth comb

BLOOD AND CIRCULATORY DISORDERS

CONGENITAL HEART DEFECTS are the most common serious birth defects, but, in most cases, their causes remain unknown. Fortunately, many are now curable. High cure rates are also now usual for most serious blood disorders, even those such as leukaemia that formerly were fatal. However, the early recognition of the symptoms of these blood disorders is still important to maximize the chance of a cure.

CONGENITAL HEART DISEASE

A child with congenital heart disease is born with one or more malformations of the heart. The risk of a woman having a child with a heart defect is increased if she has RUBELLA (p.119) in early pregnancy, has poorly controlled diabetes, takes certain drugs during pregnancy, or has had another child with a heart defect. About 1 child in 140 is born with a heart defect. Some get better without treatment, but others need surgery.

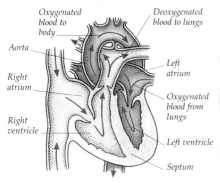

Oxygenated blood to body
Aorta
Right atrium
Right ventricle
Deoxygenated blood to lungs
Left atrium
Oxygenated blood from lungs
Left ventricle
Septum

NORMAL

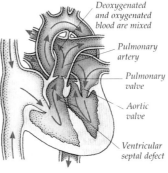

Deoxygenated and oxygenated blood are mixed
Pulmonary artery
Pulmonary valve
Aortic valve
Ventricular septal defect

ABNORMAL

What are the types of heart defect?
The most common type of congenital heart abnormality is a ventricular septal defect (see illustrations above). Another relatively common defect is patent ductus arteriosus, in which the ductus arteriosus (a blood vessel that acts as a bypass in a baby's circulation before birth) fails to close after birth.

Other common heart abnormalities are atrial septal defect, a hole between the atria (upper heart chambers); aortic stenosis, narrowing of the aortic valve; and pulmonary stenosis, in which the pulmonary valve is narrowed.

Ventricular septal defect
A hole in the septum allows blood to flow from left to right ventricle. Oxygenated blood that should flow into the aorta and out to body tissues instead returns to the lungs.

Other rarer defects, which may be more serious, include: transposition of the great arteries, in which the position of the aorta and pulmonary artery are reversed; coarctation of the aorta, which is narrowing of the aorta; and tetralogy of Fallot, a combination of four defects including a ventricular septal defect, pulmonary stenosis, a displaced aorta, and a thickened right ventricle.

What are the symptoms?
Symptoms of congenital heart disease depend on the nature and severity of the defect or defects that a child has. In some cases, symptoms are detected when a doctor carries out his or her routine examination of the newborn baby. In other cases, symptoms of heart disease are not apparent until later in childhood or even until adult life.

Among the various possible features of congenital heart disease are:
- A heart murmur (abnormal heart sounds). A doctor will be able to hear the heart murmur when he or she listens to the child's heart through a stethoscope. Most murmurs do not indicate congenital heart disease, but in some cases the murmur is due to a narrowed pulmonary or aortic valve or some other form of heart defect.
- Feeding problems and loss of weight. In some babies with congenital heart disease, heart failure (inability of the heart to pump efficiently) causes slow feeding and inability to finish feeds. An affected baby may breathe rapidly and sweat, especially after feeding.
- Bluish discoloration of the tongue and lips (cyanosis). Several heart defects prevent effective circulation of the blood through the lungs. This means that the blood supplied to the body by the heart carries less oxygen than it should, which causes some tissues to appear blue.
- Breathlessness on exertion.
Children with congenital heart disease grow at a slower rate than children who have healthy hearts.

What are the complications?

Children with congenital heart disease, even if it is mild, may be susceptible to bacterial endocarditis. In this condition, the heart valves become inflamed due to infection by bacteria that have entered the bloodstream, usually during dental treatment or a surgical operation.

Should I consult a doctor?

Your child should be seen by a doctor if you suspect that he or she might have a congenital heart abnormality.

If you are aware that your child has congenital heart disease, consult a doctor without delay if he or she has a fever, lacks energy, and has a poor appetite; these symptoms indicate that your child might have bacterial endocarditis.

What might the doctor do?

The doctor will examine your child. If he or she suspects that your child might have congenital heart disease, your child will be referred to a paediatrician or paediatric cardiologist. The specialist will arrange for a chest X-ray, an electrocardiogram (a recording of heart rate and rhythm), and also an ultrasound heart scan to be carried out in hospital. These investigations will reveal the nature and the severity of any congenital heart abnormality.

In many cases of congenital heart disease, the defects get better on their own without the need for surgery.

In some cases, however, emergency surgery needs to be performed to save a child's life. In other cases, surgery to correct a defect can be delayed until later in childhood. Sometimes, more than one operation may be necessary.

Your child will be monitored by a paediatrician or cardiologist and will also have periodic hospital assessments Your family doctor can provide you with any immediate advice you require. In order to minimize the risk of your child contracting bacterial endocarditis, preventive antibiotics will be prescribed whenever dental treatment is required or if your child needs surgery.

Listening to a child's heart
The doctor will use a stethoscope to listen to your child's heart. Abnormal sounds may indicate the presence of a defect.

What can I do to help?

Unless the doctor tells you otherwise, you should encourage your child to lead a completely normal life, with a normal amount of exercise. In a very few cases, particularly if your child has a heart abnormality that causes bluish discoloration of the tongue and lips, the doctor may tell you to restrict the amount of exercise taken by your child.

You should always make sure that your child takes the full course of any antibiotics that have been prescribed to prevent bacterial endocarditis. You should also make sure that your child always carries a card (obtained from the doctor) stating that he or she has congenital heart disease.

What is the outlook?

The outlook depends on the type of heart defect and on its severity. In most cases, ventricular septal defects close on their own before the child is 5 years old. Those that do not close and many other heart abnormalities, such as atrial septal defect, patent ductus arteriosus, or narrowing of a pulmonary or aortic valve, are treatable by surgery. As a result of surgical advances over the last 20 years, children with heart disease, even those with very severe defects, usually grow up to lead normal lives.

ANAEMIA

The term anaemia refers to a deficient amount of haemoglobin in the blood. Haemoglobin is the pigment in red blood cells that carries oxygen from the lungs to body tissues. If haemoglobin is deficient, the tissues receive an insufficient oxygen supply.

How is it caused?

Red blood cells are manufactured in the bone marrow, then released into the bloodstream. They normally circulate for about 120 days before they become defective and are destroyed. Anaemia can result from inadequate production or excessive destruction of red cells.

Inadequate red cell production usually results from deficiency of a substance that is essential for healthy red blood cell formation. The most common type is IRON-DEFICIENCY ANAEMIA (p.146).

Excessive destruction of red blood cells is often due to a genetic fault. The fault causes the production of abnormal red cells that are destroyed at a high rate. Examples are SICKLE-CELL ANAEMIA (p.199) and THALASSAEMIA (p.200).

What are the symptoms?

A child may have no symptoms if the anaemia is mild. In more severe cases, the following symptoms are typical:
• Pale skin.
• Lack of energy.
• Breathlessness on exertion.
Other symptoms may occur, depending on which type of anaemia the child has.

Should I consult a doctor?

Your child should be seen by a doctor if you think that he or she might have anaemia. The doctor will ask about your family history and your child's general health and diet. If the doctor suspects that your child has anaemia, he or she will arrange for blood tests to confirm the presence of the condition and its severity. Your child's blood will be analysed to determine the number, shape, size, and colour of the blood cells. The analysis reveals which type of anaemia is present. Subsequent tests, such as iron measurements, might be required to make a precise diagnosis. The treatment will depend on the cause of your child's anaemia. If the anaemia is due to a genetic fault, your child will require lifelong treatment.

NORMAL RED
BLOOD CELL

THALASSAEMIA

IRON-DEFICIENCY
ANAEMIA

SICKLE-CELL
ANAEMIA

Red blood cells
In many types of anaemia, red blood cells are small and pale. In sickle-cell anaemia, however, the shape of the red blood cells is distorted.

IRON-DEFICIENCY ANAEMIA

This type of ANAEMIA (p.145) is the result of a deficiency of iron, which is one of the essential components of haemoglobin, the oxygen-carrying pigment in red blood cells. Iron-deficiency anaemia is the most common form of anaemia affecting children.

What are the symptoms?
Mild iron-deficiency anaemia may not produce any symptoms. In more severe cases, symptoms may include:
• Pale skin.
• Lack of energy.
• Breathlessness on exertion.
• Brittle fingernails.
• Sore mouth or tongue.
Long-term iron-deficiency anaemia in children may cause impaired mental development and function.

Should I consult a doctor?
Consult a doctor if you think that your child might be anaemic. The doctor can arrange for blood tests to find out whether your child has anaemia, and to assess its severity. The type of anaemia may be identified by examination of red blood cells: in iron-deficiency anaemia, they are smaller and paler than normal.

What is the treatment?
The doctor will probably ask about your child's diet, and may give you advice on foods to offer your child.

Your child may be prescribed iron in medicine form, typically for about 3 months, in order to build up your child's iron stores.

If your child is under the age of 6 months and was born prematurely, he or she will probably already have been prescribed supplements of iron. If not, the doctor may prescribe them at this time. Typically, premature babies are not born with sufficient iron stores to compensate for the low iron content of a milk-only diet during the first 6 months of life, before they start on solids.

What can I do to help?
Try to ensure that your child receives adequate iron in his or her diet (by giving plenty of green vegetables and meat, for example). If your baby is not eating solids by the age of 6 months, he or she should be given milk formula that is enriched with iron. Otherwise, your baby will be at risk of developing iron-deficiency anaemia, particularly between the ages of 12 and 18 months. If your child refuses to eat iron-rich foods, talk to the doctor about whether he or she should be taking iron supplements.

What is the outlook?
Children are less likely to develop iron-deficiency anaemia as they grow and eat a varied diet.

An iron-rich diet
Give your child foods that are rich in iron, including meat and green vegetables. A child who does not eat meat should eat plenty of green vegetables.

LEUKAEMIA

In leukaemia, a form of cancer, the bone marrow produces many abnormal (leukaemic) white blood cells, and a reduced number of normal white cells, red cells, and platelets. The leukaemic cells infiltrate the liver, spleen, and lymph glands. The main form of leukaemia in childhood is acute lymphoblastic leukaemia.

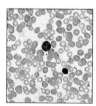 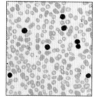

NORMAL   LEUKAEMIA

Acute lymphoblastic leukaemia
Seen under a microscope, blood taken from a person with leukaemia shows a large number of abnormal white blood cells (dark purple).

What are the symptoms?
Acute lymphoblastic leukaemia may produce the following symptoms:
• Pale skin.
• Pink or purple flat spots on the skin.
• Easily bruised skin.
• Lack of energy.
• Swollen lymph nodes in the neck, armpits, and groin.
• Fever.
• Pain in limb bones and joints.
• Bleeding gums.
Consult a doctor at once if you suspect that your child might have leukaemia.

What might the doctor do?
The doctor will examine your child and may arrange for blood tests. If the tests cannot exclude leukaemia, your child will be admitted to hospital for a bone marrow biopsy. This procedure, which involves removing cells from the bone marrow for analysis, can show whether your child has leukaemia.

Treatment for acute lymphoblastic leukaemia is divided into two phases.

During the first phase, which generally lasts for several weeks, drugs are given to destroy the leukaemic cells. This phase continues until a bone marrow biopsy indicates that no abnormal cells are present. At this point, your child is described as being in remission.

The second phase of treatment lasts for a further 2 years. During this time, your child will undergo periods of intensive drug treatment that are aimed at destroying any leukaemic cells that might still be present in the body.

What can I do to help?
Your child should lead as normal a life as possible. Because drug treatment increases susceptibility to infection, he or she should, however, be kept away from anyone who has a viral infection, such as chickenpox or measles.

What is the outlook?
Treatments currently available lead to full recovery in about 60 to 70 per cent of children diagnosed as having acute lymphoblastic leukaemia.

HENOCH-SCHÖNLEIN PURPURA

In Henoch-Schönlein purpura, small blood vessels become fragile and allow blood to leak from them. Bleeding into the skin results in an easily identifiable rash, while leakage of blood into joints, the kidneys, or the digestive tract causes various other symptoms. The disease is fairly common in children between the ages of 2 and 10 years, and is not usually serious. The cause is unknown, but may involve an allergic reaction or bacterial infection.

What are the symptoms?
Henoch-Schönlein purpura may cause the following symptoms:
- Rash (present in all cases), made up of pink, red, or purplish, blood-filled spots that do not fade when pressed. The rash appears first on the buttocks and the backs of the arms and legs, especially around the ankles and elbows, then spreads to the fronts of the limbs (see illustration right).
- Joint pain and swelling.
- Abdominal pain, in many cases with vomiting and diarrhoea.
- Blood in the faeces.

Inflammation of the kidneys (see GLOMERULONEPHRITIS, p.194) is a possible complication. It does not usually cause symptoms.

Should I consult a doctor?
You should consult a doctor within 24 hours of the onset of symptoms that might indicate your child has Henoch-Schönlein purpura.

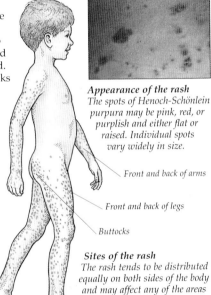

Appearance of the rash
The spots of Henoch-Schönlein purpura may be pink, red, or purplish and either flat or raised. Individual spots vary widely in size.

— Front and back of arms

— Front and back of legs

— Buttocks

Sites of the rash
The rash tends to be distributed equally on both sides of the body and may affect any of the areas that are indicated here.

What might the doctor do?
The doctor will examine your child. If a diagnosis cannot definitely be made from your child's symptoms, he or she will arrange for blood tests to rule out other possibilities. A sample of your child's urine will be sent for laboratory examination. The presence of red blood cells and protein in the urine indicates that the kidneys are inflamed.

If symptoms are mild, no treatment is required. Corticosteroids may be given for severe abdominal pain and may bring about rapid improvement. If the kidneys are affected, the doctor may carry out repeat urine and blood tests to ensure the condition is improving.

What can I do to help?
If your child's symptoms are causing pain or discomfort, you may give him or her paracetamol. Your child may stay in bed if he or she wants to.

What is the outlook?
Henoch-Schönlein purpura may last from only a few days to up to a month, during which time the symptoms may come and go. Most children who have the illness make a complete recovery, and there are no long-term ill effects. In most cases, any inflammation of the kidneys disappears in a few days, but in some children the kidneys remain inflamed for up to 2 years.

THROMBOCYTOPENIA

In this condition, there is an abnormally low number of platelets in the blood. In children, thrombocytopenia most frequently occurs as part of a disorder called idiopathic thrombocytopenic purpura (ITP). The cause of this disorder is unknown, but it usually develops within 2 weeks following a viral infection.

What are the symptoms?
The symptoms of ITP are caused by abnormal bleeding due to the reduced number of platelets (which are essential for blood clotting). They may include:
- A widespread, flat purple rash caused by bleeding into the skin; the rash does not fade when pressed.
- Bruising from only minor pressure.
- Nosebleeds.
- Bleeding in the mouth.
- Blood in the urine as a result of bleeding in the kidneys.

Brain haemorrhage (bleeding around or within the brain) is a rare possible complication of the condition.

Should I consult a doctor?
You should consult a doctor at once if your child has symptoms that might be caused by ITP. If the doctor has any doubts about the diagnosis, admission to hospital may be arranged so that tests can be performed to confirm that your child has ITP and not another illness that produces similar symptoms.

What is the treatment?
Most children do not require treatment. However, strenuous activities should be avoided until symptoms clear up, which is usually within a few weeks.

If your child has bleeding from the nose or mouth or a very low blood platelet count, he or she will be treated in hospital. Your child may be given a short course of corticosteroid drugs or, in some cases, intravenous gamma-globulin in order to speed recovery and reduce the risk of severe bleeding.

What is the outlook?
Most children are free from symptoms within about 2 weeks. However, in a few children, blood platelet levels may take up to 6 months, or occasionally longer, to return completely to normal.

RESPIRATORY SYSTEM DISORDERS

INFECTION BY BACTERIA or viruses is the most common cause of respiratory tract disorders in children. Young children are particularly prone to infection because they have not had time to build up immunity. Allergic disorders, such as asthma and allergic rhinitis (hay fever), are the other main respiratory problems affecting children. Asthma is becoming increasingly common.

COMMON COLD

A viral infection of the nose and throat, the common cold is a minor contagious illness that occurs frequently in children. Most children have at least six colds a year, with the frequency usually increasing when they start playgroup or nursery. Some children, who are otherwise healthy, have up to 10 colds a year.

What are the symptoms?
Symptoms typically begin 1 to 3 days after infection, usually starting with a tickly or scratchy feeling in the throat. Symptoms that follow may include:
- A runny nose.
- Sneezing.

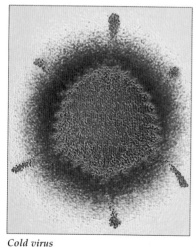

Cold virus
The adenovirus shown in this micrograph is one of more than 200 strains of virus that are known to cause the common cold.

- A blocked nose, which may make feeding difficult for a baby.
- A cough and sore throat.
- Watering eyes.
- Muscular aches.
- Sometimes, a fever.

What are the complications?
Cold viruses may spread to the lungs, causing BRONCHIOLITIS (p.155), BRONCHITIS (p.154), or PNEUMONIA (p.156), which may be complicated by secondary bacterial infection. Bacterial infection may also affect the ears, causing OTITIS MEDIA (p.162) or the sinuses, causing SINUSITIS (opposite). In children who suffer from ASTHMA (p.153), a cold may trigger an asthmatic attack.

How is it caused?
Many different viruses can cause the common cold. Immunity gained as a result of infection with one strain does not provide protection against another, so that infections can occur repeatedly. Children attending nursery or school are particularly susceptible to colds because they are exposed to a wide variety of viruses to which they have not yet become immune.

Cold viruses are spread in droplets that are sneezed or coughed out and inhaled by others. The viruses may also be spread through direct contact with an infected person or object.

What can I do to help?
Most colds clear up within a week. Meanwhile, the following measures should help relieve the symptoms.

Keep your child's room warm (but not too hot) and increase the moisture in the atmosphere (see illustration: *Humidifying the air*, p.150).

Make sure that your child drinks plenty of fluids. A baby with a cold should be given feeds in small amounts at more frequent intervals than usual. You may give paracetamol liquid to relieve a sore throat and any aches.

Should I consult a doctor?
Your baby should be seen by a doctor within 24 hours if he or she is refusing feeds, has a fever over 39°C (102°F), or seems very unwell. The doctor should also be consulted if a cough has not improved after 5 days, other symptoms have lasted longer than 10 days, or new symptoms, such as earache, develop.

How can colds be prevented?
There is no method of preventing colds apart from avoiding contact with infected individuals. To reduce the risk of infection, avoid taking babies into crowded places, such as supermarkets.

ENLARGED ADENOIDS

The adenoids are pads of tissue at the back of the nose that form part of the body's defences against infection. In some children, the adenoids become enlarged following repeated infections. As a result, they may block the passage of air or obstruct drainage of the middle ears through the eustachian tubes.

What are the symptoms?
The symptoms may include:
- Snoring.
- Frequent waking at night due to breathing problems, leading to excessive tiredness the next day.
- Breathing through the mouth.
- Nasal voice.

If the eustachian tubes are blocked by the enlarged adenoids, your child may suffer from recurrent ear infections (see OTITIS MEDIA, p.162), which may lead to GLUE EAR (p.163) and hearing loss.

Should I consult a doctor?
If your child's symptoms are mild, no treatment is usually required, because the adenoids shrink naturally with age.

If your child suffers from severe snoring or speech problems, or has frequent ear infections, you should make an appointment to see a doctor.

The doctor may refer your child to an ear, nose, and throat specialist, who will assess the size of the adenoids from an X-ray picture taken of the area. Surgical removal of the adenoids may be recommended. The operation, called an adenoidectomy, is performed in hospital under a general anaesthetic.

What can I do to help?
To relieve a dry mouth caused by persistent mouth breathing, keep the air in your child's room moist (see illustration: *Humidifying the air*, p.150). Encourage your child to sleep on his or her side or front; snoring is less likely to occur in these positions.

What is the outlook?
In children whose adenoids have not been removed, symptoms usually start to diminish around the age of 7 years, when the adenoids begin to shrink. By the time your child has reached adolescence, the adenoids will probably have disappeared completely.

A child whose adenoids have been removed should have fewer respiratory infections and is less likely to suffer from ear infections.

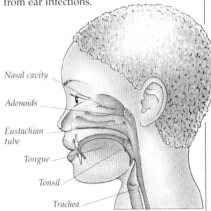

Nasal cavity

Adenoids

Eustachian tube

Tongue

Tonsil

Trachea

Location of the adenoids
Made up of lymphatic tissue, the adenoids are located at the back of the nasal cavity above the tonsils. Lymphatic tissue is rich in white blood cells, which fight infection.

SINUSITIS

Most commonly affecting adolescents, sinusitis is inflammation of the lining of the sinuses (air-filled cavities in the bones that surround the nose). It is most often caused by bacterial infection that occurs as a complication of a COMMON COLD (opposite).

What are the symptoms?
The first indication of sinusitis may be symptoms of a common cold, such as a runny nose and coughing, that persist for longer than usual. Your child may then develop the following specific symptoms of sinusitis:
- A yellowish-green nasal discharge.
- A feeling of fullness or pain in the cheeks and sometimes the forehead.
- Sometimes, severe pain in the upper back teeth.

Some children with sinusitis also have a persistent fever.

How is it caused?
Mucus produced in the sinuses traps bacteria. Cilia (hair-like structures) that project from the lining of the sinuses move the mucus along until it drains through narrow passages into the nose and throat. If a viral infection, such as a cold, causes inflammation of tissues, these passages may be blocked. As a result, mucus collects in the sinuses, enabling the bacteria in it to multiply.

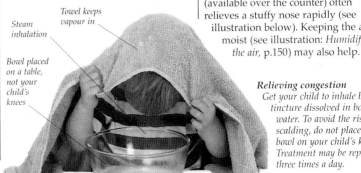

Steam inhalation

Towel keeps vapour in

Bowl placed on a table, not your child's knees

Should I consult a doctor?
Make an appointment to see a doctor within 24 hours. The doctor will examine your child and, if sinusitis is likely, will prescribe antibiotics. With antibiotic treatment, the infection usually clears up within 7 days.

What can I do to help?
Give your child paracetamol to relieve the pain, and plenty of fluids. A steam inhalation containing benzoin tincture (available over the counter) often relieves a stuffy nose rapidly (see illustration below). Keeping the air moist (see illustration: *Humidifying the air*, p.150) may also help.

Relieving congestion
Get your child to inhale benzoin tincture dissolved in boiling water. To avoid the risk of scalding, do not place the bowl on your child's knees. Treatment may be repeated three times a day.

CROUP

Usually caused by a viral infection, croup is inflammation and narrowing of the main airway to the lungs. It most commonly affects children aged between 6 months and 3 years. Croup is usually a mild illness; occasionally, however, it causes severe breathing difficulties and requires emergency treatment.

What are the symptoms?
Croup starts with the symptoms of a COMMON COLD (p.148), including a runny nose and sneezing. After 1 or 2 days, the following symptoms develop:
• Noisy breathing.
• Persistent, barking cough.
• Hoarse voice.
In severe cases, a child may have:
• Difficulty breathing.
• Abnormally fast breathing.
• Bluish tongue and sometimes skin.
Episodes of croup tend to occur in the early morning and last for a few hours.

If your child has an attack of croup, phone a doctor at once. If symptoms worsen or severe symptoms develop, call an ambulance or take your child to an accident and emergency department.

What might the doctor do?
After assessing the severity of the croup and excluding other conditions, such as EPIGLOTTITIS (below), the doctor may treat mild croup with oral, inhaled, or injected steroids. Self-help measures (right) may relieve the symptoms.

Children who are severely affected are usually admitted to hospital. To ease breathing, oxygen and medicated inhalations are given. If the airways are severely obstructed, a tube may be inserted through the nose into the windpipe. A child with severe croup usually takes a few days to recover.

What can I do to help?
Give paracetamol syrup and frequent warm drinks, and keep the air in your child's room moist (see illustration below). To ease the symptoms of an acute attack, take your child into the bathroom and turn on the hot taps to humidify the air rapidly. Your child should be better within 5 days.

What is the outlook?
Most children do not have a recurrence of croup. However, those with ASTHMA (p.153) may be prone to further attacks. For these children, treatment with drugs for preventing asthma may be recommended. The doctor may also prescribe inhalations of corticosteroids to be taken at the first signs of an attack of croup.

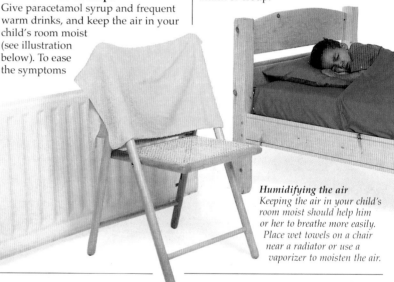

Humidifying the air
Keeping the air in your child's room moist should help him or her to breathe more easily. Place wet towels on a chair near a radiator or use a vaporizer to moisten the air.

EPIGLOTTITIS

A serious, potentially fatal infection, epiglottitis mainly affects children aged between 2 and 6 years. Caused by the bacterium *Haemophilus influenzae*, the infection results in inflammation of the epiglottis, the flap of cartilage located at the entrance to the larynx. The epiglottis swells and obstructs the passage of air.

What are the symptoms?
Epiglottitis comes on suddenly. The main symptoms are:
• Difficulty and pain on swallowing.
• Drooling because the child cannot swallow his or her saliva.
• Fever.
• Noisy breathing that becomes quieter as the illness worsens.
• Increasing difficulty in breathing. The child will probably want to sit upright in order to ease breathing.
• Bluish discoloration of the tongue and sometimes the skin.
If your child has difficulty swallowing and breathing, call an ambulance or take him or her to a hospital accident and emergency department: there is a risk of complete airway obstruction.

You should not attempt to look down your child's throat, because he or she may start to cry. Crying increases the production of secretions, which may totally block the narrowed airway.

What is the treatment?
Your child will be examined and an X-ray may be taken to confirm the diagnosis. Antibiotics will be given intravenously. In some cases, it may be necesssary to bypass the swollen epiglottis by inserting a tube through the nose and into the windpipe.

Children who are treated promptly make a complete recovery, usually within a week. A child who has had epiglottitis becomes immune to the infection, and it should not recur.

How can I prevent epiglottitis?
Infection with *Haemophilus influenzae* can be prevented by IMMUNIZATION (p.30). Children are routinely offered immunization against the bacterium.

PHARYNGITIS AND TONSILLITIS

Often occurring as part of a COMMON COLD (p.148), pharyngitis is inflammation of the throat. It is the most common cause of a sore throat. Tonsillitis (inflammation of the tonsils) often occurs with pharyngitis in children aged up to 8 years. Both conditions may be caused by viruses or streptococcal bacteria.

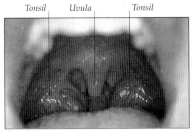

Tonsil   Uvula   Tonsil

Swollen tonsils
In tonsillitis, the tonsils are swollen and fiery red (as seen here) and are sometimes flecked with yellow or white pus. Rarely, the tonsils become so enlarged that they block the airway.

What are the symptoms?
Both pharyngitis and tonsillitis have similar symptoms, although those of tonsillitis are usually more severe. The main symptoms are:
• Sore, inflamed throat.
• Fever.
• Discomfort during swallowing (young children may refuse to eat).
• Enlarged, tender glands in the neck.
• Earache.
• In tonsillitis, red, swollen tonsils.
In the majority of cases, the symptoms disappear within 3 days. Rarely, an abscess, known as a quinsy, may form around a tonsil. It causes a high fever and increasing difficulty in swallowing.

Should I consult a doctor?
If the symptoms persist for more than 24 hours or get worse, phone a doctor at once. The doctor will examine your child and, if a bacterial infection is likely, may prescribe antibiotics. To confirm the diagnosis, a throat swab may be sent for analysis. A quinsy may need surgical drainage in hospital.

What can I do to help?
Give your child liquid paracetamol (see also panel: *Relieving a sore throat*, p.91) and plenty of fluids. Your child is infectious for about 3 days after a sore throat starts and should be kept away from other children during this time.

What is the outlook?
Most children stop having problems because they develop immunity to the common viruses. Occasionally, surgical removal of the tonsils is recommended for children who have recurrent bouts of tonsillitis due to bacterial infection (more than three attacks a year).

INFLUENZA

Commonly known as flu, influenza is a viral infection of the upper respiratory tract that may affect children of all ages. The influenza virus is spread by coughing and sneezing, and by direct contact. There are small outbreaks of influenza every year.

What are the symptoms?
The symptoms develop 1 to 3 days after infection, and usually come on rapidly. They may include:
• Fever, usually above 39°C (102°F).
• Dry cough.
• Muscular aches.
• Stuffy nose.
• Tiredness and weakness.
• Headache.
• Sometimes, a sore throat.
The symptoms are usually most severe during the first 2 to 5 days of the illness. In most cases, influenza clears up completely within about 10 days.

What are the complications?
The influenza virus may spread to the lungs, causing PNEUMONIA (p.155) or BRONCHITIS (p.154), often complicated by secondary bacterial infection. Bacterial infection may also affect the sinuses (see SINUSITIS, p.149) or ears (see OTITIS MEDIA, p.162). Children at high risk of such complications include those with chronic heart, lung, or kidney disease; DIABETES MELLITUS (p.190); CYSTIC FIBROSIS (p.201); or a depressed immune system. A possible complication in babies is FEBRILE CONVULSIONS (p.156).

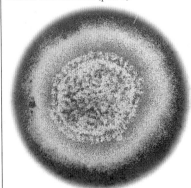

Influenza virus
The influenza virus can change its structure, producing new strains to which a child has not developed immunity. For this reason, repeated attacks of influenza can occur.

Should I consult a doctor?
Phone a doctor at once if your child is under the age of 2 years or is at high risk of complications. You should also contact a doctor immediately if your child develops any of the following symptoms: a temperature above 40°C (104°F); abnormally fast breathing; drowsiness; unwillingness to eat.

What is the treatment?
If a bacterial infection is present, the doctor may prescribe antibiotic drugs. Your child may be admitted to hospital if the symptoms are severe, or if he or she is at high risk of complications, for example, because of a chronic disorder.
   A child who is receiving care at home should stay in bed in a warm, well-ventilated, and humidified room (see illustration: *Humidifying the air*, p.150) until his or her temperature returns to normal. Liquid paracetamol may be given for aches and fever. You should offer warm drinks at frequent intervals.

How can I prevent influenza?
Annual vaccination against influenza may be recommended for children with a chronic disorder, such as lung disease, or any defect of the immune system.

ALLERGIES

An allergy is a condition in which the immune system responds to a substance inappropriately. The result is an allergic reaction that may produce a wide range of symptoms, such as a rash, coughing, or vomiting. A child is more likely to suffer from an allergy if there is a family history of allergic disorders.

How is an allergic reaction caused?
The body's immune system responds to foreign material (such as bacteria or viruses) by producing antibodies and sensitized white blood cells that can recognize and then destroy the foreign substance. An allergic reaction is similar except that it is misdirected at normally harmless substances (called allergens), such as dust or a food.

The initial exposure to an allergen sensitizes the immune system to the substance. On subsequent exposures, the immune response to the allergen is fast and strong, producing an allergic reaction. This reaction may occur when a chemical comes into contact with the skin (see CONTACT DERMATITIS, p.136); a particular food is swallowed; or airborne particles, such as pollen, are inhaled (see ALLERGIC RHINITIS, below; ASTHMA, opposite). Insect venom (see INSECT BITES AND STINGS, p.138) and injections or tablets of certain drugs (for example, penicillin or penicillin-based drugs) may also cause an allergic reaction. In a few cases, a very severe, life-threatening allergic reaction may occur (see ANAPHYLACTIC SHOCK, p.154).

What are the symptoms?
The symptoms of allergies range from mild to severe, and may affect one area or part of the body (such as the skin, the lining of the nose, or the eyes), or may be more widespread. Symptoms of an allergic reaction may include:
• Rash.
• Sore, itchy eyes.
• Blocked, runny nose.
• Coughing.
• Faintness.
• Abdominal pain.
• Nausea and vomiting
• Diarrhoea.

What is the treatment?
The most effective treatment for many allergies is to identify the causes (the allergens responsible) and to remove or avoid them; for instance, by keeping your house as free of dust as possible or by not eating certain foods.

Allergic symptoms are often treated with drugs, the most common of which are antihistamines and corticosteroids. Some allergies become less severe or disappear altogether with time.

ALLERGIC RHINITIS

Inflammation of the lining of the nose due to an allergic reaction (see ALLERGIES, above) is called allergic rhinitis. Allergic rhinitis takes two forms. The seasonal variety, commonly known as hay fever, causes symptoms only in the spring and summer months, while the perennial variety affects people throughout the year. Allergic rhinitis often runs in families and is most common among children with other allergies.

How is it caused?
Allergic rhinitis occurs when a person inhales an allergen (a substance that causes an allergic reaction). Allergens that most often cause hay fever are grass, tree, and weed pollens. Perennial allergic rhinitis is most often caused by house-dust mites, animal dander (flakes of dead skin), or mould spores.

What are the symptoms?
The symptoms of both forms of allergic rhinitis are similar, although those of the perennial type tend to be less severe. The main symptoms are:
• Initially, an itchy feeling in the eyes, nose, and throat.
• Blocked, runny nose.
• Sneezing.
• Red, sore, watery eyes.
• Occasionally, dry skin.

What can I do to help?
If the allergen is known, try to reduce or eliminate exposure to it. A child who has hay fever should stay indoors as much as possible during the pollen season. Keep the windows closed, especially on hot, dry, breezy days, when pollen counts may be high. Animals should be kept away from a child who is allergic to animal dander. If house-dust mites are causing the problem, keep house dust to a minimum. Dust all surfaces with a damp cloth, and treat carpets with insecticide to kill mites. Enclose your child's mattress in a plastic cover, and avoid feather-filled bedding. If your child has an allergy to mould spores, make sure his or her bedroom is well ventilated, and free of mould and dust.

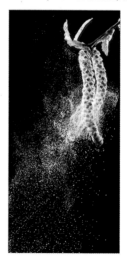

Pollen grains
Pollen from trees (shown here), grass, or weeds is the most common cause of hay fever. Tree pollens are most prevalent in the spring.

Oral antihistamines may help if your child's hay fever is severe or if he or she cannot avoid going outside. Antihistamines have little or no effect on perennial allergic rhinitis.

Should I consult a doctor?
Make an appointment to see a doctor if your child has severe or persistent symptoms not relieved by self-help measures.

The doctor will probably prescribe a nasal spray that contains either sodium cromoglycate or a cortico-steroid drug to alleviate the symptoms of rhinitis.

What is the outlook?
In many children, allergic rhinitis becomes less severe as they grow older and eventually disappears.

ASTHMA

The most common chronic lung disease of childhood, asthma is a distressing condition in which there are recurrent episodes of wheezing and breathlessness. The disease has become more prevalent in recent years: one out of seven children in the UK is affected. Most children who develop asthma have had their first attack by the age of 4 or 5 years. Untreated, asthma may slow down a child's growth and is potentially fatal.

How is it caused?

The cause of asthma is unclear. Many affected children have other allergic conditions, such as ALLERGIC RHINITIS (opposite) or ATOPIC ECZEMA (p.135). There is also often a family history of asthma and other allergic disorders. Individual attacks of asthma may be triggered by infection with a virus or

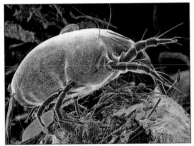

House-dust mite
For many children who have asthma, attacks may be triggered by exposure to house-dust mites. The mites live in soft furnishings, mattresses, bedding, carpets, and soft toys.

by allergens (see ALLERGIES, opposite), such as house-dust mites or food. Exercising, particularly in cold air, may bring on an attack. Attacks may also be brought on or made worse by anxiety.

The symptoms of asthma are caused by narrowing of the airways in the lungs as a result of inflammation and swelling of the walls, contraction of the muscles within the walls, and an increase in the secretion of mucus.

What are the symptoms?

In young children, the first sign of asthma is often a recurring cough, especially with a cold or after exercise. Sometimes, the first sign of asthma is coughing that occurs only at night. Other symptoms, which are similar to those of BRONCHITIS, (p.154) include:
• Wheezing.
• Shortness of breath.
• Tightness in the chest.

During severe attacks of asthma, the symptoms may include:
• Difficult and noisy breathing.
• Difficulty speaking.
• Drowsiness.
• Disturbed sleep.
• Blue lips and tongue.
• Refusal to eat or drink.

Should I consult a doctor?

If you think that your child has asthma, he or she should be seen by a doctor within 24 hours. If the symptoms are severe, call an ambulance or take your child to the nearest hospital accident and emergency department.

What might the doctor do?

The doctor will ask about any possible exposure to allergens and if there are factors that could be causing your child anxiety, such as difficulties at school.

To assess the severity of the disease, the doctor will use a peak-flow meter, which measures the capacity to exhale air. A chest X-ray may be carried out to check for any associated infection.

If your child's asthma is mild, the doctor will prescribe a bronchodilator drug. The bronchodilator is inhaled to ease breathing during asthma attacks. If your child's asthma is more severe,

Taking inhaled drugs
Children over about 8 years old can use an inhaler. A spacer makes it easier for younger children to inhale the drug. The drug is usually delivered as a spray, but for children over 5 years old a powder may be used.

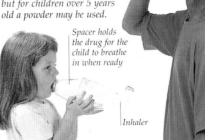

Inhaler

Spacer holds the drug for the child to breathe in when ready

Inhaler

the doctor may also prescribe sodium cromoglycate or, sometimes, a corticosteroid. These drugs have to be inhaled regularly to help prevent attacks. Some children require oral corticosteroids or regular treatment with an inhaled, long-acting bronchodilator drug.

Children may take inhaled drugs with an inhaler (see illustration below). For infants, a nebulizer is used. This device has a pump that disperses the drug as a fine mist into a face mask.

What can I do to help?

If your child is over the age of 6 years, the doctor may suggest that you use a peak-flow meter in order to monitor the asthma; the meter should warn of an impending attack. Keep an asthma diary to chart the symptoms and the peak-flow meter readings from day to day. This record will help the doctor to modify your child's treatment as the disease changes, develops, or subsides.

You or your child should always have a bronchodilator available to use in case of an attack. If your child has a severe attack of asthma and the normal bronchodilator does not work, a repeat dose should be taken. If that fails to ease the condition, phone your doctor at once or take your child to a hospital accident and emergency department.

How can I prevent asthma?

You cannot prevent your child from developing asthma, but you may be able to reduce the condition's severity by encouraging your child to avoid any known allergens or reducing his or her exposure to them. Helping your child to avoid stressful situations and being supportive during times when your child feels anxious may also be effective. Some children find that taking their bronchodilator drug half an hour before vigorous exercise prevents an attack.

What is the outlook?

At least half the children who develop asthma before they reach the age of 5 years stop having attacks by the time they reach adulthood. If your child still has asthma at the age of 14 years, however, there is a strong chance that it will persist into adulthood.

ANAPHYLACTIC SHOCK

A rare, severe, widespread allergic reaction, anaphylactic shock causes constriction of the airways and a sudden drop in blood pressure. Without immediate medical attention, it can be fatal. Stings from insects (such as bees) and reactions to certain drugs (particularly those based on penicillin) are the most common causes of anaphylactic shock. Some foods (for example, peanuts, shellfish, eggs, and cow's milk) may also trigger the reaction.

What are the symptoms?
People who are sensitive to a substance usually start having a reaction a few minutes after they have been exposed to it. Initially, they may experience an itching or burning feeling in the lips, mouth, or throat. Other symptoms that soon follow may include:
- Blotchy, itchy, raised rash.
- Paleness of the skin and sweating.
- Anxiety.
- Swollen eyelids, lips, and tongue.
- Puffy face and neck.
- Difficulty breathing.
- Abdominal pain and sometimes vomiting or diarrhoea.
- Faintness, abnormal drowsiness, or loss of consciousness.
- In infants, refusal to drink and sometimes dribbling as a result of an inability to swallow.

If your child has any of the symptoms listed above, call an ambulance or take him or her to a hospital accident and emergency department immediately.

What can I do to help?
While waiting for the ambulance to arrive, you should place your child in a semi-sitting position to make breathing easier (see illustration right). Your child should not eat or drink anything. If your child starts to vomit, place him or her in the RECOVERY POSITION (p.203). If your child loses consciousness, you should follow the ABC of resuscitation (see PRINCIPLES OF FIRST AID, p.202).

What might the doctor do?
The doctor will immediately give your child an injection of adrenaline to raise low blood pressure. He or she will check whether your child has breathing problems, and may pass a tube into the windpipe for mechanical ventilation. If the heart has stopped, the doctor may give your child heart massage. To reduce swelling and relieve itching, the doctor may inject a corticosteroid or antihistamine drug. Intravenous fluids may be given to help bring the blood pressure back to normal.

How can I prevent anaphylactic shock?
Your child should avoid the substance that caused the reaction. Your doctor may prescribe a syringe of adrenaline for use in an emergency. Tell your child's school about the allergy and give your child a bracelet to wear that alerts other people to the allergy.

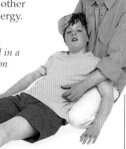

Easing breathing
Support your child in a semi-sitting position to help ease breathing.

BRONCHITIS

Inflammation of the bronchi (the main airways to the lungs) is known as bronchitis. The condition is usually a complication of a viral infection such as a COMMON COLD (p.148) or INFLUENZA (p.151), but is sometimes caused by bacterial infection.

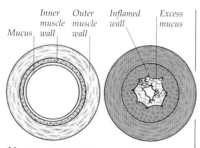

Inner muscle wall · Outer muscle wall · Inflamed wall · Excess mucus · Mucus

NORMAL BRONCHUS (CROSS-SECTION) · **AFFECTED BY BRONCHITIS**

How bronchitis affects the airways
In bronchitis, the walls of the bronchi become inflamed, and the glands that line the walls produce excess mucus. The air channel is narrowed, causing difficulty breathing.

What are the symptoms?
Your child may have a runny nose for 2 or 3 days before bronchitis appears. The main symptoms are:
- Persistent cough. Although the cough is usually dry at first, it may later produce yellowish-green phlegm if there is a bacterial infection.
- Wheezing and shortness of breath.
- Sometimes, a fever.

What can I do to help?
Keeping the air in your child's room moist (see illustration: *Humidifying the air*, p.150) or giving steam inhalations may help decongest the airways. Give warm drinks to relieve the cough, and liquid paracetamol to reduce a fever.

Most children feel better after a few days and have completely recovered within a week. If, however, there is no improvement after 24 hours, your child should be seen by a doctor. Phone a doctor at once if breathing becomes abnormally fast or the fever rises above 39°C (102°F). Call an ambulance if your child becomes drowsy or refuses to eat.

What might the doctor do?
Your child will be examined to make sure he or she does not have a more serious condition, such as PNEUMONIA (opposite) or BRONCHIOLITIS (opposite).

The doctor may prescribe antibiotics if a bacterial infection is suspected. To relieve the wheezing, a bronchodilator drug may be prescribed.

What is the outlook?
Some children have recurrent bouts of bronchitis, but they are likely to grow out of the condition by 5 years of age.

BRONCHIOLITIS

This acute viral infection of the lungs causes inflammation of the bronchioles (the smallest airways in the lungs). Bronchiolitis mainly affects children under 1 year and can be a serious illness. It usually occurs in epidemics during the winter months.

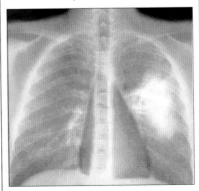

Easing the cough
Place your child across your lap and slap him or her gently on the back to help loosen thick mucus.

What are the symptoms?
Initially, your child may have symptoms resembling those of the COMMON COLD (p.148). After 2 or 3 days, the following symptoms may develop:
• Dry, rasping cough.
• Wheezing and/or rapid, difficult breathing. In some infants, long pauses (more than 10 seconds) occur between each breath.
• Reluctance to feed.
• Bluish lips and tongue.
• Abnormal drowsiness.
If your child is under 1 year and is coughing and/or wheezing, phone a doctor. Call an ambulance if breathing is difficult, if the lips and tongue are blue, or if your child becomes drowsy.

What is the treatment?
For mild bronchiolitis, the doctor may prescribe a bronchodilator drug and advise you to look after your child at home. Give your child plenty of fluids and feed him or her small amounts frequently. Liquid paracetamol can help to bring down the fever. Thick mucus in the lungs may be loosened by slapping your child's back (see illustration right). Mild bronchiolitis usually improves within about a week.

A child who needs hospital treatment may be given oxygen in a plastic head box. He or she may be fed by means of a tube inserted through the nose or, sometimes, intravenously. In severe cases, mechanical ventilation may be required. The child will be allowed home when he or she is feeding normally again, usually within 7 days. The cough, however, may persist for up to 6 weeks.

What is the outlook?
Bronchiolitis does not cause permanent damage to the lungs. For the next few years, however, many children who have had the illness tend to suffer from wheezing when they have a cold.

PNEUMONIA

Inflammation of the lungs, known as pneumonia, is usually due to a viral or bacterial infection. It is most often a complication of an upper respiratory tract infection, such as a COMMON COLD (p.148), or of an infectious disease, such as CHICKENPOX (p.120). Children with CYSTIC FIBROSIS (p.201) are particularly prone to pneumonia.

What are the symptoms?
Pneumonia may start with symptoms of a common cold, such as sneezing and a runny nose. The following symptoms then develop:
• Coughing, which in older children produces yellowish, greenish, or blood-flecked phlegm.
• Rapid, difficult breathing.
• Fever.
• Headache.
• In severe pneumonia, drowsiness, blueness of the lips and tongue, and refusal to eat or drink.

Should I consult a doctor?
Phone a doctor at once if your child is breathing fast while resting in bed; if a cough and fever last for more than a few days; or if your child seems far more ill than an ordinary cold would warrant. You should call an ambulance if your child has any of the symptoms of severe pneumonia listed above.

What might the doctor do?
The doctor will listen to your child's chest through a stethoscope and may send a throat swab or blood sample for tests to identify the cause of infection.

Chest X-ray showing pneumonia
Pneumonia causes some of the air sacs in the lungs to fill with fluid. The affected part of the lung shows as a white shadow.

Antibiotics may be prescribed. Most children can be treated at home (see "What can I do to help?").

If your child's pneumonia is severe, he or she may be admitted to hospital. A chest X-ray will be taken to confirm the diagnosis and antibiotics will be given. Your child may receive oxygen; rarely, mechanical ventilation will be required. Your child should be able to go home after about 4 days.

What can I do to help?
If treating your child at home, make sure he or she has plenty of warm fluids to drink. Feed your baby small amounts at frequent intervals. You may give liquid paracetamol to reduce your child's fever and relieve a headache. Most children recover within a week.

After discharge from hospital, your child should not take vigorous exercise for about a week. Going outside will not harm your child, provided that the weather is not damp or very cold.

What is the outlook?
A cough may continue for a further 2 weeks after your child has otherwise recovered. Pneumonia does not result in any permanent damage to the lungs.

NERVOUS SYSTEM DISORDERS

MOST OF THE GROWTH AND DEVELOPMENT of the brain – the nervous system's control centre – is complete by the age of about 5 years. Any brain injury or infection that occurs in a child's early years (or in some cases before birth), when the brain is still immature, may have serious long-term consequences. Early recognition and treatment of brain disorders is, therefore, extremely important. On the other hand, children's brains have a much greater capacity for recovery than do those of adults. However, a few nervous system disorders, such as cerebral palsy, are incurable.

FEBRILE CONVULSIONS

A febrile convulsion is a type of seizure associated with a high temperature – over 39°C (102°F) – that accompanies an infection in a part of the body other than the brain. Febrile convulsions may occur in children between the ages of 6 months and 5 years. Although frightening, the seizures are not usually serious.

How are they caused?
Febrile convulsions are triggered by an abrupt rise in body temperature and usually occur at the onset of a feverish illness. The convulsions are most often associated with upper respiratory tract infections, such as a cold. Children are susceptible to the seizures because their brains are not yet mature.

What are the symptoms?
The first stage of the seizure lasts about half a minute. Symptoms may include:
- Loss of consciousness.
- Rigidity of the body.
- Cessation of breathing for up to half a minute; when it starts again, breathing may be shallow and barely detectable.
- Passing urine and/or faeces.
The second stage usually lasts for less than 5 minutes. The child remains unconscious and there may also be:
- Twitching of the limbs and/or face.
- Rolling back of the eyes.
At the end of the second stage, the child regains consciousness and may then fall into a deep sleep for an hour or two. He or she may be confused, sleepy, and irritable on waking.

Should I consult a doctor?
If your child has a seizure or his or her temperature is above 39°C (102°F), you should phone a doctor at once. If a seizure lasts for more than 5 minutes (or 15 minutes if diazepam has been given; see "What might the doctor do?"), you should call an ambulance.

What can I do to help?
If your child has a raised temperature, you should try to reduce it (see panel: *Bringing down a high temperature*, p.37, and illustration above right) in order to prevent febrile convulsions.

Your child should be placed in the RECOVERY POSITION (p.203) if he or she has had a febrile convulsion. Carry on with action to reduce your child's fever to prevent another seizure.

What might the doctor do?
If this is a first attack, your child may be admitted to hospital for tests so that the possibility of MENINGITIS (p.158) may be excluded. Other tests may also be carried out to identify the cause of the fever; antibiotics may be prescribed if there is a bacterial infection.

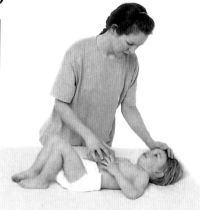

Reducing your child's temperature
Sponge your child with lukewarm water to reduce a fever. Do not place a child who has had a seizure in a bath; he or she could drown.

You will be given advice on how to deal with future attacks. The doctor will prescribe diazepam (an anticonvulsant drug) for use at home; squirted into the child's rectum during an attack, it shortens the duration of convulsions.

What is the outlook?
About a third of children who have had one attack will have a second one, usually within 6 months. However, children older than 5 years are unlikely to have attacks. A small minority of those who have had febrile convulsions later develop EPILEPSY (opposite).

EPILEPSY

Recurrent seizures (or fits), a condition called epilepsy, occur in about 1 in 200 children. During a seizure, there is chaotic and unregulated electrical brain activity, which causes an alteration in consciousness and sometimes uncontrollable movements of the limbs and/or head. There are many causes of seizures other than epilepsy (see, for example, FEBRILE CONVULSIONS, opposite). A child who has a single seizure is not considered to have epilepsy.

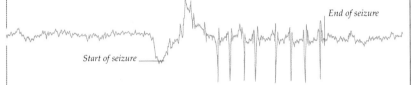

Start of seizure

End of seizure

How is it caused?
Children with epilepsy sometimes have a structural abnormality in the brain, but in most cases no obvious cause can be found. In some children, individual attacks may be brought on by a trigger, for example, flashing lights; in others, the attacks have no apparent trigger.

What are the symptoms?
There are a number of different types of epileptic seizure. In children, grand mal seizures are most common: more than three-quarters of children with epilepsy suffer from this type. Petit mal (absence) seizures are the second most common type in children. The main features of these seizures are:

Grand mal seizures
• Irritability or unusual behaviour for a few minutes before the seizure.
• A rigid spasm, which lasts for up to 30 seconds, during which the child usually falls unconscious to the floor and breathing becomes irregular.
• Jerky movements of the limbs or face which may last from 20 seconds to several hours. The child may bite his or her tongue and there may be loss of bladder or bowel control.
• After convulsions stop, the child may stay unconscious for a few minutes or, more rarely, for up to 10 minutes.
• When the child regains consciousness, he or she often feels disoriented and confused, may have a headache, and will probably want to sleep.

Petit mal (absence) seizures
• Child stops normal activities and stares into space, unaware of the surroundings, for 10 to 15 seconds, but does not fall to the floor.
• Child has no memory of the seizure.

Brain activity during a seizure
This EEG recording of the brain's electrical activity was made during a petit mal seizure. This type of seizure is very brief, typically lasting for just 10 to 15 seconds.

A less common form of epilepsy, called benign focal epilepsy, causes jerking of one side of the face or of one limb. The child may also lose consciousness.

In most cases, a child will have only one type of seizure. However, some children have more complex forms of epilepsy, which combine two or more different types of seizure.

What can I do to help?
If your child has a grand mal seizure, place him or her in the recovery position (see photograph below right and RECOVERY POSITION, p.203) and stay until he or she has fully recovered.

For other types of seizure, sit your child down in a quiet spot, and stay until he or she is fully recovered and alert. Talk calmly and reassuringly to your child. Do not slap or shake your child in an attempt to stop the seizure.

Should I consult a doctor?
If your child has never had a grand mal seizure before, phone a doctor at once. You should call an ambulance or take your child to the nearest accident and emergency department if he or she remains unconscious for longer than 10 minutes, whether the attack is the first one or not. Although other types of seizure are less serious, make an appointment to see a doctor. Notify the doctor of any subsequent seizures that your child has.

What might the doctor do?
You will probably be asked to describe your child's behaviour and symptoms before, during, and after any seizure. To identify possible triggers, the doctor may also ask what your child had been doing just before the seizure.

An electroencephalogram (EEG) is usually performed to help determine the type of epilepsy. Brain scanning may be carried out to find out whether a structural brain abnormality might be causing the seizures. Blood may be tested to rule out other possible causes of the seizure, such as low blood sugar.

What is the treatment?
Children with epilepsy normally need regular anticonvulsant drug therapy. Anticonvulsants are usually given until 2 to 4 years have passed since the last seizure, and may then be gradually stopped over several months.

If medication does not control your child's seizures, and scans indicate a structural brain abnormality, surgery may, extremely rarely, be considered to correct the problem.

The doctor will advise you on any precautions that you or your child should take, and whether there are any activities that should be avoided.

What is the outlook?
The outlook varies, depending on the type of epilepsy. Over three-quarters of children with grand mal epilepsy who have been free of seizures for 2 years do not have a recurrence. Most children with benign focal epilepsy outgrow the condition and need no medication after puberty. The outlook is less predictable for children with petit mal epilepsy. Most children, even those who do not outgrow their epilepsy, have no other disability, and can go to normal schools and participate in most sports.

Dealing with a grand mal seizure
Place your child on the floor in the recovery position, with the head on the same level or slightly lower than the body. You should not try to force anything into the child's mouth to prevent a bitten tongue.

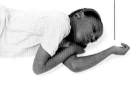

MENINGITIS

Inflammation of the meninges (the membranes covering the brain and spinal cord) is known as meningitis. It is caused by infection with bacteria or viruses. The symptoms of viral meningitis are mild, but bacterial meningitis can be life threatening. Bacterial meningitis is most common in children under the age of 5 years, although it can occur at any age. It usually appears as isolated cases. Viral meningitis tends to occur in epidemics in the winter months and is most common in children over 5 years old.

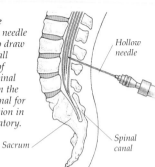

Lumbar puncture
A hollow needle is used to draw out a small amount of cerebrospinal fluid from the spinal canal for examination in the laboratory.

Hollow needle

Sacrum

Spinal canal

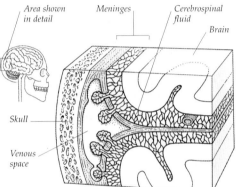

Area shown in detail

Meninges

Cerebrospinal fluid

Brain

Skull

Venous space

The meninges
Three layers of protective membranes, known as the meninges, cover the brain and spinal cord. Meningitis is caused by infection of the meninges by viruses or bacteria.

How is it caused?
Bacterial meningitis in children is most often caused by *Neisseria meningitidis* bacteria, and is called meningococcal meningitis. The *Neisseria* bacteria are normal inhabitants of the nose and throat, and usually cause no ill effects. Why they cause meningitis in some children is unknown. Another common cause of meningitis was infection with *Haemophilus influenzae* bacteria, but this has become a rare cause since the introduction of routine IMMUNIZATION (p.30) of babies in 1993.

There are many different viruses capable of causing meningitis, including those responsible for influenza, chickenpox, infectious mononucleosis (glandular fever), and AIDS. As with meningitis due to bacterial infection, it is not known what leads these viruses to infect the meninges and cause meningitis.

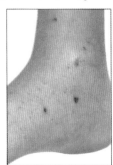

Meningitis rash
Development of this rash is a serious symptom of meningitis and indicates that immediate medical treatment is vital.

What are the symptoms?
The symptoms of the bacterial and viral forms of meningitis are similar in the early stages. However, those of bacterial meningitis are usually more severe and tend to develop rapidly, sometimes within a few hours. In infants the early symptoms are often vague, and may include:
• Abnormal drowsiness.
• Fever.
• Vomiting.
• Reluctance to feed.
• Increased crying; restlessness.
In older children, the symptoms may include all of the above, as well as:
• Severe headache.
• Dislike of bright light and loud noise.
• Rigidity of muscles, particularly the muscles of the neck.
In children of all ages with bacterial meningitis, the initial symptoms may be followed by increasing drowsiness and, occasionally, by loss of consciousness or convulsions. Some children with meningitis develop a characteristic rash (see photograph below) consisting of flat, pink or purple spots that do not fade when pressed.

Should I consult a doctor?
If your child is abnormally drowsy or develops any two of the symptoms listed above, he or she should be seen by a doctor at once or taken to the nearest hospital accident and emergency department. The child will be admitted to hospital, where a lumbar puncture (see illustration above right) may be performed. This test can confirm the diagnosis of either viral or bacterial meningitis and, in some cases, enables identification of the particular infectious organisms. Blood samples may also be taken for culture in the laboratory to identify bacteria.

What is the treatment?
A course of high-dose antibiotics will be started immediately, even before the laboratory results are available.

If tests confirm viral meningitis, the antibiotics can be discontinued. No form of treatment other than painkillers is necessary, and the infection usually clears up in 5 to 14 days, depending on the particular virus involved.

If bacterial meningitis is confirmed, antibiotics will be continued (or, they may be changed, if necessary, to target the particular bacteria that have been identified). Your child may be given intravenous fluids, and anticonvulsant drugs may be prescribed if he or she is having convulsions. Treatment with antibiotics may last for up to 10 days.

How can meningitis be prevented?
Routine immunization gives protection against *Haemophilus influenzae*. Short-term protection against one type of meningococcal meningitis is provided by immunization, which may be given during local outbreaks. The only other way to prevent the spread of bacterial meningitis is to give antibiotics to those in close contact with an affected child.

What is the outlook?
Viral meningitis rarely has after-effects. Prompt treatment with antibiotics in the early stages of bacterial meningitis usually leads to complete recovery. A few children may have some brain damage, resulting in deafness, seizures, or learning difficulties, especially if treatment is delayed. Rarely, the illness may be fatal, even if treated promptly.

ENCEPHALITIS

Inflammation of the brain is called encephalitis. A rare condition, it can be caused by any viral infection. For unknown reasons, the viruses spread through the bloodstream to the brain from sites elsewhere in the body. Encephalitis can vary in severity from being mild and harmless to a serious and life-threatening illness.

How is it caused?
In newborn babies, the herpes simplex virus (the virus responsible for cold sores) is the most common cause of encephalitis. Rarely, encephalitis can also occur following measles, rubella (German measles), or chickenpox. The live viruses contained in some vaccines (for example, the measles vaccine) may, very rarely, cause encephalitis.

What are the symptoms?
In mild encephalitis, the symptoms may be barely noticeable. Chickenpox encephalitis, for example, may cause only slight unsteadiness in walking for a few days. In more serious forms of encephalitis, the most important symptom is abnormal drowsiness that progressively worsens, possibly leading to coma. There may also be:
- Fever.
- Irritability.
- Vomiting.
- Double vision or an obvious squint.
- Weakness of a limb.
- Convulsions.

Should I consult a doctor?
Phone a doctor at once if your child is abnormally drowsy or if he or she has a fever plus any two of the symptoms above. The diagnosis will be based on the child's symptoms and the results of brain scans. In the early stages of the illness, the tests may not show anything wrong, even if the child is later shown to have encephalitis. A lumbar puncture may be carried out to exclude bacterial MENINGITIS (opposite).

The antiviral drug acyclovir is used to treat herpes simplex infection. There are no drugs to treat other viral infections. Mechanical ventilation may be needed for breathing difficulties.

What is the outlook?
The outlook depends on the causative virus and the severity of the symptoms. Most children recover completely. In a few cases, there is permanent brain damage, which may cause weakness of an arm or leg, learning difficulties, behavioural problems, or epilepsy. Very rarely, encephalitis is fatal.

HEAD INJURY

Bangs or knocks to the head are common in childhood and are rarely serious. Common causes include falling out of a cot or bed, falling from a tree or climbing frame, or a traffic accident. Even a small cut on the scalp or forehead can cause severe bleeding. The main risk of a head injury, however, is bleeding inside the skull (brain haemorrhage), which can lead to brain damage. In rare cases, a head injury can be fatal.

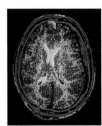

Blood clot

CT scan of brain
Bleeding inside the skull can result in a blood clot, which may put pressure on and damage brain tissues.

What are the symptoms?
If the head injury is mild, there may be no symptoms other than a slight headache and a bump or swelling at the site of the injury. However, if there has been a blow to the head there may be concussion (brief unconsciousness, usually lasting a few seconds).

Common symptoms immediately following concussion include:
- Confusion.
- Inability to remember events that occurred just before the injury.
- Dizziness.
- Blurred vision.
- Vomiting.

With more severe head injuries, there may be unconsciousness lasting for more than a few minutes or even coma.

If straw-coloured fluid or watery blood trickles from your child's nose or ear, there may be a skull fracture.

Should I consult a doctor?
If your child is knocked unconscious even for only a few seconds, appears confused or abnormally drowsy, vomits persistently, or there is fluid or watery blood leaking from the nose or ears, call an ambulance or take your child to the nearest hospital accident and emergency department.

Your child will be examined by the doctor. A cut to the scalp may need to be stitched in order to stop bleeding. An X-ray of the skull may be taken if a fracture is suspected and a CT scan (see photograph above) may be performed. If the CT scan shows signs of a brain haemorrhage, an emergency operation may be needed to stop the bleeding and remove a blood clot. If your child has a fracture of the skull or a severe concussion, he or she will be observed in hospital for 24 hours after the injury.

What can I do to help?
If your child has a minor head injury, he or she should rest at home for 2 or 3 days. You will be asked to observe your child carefully during the first 24 hours and to take him or her back to the hospital as an emergency if any of the following symptoms of a blood clot develop: abnormal drowsiness; vomiting; irritability; confusion; slurred or incoherent speech; fluid or watery blood leaking from the nose or ears.

A child with a more severe injury that required hospital treatment may need to rest at home for several weeks.

What is the outlook?
There should be no long-lasting effects from minor head injures. More severe head injuries may cause permanent brain damage, resulting in a degree of physical or mental disability.

NEURAL TUBE DEFECTS

The neural tube is the part of an embryo that develops into the brain and spinal cord, and the back of the skull and vertebrae. If normal development fails to occur, a baby may be born with defects in any of these parts. The most common type of defect is spina bifida, which affects one or more vertebrae.

What are the symptoms?
To a greater or lesser degree, the spinal cord, the brain, or their coverings (the meninges) are exposed, making them vulnerable to damage and infection. The abnormality may be so slight that it is apparent only from a dimple or a tuft of hair over the defect, or there may be a large, fluid-filled swelling, covered by a thin membrane or by skin. The symptoms, if there are any, depend on the severity of the neural tube defect and may include:
• Weakness or paralysis of the legs.
• Deformity of the legs.
• Urinary and/or faecal incontinence.
• Insensitivity to pain of the skin below the level of the abnormality.
• Sometimes, hydrocephalus (water on the brain).
• In some cases, LEARNING DIFFICULTIES (p.172).

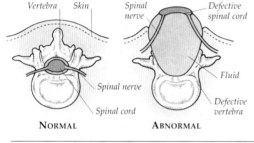

Vertebra *Skin* *Spinal nerve* *Defective spinal cord* *Fluid* *Spinal nerve* *Spinal cord* *Defective vertebra*

NORMAL ABNORMAL

Myelomeningocele
In this type of severe neural tube defect, part of the spinal cord and the vertebrae that normally protect it are defective. The defect appears as a fluid-filled sac covered by a thin membrane.

How can neural tube defects be prevented?
The causes of neural tube defects are unknown. However, the risk has been shown to be reduced substantially if a woman takes a small amount of folic acid once a day for a month before she conceives and during the first month of her pregnancy. Early in pregnancy, screening tests, such as a blood test and an ultrasound examination, usually detect a neural tube defect. The parents may choose a termination if the defect is particularly severe or if there is little chance that the baby will survive.

What is the treatment?
A child with a mild defect may have no symptoms and require no treatment. Surgical treatment may be necessary for a more severely affected child; for example, in hydrocephalus, a tube may be inserted into the brain in order to drain off fluid. Nevertheless, the child may remain permanently disabled. He or she will receive physiotherapy and help with learning to live with disability.

CEREBRAL PALSY

A general term for abnormalities of limb movement and posture, cerebral palsy results from damage to the brain in late pregnancy, at birth, in the newborn period, or in early childhood. Usually, damage occurs before birth. Cerebral palsy is most common in babies born prematurely or weighing less than 1.5 kg (3.3 lb).

What are the symptoms?
Cerebral palsy may not be recognized until your child is several months old. The earliest signs are usually:
• Stiffness of the arms and legs on being picked up.
• Reluctance to use one hand or arm.
• Feeding difficulties.
• Not sitting by the age of 1 year.
In some children, the muscles of one or more limbs are stiff (spastic), making normal movements very difficult. This problem usually starts to appear from the age of 6 months onwards. Other children have irregular and involuntary writhing movements of the body.

Many children with cerebral palsy have LEARNING DIFFICULTIES (p.172). Some also have epilepsy and problems with hearing and eyesight. SPEECH PROBLEMS (p.171) are common due to a variety of causes, including poor hearing, slow learning ability, and poor coordination of the muscles that are used in speech. Behavioural problems may occur as a result of a child's frustration with his or her disabilities, or can be due to family tension or to the brain damage itself.

Should I consult a doctor?
If you have any concerns that your baby is not developing properly, you should make an appointment to see a doctor.

Scans and tests may be carried out to make a precise diagnosis of the cause of your child's problems. Depending on the specific difficulties, your child may be seen by a consultant paediatrician, occupational and speech therapists, a psychologist, and a social worker. In some cases, deformities resulting from muscle contractures require surgery.

What is the outlook?
Although cerebral palsy is incurable, with patience and as much stimulation as possible, your child's symptoms may show improvement. Children who have mild cerebral palsy can usually attend normal schools, but those who are more severely affected may require special education. Children with mild or moderate disability should have a near-normal life expectancy.

Occupational therapy
The concentration and coordination of children with cerebral palsy can be improved by doing puzzles and playing games involving fine hand movements.

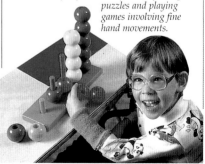

RECURRENT HEADACHES

Almost all children have occasional headaches. Some children, however, have recurrent headaches, which may be severely debilitating and interfere with schoolwork. The two main forms of recurrent headache are migraine and tension headache. Very rarely, recurrent headaches are caused by a brain disorder.

MIGRAINE

Children who suffer from migraine frequently have a family history of the disorder. The most common trigger of migraine attacks is emotional stress. Other possible triggers include certain foods, such as citrus fruits or cheese; hunger; too much sun; and tiredness.

What are the symptoms?

Attacks of migraine rarely occur more than once or twice a month. A few children have initial warning signs of seeing sparkling lights or zigzag lines. Symptoms that follow, which may last from 2 hours to 2 days, may include:
• Pain, which may affect one side of the head only or both sides of the head.
• Vomiting.
• Dislike of light and noise.
• Lightheadedness or dizziness.
• Tingling, weakness, or numbness of an arm or hand.
A doctor should see your child if the symptoms suggest migraine.

What is the treatment?

The doctor may suggest that you try to identify trigger factors, so that they can be avoided, if possible. Anti-emetic medicine may be prescribed to prevent vomiting during attacks. Propranolol, a drug that prevents migraine, may be prescribed if attacks are very frequent.

Taking paracetamol and lying down in a darkened room should help to relieve pain during a migraine attack.

What is the outlook?

Frequent attacks of migraine may be followed by long periods when there are none. If your child avoids known triggers, the number of attacks may be limited. Propranolol reduces the frequency of migraine attacks.

Stress-related headache
Migraine or a tension headache may be triggered by working too hard at school, possibly in an attempt to keep up with peers or as a result of worry over coming exams.

TENSION HEADACHE

The pain of a tension headache may be due to muscular tension in the face and neck, for example from clenching or grinding the teeth. Emotional stress is the most common trigger.

What are the symptoms?

The symptoms, which may be present every day, consist of:
• Pain, affecting any part of the head.
• Sometimes, accompanying signs of tension, such as abdominal pain.

What is the treatment?

Give your child paracetamol to relieve the pain and try to identify and reduce any causes of stress. If the headaches persist, consult a doctor, who may refer your child to a consultant.

BRAIN DISORDERS

The symptoms vary, but the following may point to the possibility of a brain disorder, such as a tumour:
• Headache that wakes a child at night, is present on waking in the morning, or is made worse by coughing.
• Convulsions.
• Changes in behaviour.
A doctor should see your child at once if you suspect a brain disorder. The doctor will examine your child and may arrange for tests in hospital. The treatment and outlook will depend on the nature of the problem.

CHRONIC FATIGUE SYNDROME

This disorder consists of a collection of symptoms, of which the most important is severe fatigue that persists for months or even years. A viral illness may, for unknown reasons, be the trigger. Sometimes, the symptoms are due to unrecognized depression.

What are the symptoms?

The symptoms may include:
• Severe fatigue that prevents the child getting up from bed at the usual time.
• A feeling of weakness in the limbs.
• Pain in the head, the abdomen, or the muscles of the limbs.
• Reluctance to eat or to take part in any social activities.
• Becoming extremely exhausted after any physical or mental exertion.
• Difficulty in concentrating.

Sometimes, chronic fatigue syndrome is preceded by a sore throat or some other viral illness, such as INFECTIOUS MONONUCLEOSIS (p.124), but not always.

Should I consult a doctor?

It is normal for a child to feel "washed out" for a week or two after a severe infectious illness. If fatigue persists for more than a month, consult a doctor. The doctor will examine your child for any physical cause for the illness and may arrange for blood tests to check for any signs of illness. In most cases, physical examination and test results are normal, although in a large number of sufferers tests show evidence of a recent or current viral infection.

What is the treatment?

There is no specific treatment. If your child has been away from school for a long time, a gradual return should be arranged. Ask teachers about possible causes of anxiety in school that could be alleviated. Your child is considered to be cured once he or she has returned to school full time. However, if one or more relapses occur, the help of a child psychiatrist may be required.

EAR AND EYE DISORDERS

JUST AS THEY CATCH COLDS EASILY, most children have several attacks of ear and eye infections caused by either viruses or bacteria. By the time they reach the age of 7 or 8 years, they have usually become immune to the more common viruses, and infections become less troublesome; bacterial infections are usually easily treated by antibiotics. Occasionally, ear and eye infections may cause severe illness, and symptoms should never be ignored. Persistent ear infections may lead to hearing difficulties, which can delay speech and learning. Early detection and treatment of vision problems is vital to enable vision to develop normally.

OTITIS MEDIA

Inflammation of the middle ear, called otitis media, is a common cause of earache in children. Otitis media most frequently affects children up to 8 years old. It is often a painful complication of an upper respiratory tract infection, such as a COMMON COLD (p.148) or a throat infection (see PHARYNGITIS AND TONSILLITIS, p.151).

How is it caused?
When bacterial or viral infection spreads up the eustachian tube (the narrow canal that connects the middle ear to the back of the throat), the tissues that line the middle ear become inflamed and produce fluid and sometimes pus. The secretions are unable to drain away because the eustachian tube is blocked by the inflammation or by ENLARGED ADENOIDS (p.149). The accumulating secretions cause pain as they press on the eardrum, which sometimes splits.

What are the symptoms?
Earache is the main symptom of otitis media. However, in a very young child, who may have difficulty in locating the site of the pain (especially if both ears are affected), fever and vomiting may be the only initial symptoms. In children of all ages, otitis media may produce the following symptoms:
• Waking at night, crying.
• Irritability.
• Tugging at or rubbing one ear.
• Partial deafness.
• A discharge from the ear, which relieves pain but signals that the eardrum has split.
Your child should be seen by a doctor within 24 hours if you think he or she has otitis media. You should phone a doctor at once if the pain is severe or if your child is very young.

What can I do to help?
To relieve the pain while waiting to see the doctor, your child should be given liquid paracetamol and should rest the painful ear on a hot water bottle that is wrapped in a towel (see illustration right). Fill the bottle with warm, not hot, water. Resting with the affected side of the head turned downwards will allow any discharge to drain out. You should not use a hot water bottle to relieve earache in a baby, because he or she will not be able to push it away if it is too hot. Instead, heat a soft cloth and hold it against the baby's ear.

What might the doctor do?
The doctor will examine your child's ear with an auriscope (a viewing instrument). If there is a discharge from the ear, a sample may be sent for tests to identify the infectious organisms. The doctor may prescribe a course of oral antibiotics, which should bring down your child's temperature and relieve the pain within 2 days. If the earache and fever do not subside after 3 days, the doctor may prescribe a different antibiotic for your child. Fluid sometimes remains in the middle ear for as long as 3 months so that your child may continue to be partially deaf. An eardrum that has split should heal within about a week.

The doctor will probably give your child a hearing test 3 months after the attack of otitis media to ensure that his or her hearing has returned to normal. If your child's hearing is still impaired, GLUE EAR (opposite) may be a cause.

What is the outlook?
As a child grows, the eustachian tube increases in width, allowing fluid to drain out more easily. The middle ear is therefore much less vulnerable to infection. Your child is not likely to have attacks of otitis media after he or she is about 7 or 8 years of age.

Easing earache
Lying flat may make earache worse. Prop your child up with pillows while he or she rests the painful ear on a hot water bottle.

GLUE EAR

This condition occurs when the middle ear becomes filled with a thick, sticky, glue-like mucus that is produced by the lining of the middle ear. Hearing is usually impaired because the mucus reduces the ability of the eardrum and the small bones in the middle ear to vibrate fully and transmit sound to the inner ear.

How is it caused?
Glue ear results from overproduction of mucus by the lining of the middle ear. The excess mucus accumulates in the middle ear, particularly if the eustachian tube (the narrow canal that connects the middle ear to the back of the throat) is blocked by inflammation. Glue ear may develop if OTITIS MEDIA (opposite) is left untreated or is not treated adequately; it may appear even if there is adequate treatment.

What are the symptoms?
If your child has glue ear, he or she may:
• Complain of partial deafness. Your child's hearing may be worse at some times than others.
• Be inattentive and slow at learning.
Pain is seldom a symptom of glue ear, so your child may be affected for some time before the condition is detected. Your child should be seen by a doctor if you think he or she has glue ear.

What might the doctor do?
The doctor will examine the ears with a viewing instrument and may refer your child to an ear, nose, and throat specialist. The specialist will carry out a hearing test; he or she may also measure the movements of the eardrum. If the test results are abnormal, they will be repeated 3 months later. If the condition of the ear has not improved, while your child is under a general anaesthetic, a hollow needle may be used to withdraw fluid from the middle ear. In some cases, a small cut is made in the eardrum, and a tiny plastic tube called a grommet is inserted (see illustration below). The grommet falls out 2 months to 2 years after insertion; the eardrum heals a few days after the grommet drops out.

What is the outlook?
The width of the eustachian tube will increase as your child grows, and fluid will drain much more efficiently from the middle ear. Glue ear is unlikely to occur after your child is 8 years of age.

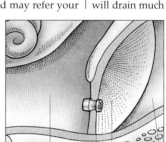

An eardrum grommet
A small tube called a grommet is inserted into the eardrum to allow air to enter, circulate, and dry out the middle ear.

Middle ear | Grommet | Eardrum | Outer ear canal

OTITIS EXTERNA

There are several causes of otitis externa (inflammation of the outer ear canal), including bacterial infection and skin conditions such as SEBORRHOEIC DERMATITIS (p.134) and ATOPIC ECZEMA (p.135). The risk of infection is increased if the sensitive skin lining the ear canal is exposed to water for too long, for example during swimming; or if the lining is scratched or irritated by a foreign body, such as a cotton swab, or by long-standing wax blockage.

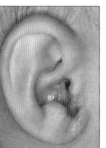

An infected ear canal
A child who has otitis externa may have a discharge from the ear canal. Although you may be tempted to wipe the discharge away, it should be left so that a doctor may send a sample for tests to determine the cause of the infection.

What are the symptoms?
The outer, fleshy part of the ear may be tender when it is touched or moved. However, the symptoms mainly affect the ear canal and may include:
• Itchiness, usually followed by pain.
• Discharge from the canal, which may be thick and white or yellowish.
• Partial deafness, if wax or a discharge is blocking the canal.
• Weeping, crusting blisters.
Your child should be seen by a doctor within 24 hours if he or she has an earache, a discharge from the outer ear canal, or difficulty hearing.

What might the doctor do?
The doctor will probably examine your child's ear with an auriscope (a viewing instrument). If there is a discharge of pus from the ear canal, a sample may be taken and sent for tests. If the doctor finds a foreign body or a plug of wax, he or she will remove it, and clean and dry the canal. Antibiotic ear drops may be prescribed. If either atopic eczema or seborrhoeic dermatitis is the cause of your child's otitis externa, the doctor may prescribe corticosteroid ear drops to relieve any itching and tenderness. With treatment, otitis externa usually clears up within 7 to 10 days.

What can I do to help?
You may give your child paracetamol to relieve the pain. A hot water bottle (which you should fill with warm, not hot, water) or a warm cloth held against your child's ear may also provide some relief. If your child has been prescribed ear drops, have him or her lie down with the affected ear uppermost. Hold your child's head still while you give the ear drops, and make sure that your child lies still for a minute or two after they have been given.

Your child should not swim or get the ear wet until the otitis externa has cleared up. Keep the affected ear dry by covering it with a shower cap during a bath or shower and by sponging your child's hair clean instead of washing it.

LABYRINTHITIS

The labyrinth (the inner ear) contains the fluid-filled chambers that are concerned with balance. Labyrinthitis (inflammation of the labyrinth) occurs as a complication of a viral infection and results in unpleasant feelings of dizziness and nausea.

What are the symptoms?
The symptoms of labyrinthitis occur in bouts, each of which lasts for between 5 and 15 minutes. Several bouts a day may occur. The main symptoms are:
• Vertigo, which is the sensation that the surroundings are spinning round and round uncontrollably.
• Unsteadiness and falling down. Your child has to lean on a wall or hold on to furniture to steady him- or herself.
• Nausea and vomiting.
Your child will probably feel extremely distressed by the condition. He or she should see a doctor within 24 hours of the symptoms developing.

What might the doctor do?
The doctor will examine your child and will ask whether he or she has had any illnesses recently. A special type of anti-histamine syrup may be prescribed to relieve the vomiting and dizziness. No other treatment is required.

What is the outlook?
Labyrinthitis usually clears up within 1 to 3 weeks, but it sometimes lasts for several months. Although labyrinthitis can be a frightening experience, it does not lead to any permanent disability.

BAROTRAUMA

This condition consists of temporary blockage of the eustachian tube (the passage that connects the middle ear and the throat) and bulging of the eardrum as a result of abrupt changes in atmospheric pressure. It is usually brought on by air travel.

How is it caused?
Air flow through the eustachian tube normally maintains equal air pressure inside and outside the middle ear. When an aircraft ascends, the air pressure in the cabin falls, and so does the pressure inside the middle ear. When the aircraft descends, pressure outside the middle ear increases, causing the eustachian tube to shut and pushing the eardrum inwards. An upper respiratory tract infection (such as a COMMON COLD, p.148), hay fever (see ALLERGIC RHINITIS, p.152), or an ear infection (see OTITIS MEDIA, p.162) makes barotrauma more likely.

What are the symptoms?
The symptoms of barotrauma are:
• Pain as the eardrum bulges in.
• Partial hearing loss.
• Ringing in the ears.
The symptoms usually disappear within 3 to 5 hours and do not cause any lasting damage. Liquid paracetamol relieves the pain.

How can I prevent barotrauma?
When an aircraft descends, sucking on a sweet, swallowing, chewing gum, or using the method shown on the right (called the Valsalva manoeuvre) all open the eustachian tube, allowing air to flow freely into the middle ear. In babies, barotrauma may be prevented by bottle- or breast-feeding during descent. A child who has a cold or another upper respiratory tract infection, hay fever, or an ear infection should not travel by air.

Preventing barotrauma
When your child begins to feel the pressure changing in the ear during descent in an aircraft, he or she should pinch the nose while keeping the mouth closed, and blow down the nose until the ears "pop".

IRITIS

Inflammation of the iris and the muscular ring that surrounds it (the ciliary body) is known as iritis. Serious attacks are rare in childhood, but children with JUVENILE CHRONIC ARTHRITIS (p.132) frequently suffer from a persistent or recurrent form of iritis.

What are the symptoms?
Iritis may affect one or both eyes at the same time. The main symptoms are:
• Pain (which may be dull or severe) in the affected eye.
• Redness of the white of the eye, particularly of the part around the edge of the iris.
• Acute sensitivity to light.
• Blurred vision.
• A swollen iris that has lost its normal colour and looks muddy.
• An irregularly shaped pupil, which (if only one eye is affected) is smaller than the pupil of the unaffected eye.
• Watering of the affected eye.
If you think your child may have iritis, you should phone a doctor at once.

What is the treatment?
The doctor may prescribe eye drops or an ointment containing a corticosteroid to reduce the inflammation. You may be able to relieve the symptoms by holding a pad of cotton wool dipped in warm water to the affected eye. Make sure that you boil the water first.

What is the outlook?
Treated promptly, iritis often clears up within 1 to 2 weeks and has no long-term ill effects. If iritis is not treated, or if it is persistent or recurrent, it can permanently damage vision.

CONJUNCTIVITIS

Inflammation of the thin, transparent membrane (conjunctiva) that covers the whites of the eyes and lines the eyelids is called conjunctivitis. A newborn baby may develop conjunctivitis as a result of infection by bacteria normally found in the birth canal; rarely, infection is transmitted by a mother who has gonorrhoea, genital herpes, or a chlamydial infection. In older children, the usual cause of conjunctivitis is viral infection. Conjunctivitis may also be a symptom of hay fever (see ALLERGIC RHINITIS, p.152).

What are the symptoms?
One or both eyes may be affected. The main symptoms are:
- Redness of the white of the eye and the inside of the eyelid.
- Itchiness and irritation of the eye.
- In bacterial conjunctivitis, yellow, sticky pus in the corner of the eye and on the eyelashes. Sticky lashes may make it hard for your child to open the affected eye in the morning.
- In allergic conjunctivitis, swollen eyelids and a clear discharge from the eye that is not sticky.

Should I consult a doctor?
Conjunctivitis affecting a baby may be detected and treated in hospital soon after birth. However, in some cases, the symptoms do not appear for several

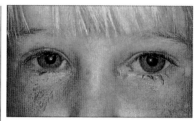

Appearance of bacterial conjunctivitis
The whites of the eyes are bloodshot and the eyelashes are gummy with yellow pus. Pus has also collected in the corners of the eyes.

weeks. If symptoms develop, contact your doctor at once. Although viral conjunctivitis in older children is not serious, your child should be seen by a doctor so that the possibility of a serious eye disorder can be excluded.

What is the treatment?
Bacterial infection is treated with an antibiotic ointment or eye drops, and usually clears up within a week. Oral or intravenous antibiotics may be given for severe bacterial infection, which may take up to 6 weeks to get better.

Viral conjunctivitis clears up without treatment within a week. To relieve the discomfort of allergic conjunctivitis, anti-inflammatory eye drops may be used. Some preparations are available over the counter; others are prescribed.

What can I do to help?
As often as needed, gently remove the sticky pus from your child's eyelashes with cotton wool that has been soaked in cooled, boiled water and squeezed out. To prevent the spread of infection, hands should be washed after touching the infected eyes, and washcloths and towels should not be shared. Viral conjunctivitis is especially contagious.

What is the outlook?
Provided treatment is given promptly, a baby infected during delivery should recover completely. In older children, infectious and allergic conjunctivitis never affect vision permanently.

BLOCKED TEAR DUCT

The tear ducts are narrow passages that drain excess fluid from the eyes to the inside of the nose. Sometimes one or both ducts are partially blocked by dead cells at birth, so that tear fluid cannot drain away. As a result, the baby's eye waters continually.

What are the symptoms?
The main symptoms are:
- Persistent watering of the eye, even when the baby is not crying.
- If the eye is infected (which is very rare), pus in the inner corner of the eye, and swelling of the side of the nose just below the eye's inner corner.

Should I consult a doctor?
In almost all cases, a blocked tear duct opens naturally by the age of 1 year. However, with treatment, the duct may open sooner than this. Therefore, make an appointment to see a doctor if your baby's eyes water continually. If there are signs of infection, your baby should be seen by a doctor within 24 hours.

What is the treatment?
The doctor will examine your child's eyes and, if there are no signs of an infection, he or she may suggest that you gently massage the upper part of the duct (see illustration right).

If the eye is infected, the doctor may prescribe an antibiotic ointment. Once the infection has cleared up (usually in a week, but check with the doctor to make sure), you may start the massage treatment to unblock the duct.

If the duct has not opened by the age of 1 year, the doctor may refer your baby to an ophthalmic surgeon. Under general anaesthetic, the specialist will clear the obstruction from your baby's tear duct using a thin metal probe.

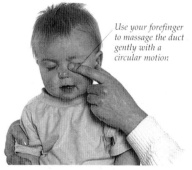

Use your forefinger to massage the duct gently with a circular motion

Unblocking a tear duct
After washing your hands, massage the skin just below the inner corner of the eye gently with your forefinger. Repeating this procedure three or four times a day for a week or two may force a blocked tear duct to open.

What is the outlook?
Once the duct is unblocked, the eyes should stop watering and your baby will be less susceptible to eye infection.

EYELID DISORDERS

Styes and blepharitis are common disorders affecting the eyelids in children. A stye is a pus-filled swelling that forms at the base of an eyelash. Blepharitis is inflammation of the eyelid edges. Although they cause discomfort, these disorders are not serious.

STYES

A stye results from an infection, usually by bacteria. Styes sometimes develop as a complication of blepharitis.

What are the symptoms?
The main symptoms of a stye are:
- A yellow head of pus on the eyelid around the base of an eyelash.
- Swollen and inflamed eyelid skin surrounding the head of pus.
- Pain or tenderness to the touch.

What is the treatment?
A stye usually clears up in a few days. Pressing a warm cloth to the infected area for about 20 minutes every hour may help to relieve the pain, and it also encourages the discharge of pus, which hastens healing. Avoid touching the stye to prevent spreading the infection.

A child with recurring styes should be seen by a doctor, who may prescribe an antibiotic ointment. Applying the ointment three or four times daily can prevent styes from recurring.

BLEPHARITIS

In many cases, blepharitis is associated with dandruff and most often affects children who suffer from SEBORRHOEIC DERMATITIS (p.134). Less commonly, it is due to viral or bacterial infection.

What are the symptoms?
The main symptoms of blepharitis are:
- A burning sensation, redness, and itching of the eyelid margins.
- Scales at the roots of the lashes. The scales in the seborrhoeic form of blepharitis are yellow and greasy.

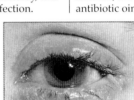
Infectious blepharitis
The eyelids are red and swollen, and crusted with scales. The white of the eye is red, indicating accompanying conjunctivitis.

- Sometimes, eyelashes that grow in the wrong direction or fall out.

In some cases infectious blepharitis is accompanied by CONJUNCTIVITIS (p.165). Your child should be seen by a doctor if you think he or she has blepharitis.

What is the treatment?
The doctor will show you how to wipe off any crusting scales from the eyelid margins using cotton wool moistened with warm water. He or she may take a swab from the lid margins for tests to determine the cause. If the eyelid is infected, the doctor may prescribe an antibiotic ointment, which you can apply after you have removed any scales. Infectious blepharitis usually clears up within 2 weeks; the ointment should be used for a further 2 weeks or more in order to prevent a recurrence. Seborrhoeic blepharitis tends to be persistent. Keeping dandruff under control helps prevent flare-ups.

SQUINT

An abnormality in the direction of the gaze of one eye is known as squint or strabismus. Most young babies squint occasionally up to the age of 2 to 4 months. However, a squint after the age of 4 months or a persistent squint at any age is abnormal.

How is it caused?
Babies squint because the mechanism that coordinates the eyes is not fully developed. A squint in older children is often due to severe longsightedness (see REFRACTIVE ERRORS, opposite), which causes the eyes to accommodate (adjust for near focus) too strongly, forcing one eye inwards. A squint can also be due to unequal refraction, which causes the two eyes to produce conflicting images. The weaker eye's image is suppressed and the eye is poorly controlled.

What are the symptoms?
The main symptoms of a squint are:
- An eye that turns too far in or out (convergent or divergent squint), or up or down (vertical squint), when a child looks directly at an object.

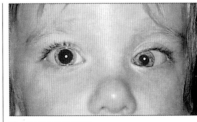
Convergent squint
This child has a convergent squint of the left eye. The normal eye looks straight ahead, while the left eye is focused inwards.

- Poor vision in the affected eye.
- Double or blurred vision, which the child may try to remedy by closing or covering the affected eye.

To prevent the double vision produced by a squint, the brain ignores the image from the weaker eye; because the eye is not used, its vision may eventually become permanently impaired.

If your child develops a squint after the age of 4 months or has a persistent squint, consult a doctor. He or she may send your child to an ophthalmologist.

What is the treatment?
The ophthalmoloigst will evaluate your child's vision. He or she may prescribe glasses if your child is longsighted or has another refractive error. Treatment may also involve covering the normal eye with a patch, which forces your child to use the affected eye. In some cases, the position of the deviating eye may be corrected by an operation. After the operation, your child will be given a series of eye exercises that encourage normal development of vision.

What is the outlook?
If treatment is provided within a few weeks of the squint appearing, a child's vision should develop normally.

REFRACTIVE ERRORS

Problems with the focusing mechanism of the eyes are known as refractive errors. There are three types of refractive error, all of which cause blurred vision to some degree. The three errors are shortsightedness (myopia), longsightedness (hypermetropia), and astigmatism. Refractive errors tend to run in families. Longsightedness and astigmatism are often present from birth. Shortsightedness is often not apparent until puberty, although it starts to develop a few years before a child reaches adolescence.

How are they caused?

Shortsightedness and longsightedness result from an incorrect relationship between the eyeball's length and the focusing power of the cornea, the front part of the eye (see illustrations below).

In shortsightedness, the images of distant objects are brought into focus in front of the retina and appear blurred.

In longsightedness, images of objects are focused behind the retina instead of on it. However, children who are mildly or moderately longsighted are able to see clearly because, in young eyes, accommodation (the process by which the eyes adjust for near focus) is strong enough to enable the focusing point to be brought forwards onto the retina.

Astigmatism occurs when the curve of the cornea is uneven. It results in an inability to focus on all the parts of an object at the same time; for example, horizontal lines may be in focus, while vertical lines appear blurred.

What are the symptoms?

If your child is shortsighted or has an astigmatism, he or she will probably not be aware that anything is wrong. However, your child may:
• Sit too close to the television set.
• Have problems with schoolwork, or appear not to be interested, because he or she cannot see what is going on at the front of the classroom.
• Complain that objects at a distance appear blurred.
If your child is severely longsighted, he or she may:
• Develop a SQUINT (opposite).
• Complain that nearby objects appear blurred.

Should I consult the doctor?

Your child should be seen by a doctor or an optician if you think that he or she might have a focusing problem. A doctor who suspects a refractive error will probably refer your child to either an optician or an ophthalmologist.

What might the optician or ophthalmologist do?

Your child's eyes will be tested one at a time. The method chosen for testing visual acuity (sharpness of vision) will depend on the age and reading ability of your child. Children who can read are usually tested using the standard adult vision-testing charts. A child who is unable to read may be tested with a chart showing the capital letter E in decreasing sizes and turned in various directions. He or she may be asked to show the orientation of the letter with a finger. A very small child's sight may be tested with charts showing images of familiar objects. Alternatively, a small child's vision may be examined using retinoscopy, which involves observing the movement of a light shone into the eye and reflected from the retina.

Once your child's visual acuity has been assessed, the severity of his or her refractive error will be established. To make sure of an accurate result, your child may be given atropine eye drops to paralyse temporarily the strong accommodation mechanism. A series of lenses is held in front of the eye, and the child is asked whether the vision improves with each lens. Once the combination of lenses that gives good vision has been found, the results are checked using retinoscopy.

The optician or ophthalmologist will prescribe glasses based on the figures obtained by retinoscopy. Contact lenses can, alternatively, be prescribed. They usually give better corrected vision than glasses and are often preferred by teenagers. The need for proper hygiene and disciplined wearing time makes them unsuitable for young children.

What is the outlook?

In most cases, refractive errors do not become any worse once body growth is complete. However, because the power of accommodation decreases with age, longsightedness that earlier did not produce any symptoms may become apparent during middle age.

SHORT- AND LONGSIGHTEDNESS

For vision to be clear, the focusing power of the cornea and the distance from the cornea to the retina must be in the correct relationship, so that the image of an object is brought into focus on the retina. Shortsightedness occurs when the cornea is too steeply curved and/or the eyeball is too long. Longsightedness occurs when the curve of the cornea is too flat and/or the eyeball is too short.

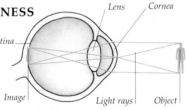

Normal vision
The shape of the eyeball and the focusing power of the cornea are correctly related. The image of an object is focused on the retina, and can be seen clearly.

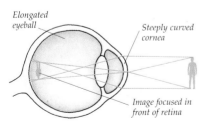

Shortsightedness
The eyeball is too long, and the focusing power of the steeply curved cornea is too strong. The image of a distant object is brought into focus in front of the retina, and appears blurred.

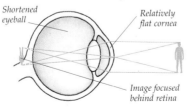

Longsightedness
The eyeball is too short and the focusing power of the relatively flat cornea is too weak. The image of an object is focused behind the retina, and appears blurred.

BEHAVIOURAL AND EMOTIONAL PROBLEMS

WHEN A CHILD BEHAVES in a way that causes concern, the problem for parents is to know whether the condition is likely to persist. Children usually grow out of upsetting or odd habits, but some require professional help. An early consultation with a doctor can help to relieve anxiety and determine whether treatment is likely to be needed.

SLEEP PROBLEMS

Children up to the age of 5 years are the group most commonly affected by sleep problems, although some older children may also be affected. The problems discussed below are usually temporary. Rarely, they are signs of anxiety (see ANXIETY AND FEARS, p.170) or, very rarely, of serious behavioural problems.

WAKEFULNESS AT NIGHT

Most children normally sleep through the night by the age of 1 year. If a child older than a year fails to settle at night or wakes during the night, you should try to identify the cause. Possible causes are lack of a fixed bedtime or putting your child to bed too early. Your child might also be afraid of the dark.

Imposing a sensible bedtime routine and being firm with your child may help him or her to settle at night. If your child is afraid of the dark, a night light may be helpful. Older children may respond to a reward system.

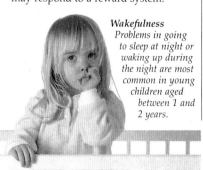

Wakefulness
Problems in going to sleep at night or waking up during the night are most common in young children aged between 1 and 2 years.

Should I consult a doctor?

Consult a doctor if the wakefulness is becoming unbearable. You may be asked to monitor your child's bedtime routine and sleep patterns, then make changes in order to establish a regular sleep pattern. This approach usually succeeds in establishing a normal sleep routine within a few weeks.

NIGHTMARES

Frightening dreams are most common in children aged 5 to 6 years. Usually, nightmares are triggered by disturbing experiences, for example, a frightening video. Sometimes, they indicate anxiety.

What can I do to help?

When your child is woken up by a nightmare, comfort him or her until sleep returns. Sometimes, nightmares can be prevented by vetting what your child watches on television. It may help to leave the bedroom door open or a light on. For some children, discussing the nightmares is helpful. If nightmares are persistent or frequent, your child should be seen by a doctor.

Nightmares usually occur less often after the age of 6 years, but people of all ages have them occasionally.

NIGHT TERRORS

Children aged 4 to 7 years seem most susceptible to night terrors, which tend to occur about 2 hours after falling asleep. Before a terror, the child becomes increasingly restless. During a terror, he or she seems to be awake and terrified, and is likely to scream, shout, and moan. However, the child is not awake and cannot be woken easily; he or she does not respond to comforting.

If you know when a night terror is likely to occur, you can wake your child in the restless period that precedes it or about 15 minutes before. There is very little you can do once a terror is under way apart from staying with your child.

Should I consult a doctor?

Consult a doctor if night terrors occur more than a few times a week. Sleeping medicine may be prescribed for a few weeks to alter the depth of sleep. Your child will outgrow night terrors.

SLEEPWALKING

This problem occurs most commonly in children aged 6 to 12 years. The child gets out of bed and wanders around, often finding his or her own way back to bed in a few minutes. There is no need to do anything except to make sure that your child is safe. Do not attempt to wake your child, but gently guide him or her back to bed if necessary.

Most children outgrow sleepwalking by puberty, but a minority continue to have episodes throughout their lives.

HABITUAL BEHAVIOUR

Many childhood habits are so common that they should be seen as normal. Habits may provide comfort for stress or anxiety or may be a means of expressing anger, frustration, or boredom. The most common habits of infancy are thumb-sucking, head-banging, and breath-holding attacks. Tics and compulsions affect mainly schoolchildren. Nail-biting and twirling or pulling hair can affect children of any age. Most habits do little harm.

THUMB-SUCKING

A child may suck his or her thumb when bored, nervous, or in need of comfort. Thumb-sucking is most common in children up to 3 years old, and is harmless. Some children continue until they are aged 6 or 7 years. In these cases, discuss trying to stop with your child. A reward system may help your child to give up.

Comforting habit
Thumb-sucking is the most common childhood habit. About half of all 3-year-olds suck their thumbs.

NAIL-BITING

About a third of all children bite their nails. The habit usually starts during a child's early years at school, and may persist into adulthood. Nail-biting may make the nails unsightly and painful. A young child may give up the habit if distracted when nail-biting occurs; older children may respond to a gift of a nail file and clippers or scissors.

HEAD-BANGING

A child who is frustrated, angry, or bored may bang his or head against a hard surface. Such behaviour occurs in a small number of preschool children, and usually disappears by the age of 4 years. Although alarming, it seldom harms the child. You may offer the child a cushion or pillow to soften the impact, but otherwise it is usually best to ignore the habit. If head-banging is severe or persistent, consult a doctor.

BREATH-HOLDING ATTACKS

A small number of preschool children habitually hold their breath for periods of up to 30 seconds. Rarely, a child passes out as a result. An attack may be brought on by pain or frustration, and may be used as a way of manipulating parents. You should ignore the attacks as much as possible. They usually disappear by the age of 4 years, but if you are concerned, consult a doctor.

TICS

Repetitive, involuntary movements, tics mainly affect schoolchildren. The head and face are most often involved; for example, rapid, repetitive blinking may occur. Tics are usually a result of stress and, in most cases, disappear on their own within a few months.

If a tic is severe or is accompanied by disturbing behaviour, consult a doctor. Your child will probably be referred to a child psychiatrist or a paediatrician for advice and treatment.

COMPULSIONS

Schoolchildren often have compulsions, in which they feel the need to perform a particular action, such as avoiding cracks in the pavement. Compulsions usually disappear if ignored. If they persist or get worse, consult a doctor.

TWIRLING OR PULLING HAIR

Children of all ages may twirl or pull their hair from frustration or anxiety. In most cases, these habits are not a cause for concern. Rarely, serious emotional disturbance may result in such severe hair-pulling that bald patches develop. Consult a doctor if your child is pulling out his or her hair.

Bald patch
The large, bald patch on this child's scalp was caused by repetitive hair-pulling.

SOILING

Most children achieve bowel control by the age of 3 years. An occasional accident after this age is usually nothing to worry about. However, persistent soiling or soiling that starts after a child has been toilet-trained indicates a problem.

What are the causes?

Soiling is most often a result of chronic CONSTIPATION (p.181). Hard faeces cannot be passed, and faecal liquid leaks out. Some illnesses occasionally cause soiling due to diarrhoea. Slowness in achieving bowel control, poor toilet-training, or stress are other possible causes. Soiling in which the child passes faeces in inappropriate places (encopresis) is a sign of serious emotional disturbance.

Should I consult a doctor?

Consult a doctor if your child is soiling after the age of 3 years, he or she starts soiling after having achieved bowel control, or has encopresis. The doctor will examine your child and treat him or her for any physical causes of soiling. For other cases of soiling, the doctor may suggest the measures on the right. A child with encopresis will probably be referred to a child psychiatrist.

What can I do to help?

Punishing your child for soiling may make the problem worse. Gently but firmly encourage frequent defecation. Your child should sit on the toilet after every meal for about 5 minutes; give him or her a book to read. Every time your child defecates into the toilet, give praise and perhaps a treat. To prevent relapse, you may need to continue this treatment for 3 to 6 months after soiling has stopped. Try to identify sources of anxiety for your child and remove or alleviate them as far as possible.

With appropriate treatment, most soiling problems disappear within a few weeks. If they persist, see a doctor.

ANXIETY AND FEARS

All children experience anxiety and fears. A degree of anxiety is normal in many situations; for example, a child may cry for a few minutes when separated from a parent. Short-lived specific fears of the dark, animals, thunder, or places, such as school, are also common. Anxiety and fears only become a cause for concern when they last longer than a few months, are so severe that they amount to a phobia, and/or disrupt a child's life.

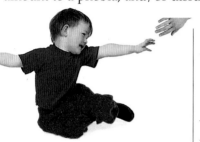

Separation anxiety
Preschool children often feel frightened and anxious when they are separated, even briefly, from their parents, especially their mothers.

What are the symptoms?
In children, the presence of anxiety or specific fears may be indicated by:
• Prolonged or persistent crying.
• Irritability and temper tantrums.

• Poor appetite and sleep disturbance.
• ENURESIS (p.192) and SOILING (p.169).
• Unexplained physical symptoms, such as recurrent stomach pains, headaches, and limb or joint pains.
• Tics and compulsions (see HABITUAL BEHAVIOUR, p.169).

What are the causes?
Anxiety and fears are often a result of insecurity. There may be an obvious trigger or cause of distress, such as being parted from a parent (known as separation anxiety), problems at school or at home, or difficulties with a peer group. Children may pick up anxiety or specific fears from other people. For example, fear of loud noises or insects may develop because a child is aware that his or her mother dislikes them.

What can I do to help?
Talking to your child about his or her worries and fears may help. If possible, take steps to remove or limit the causes.

Making a fuss about fears may only increase them. In general, it is best to adopt a calm and reassuring attitude, acknowledging and accepting a child's concern. Try to help your child gain the confidence to deal with his or her particular fear. For example, you may cuddle your child while you both look at pictures of animals he or she fears.

Should I consult a doctor?
There is no need to worry about short-lived episodes of anxiety or fearfulness, especially in toddlers. However, if a child's anxieties or fears persist, or are so intense that they interfere with daily life, consult a doctor. He or she will try to identify underlying problems, and may suggest using reward schemes and relaxation techniques. If a problem is particularly troublesome, your child may be referred to a child psychiatrist.

Anxiety and fears usually disappear within a few months. However, a child who has experienced severe problems may have recurrences later in life.

ATTENTION DEFICIT DISORDER

Young children are normally very active and, in most cases, nothing is likely to be wrong. However, a child who is restless, impulsive, and unable to concentrate may have attention deficit disorder (ADD). If the child is very hyperactive or restless and performs poorly in school, the disorder is called Attention Deficit Hyperactivity Disorder (ADHD). Diagnosis is best made by a child psychiatrist.

What are the causes?
The cause of ADD is usually unknown, but in a small minority the cause may be brain damage, psychological stress, or FOOD INTOLERANCE (p.182). Severe cases may have a genetic component.

The condition occurs more often in boys than girls, and tends to appear between the ages of 3 and 7 years.

What are the symptoms?
Symptoms of ADD may not be noticed until a child goes to school and his or her behaviour is seen in comparison with that of other children.

A child with ADD may be:
• Unable to concentrate.
• Excessively restless.
• Impulsive and excitable.
• Destructive, disruptive, and accident prone.
• Irritable and aggressive.
Consult a doctor if you are concerned that your child's behaviour is abnormal.

What is the treatment?
The doctor may refer your child to a child psychologist, a child psychiatrist, or a

paediatrician for assessment. If ADD is diagnosed, treatment will depend on its severity and cause. You may receive advice about giving your child opportunities to expend energy. If tests suggest food intolerance is a factor, a special diet may be advised. Some children need specialist educational help. Severe ADD may be treated with stimulant drugs which, oddly, have a calming effect and improve concentration.

What is the outlook?
Most children with ADD improve with treatment and as they get older. In a few cases, antisocial behaviour appears later in childhood.

Hyperactive child
A child who has ADD is very restless and tends to change activities frequently.

AUTISM

This disorder affects a child's ability to relate to others. Autism is usually noticeable by the age of 3 years and tends to affect boys more than girls. The cause is unknown, but the disorder has a genetic predisposition and may also be associated with minor brain damage before, during, or shortly after birth.

What are the symptoms?
Autism varies in severity, but a child with the disorder may:
- Fail to make eye contact or point to objects in order to draw people's attention to them.
- Engage in repetitive behaviour, such as flapping the hands or moving a toy.
- Be later than expected for his or her age in developing speech or language skills (see SPEECH PROBLEMS, below).
- Appear indifferent to other people.
- Prefer solitary activities.
- Show no interest in creative play.
- Be upset by changes in routine.
- Have LEARNING DIFFICULTIES (p.172).

You should consult a doctor if you are concerned about your child's speech or language development, or if he or she is having learning difficulties or seems to have difficulty relating to others.

What is the treatment?
If autism is suspected, your child may be referred to a child psychologist or psychiatrist, who will assess your child.

There is no curative treatment for autism. Your child may be helped by communication and language therapy and special education. Most autistic children attend schools for children with learning difficulties. A minority can go to ordinary schools, where they receive specialist support. Parents can help by teaching their children as many self-help skills as possible.

What is the outlook?
Autistic children who receive treatment tend to improve gradually throughout childhood and adolescence. Although some autistic children achieve a degree of independence as adults, almost all remain disabled to a certain extent and continue to find relating to other people difficult throughout their lives.

SPEECH PROBLEMS

Problems with speech are common in childhood, especially in boys. The most common problem is delay in speaking, which may result from a problem with understanding language or with speech production. Other common difficulties are stammering and lisping. Specific speech or language problems are common in children whose development is normal. In some cases, they may be associated with LEARNING DIFFICULTIES (p.172) or AUTISM (above).

DELAY IN SPEAKING
Impaired hearing, which is most often due to recurrent ear infections (see OTITIS MEDIA, p.162) or GLUE EAR (p.163), is a major cause of speech delay. There may be a familial tendency to speak late or a physical disorder, such as CEREBRAL PALSY (p.160), that makes it difficult for a child to control the various parts used in speech. A child may learn to speak later than other children if there is little conversation or interaction with parents. Children from bilingual families or who are left-handed or ambidextrous are sometimes late in speaking.

Should I consult a doctor?
If, by the age of 2 years, your child has not spoken any words or is not able to follow even simple commands, consult a doctor. The doctor will probably ask questions about the family background and will arrange for a hearing test. A speech therapist or child development team may be asked to assess your child.

Speech production
Air from the lungs vibrates the vocal cords to produce noise. Controlled and coordinated by the brain, movements of the mouth, lips, and tongue modify the noise to produce speech; contact of the tongue with the teeth or palate allows articulation of certain sounds.

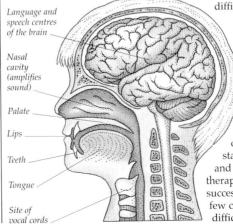

Language and speech centres of the brain

Nasal cavity (amplifies sound)

Palate

Lips

Teeth

Tongue

Site of vocal cords

What is the treatment?
A hearing problem will be dealt with first. The speech therapist may give you advice on techniques for encouraging your child to speak and may also work directly with your child. A child who has learning difficulties or a permanent hearing problem will probably require specialist educational help.

What is the outlook?
Children with verbal skills only slightly below those expected for their age, and who are not slow in other areas, tend to catch up with their peers. Those who are more behind should improve with treatment, but some may later develop difficulties with reading and writing.

SPEECH DIFFICULTIES
Children who are learning to speak often lisp or leave out consonants because they are not yet physically able to articulate sounds, and many children aged between 2 and 4 years go through a period of stammering. These problems often disappear before a child starts school. If they are persistent and severe, consult a doctor. Speech therapy may be needed, and is usually successful in curing the problem. In a few cases, stammering or other speech difficulties persist into adult life.

LEARNING DIFFICULTIES

A child with learning difficulties functions at a level below that expected for his or her age. Difficulties that affect all aspects of learning are known as general learning difficulties. A difficulty that affects only one particular sphere of learning, such as reading or writing, is termed a specific learning difficulty.

GENERAL LEARNING DIFFICULTIES

This term has now replaced "mental retardation" because it is felt to carry less stigma. A physical disability, such as CEREBRAL PALSY (p.160), is sometimes associated with the difficulties.

What are the causes?
The known causes of general learning difficulties include genetic disorders, such as DOWN'S SYNDROME (p.198), PHENYLKETONURIA (p.201), and FRAGILE X SYNDROME (p.199); impaired hearing or vision; and brain damage that occurred before, during, or shortly after birth. For many children, no specific cause can be identified. In rare cases, severe emotional problems are the cause.

What are the symptoms?
There is a wide range of disability so the symptoms are varied. A child may have been diagnosed at birth with a disorder, such as Down's syndrome, that includes learning difficulties. It may become clear early in life that a seemingly normal child has learning difficulties, or no signs may appear until a child starts school. A child with general learning difficulties may:
• Sit up and walk later than expected for his or her age.
• Be slow in developing speech (see SPEECH PROBLEMS, p.171).
• Fail to notice and respond to sounds and so appear to be deaf.
• Fail to make progress at school.
Some children may, additionally, show signs of ANTISOCIAL BEHAVIOUR (p.174) or ATTENTION DEFICIT DISORDER (p.170).

What is the treatment?
Treatment is aimed at helping a child achieve his or her maximum potential. A specialist will assess your child by using a series of psychological and/or developmental tests. Your child may be offered educational assistance (either in a normal school or in special classes or units), speech therapy, occupational therapy, and/or psychotherapy.

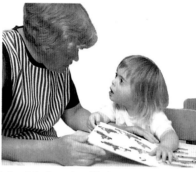

Special educational help
Children who have general learning difficulties need special educational help to enable them to achieve their maximum potential. They are often taught individually or in small classes.

What is the outlook?
With appropriate educational support, a child with mild or moderate general learning difficulties may achieve some degree of independence by adulthood. A child who has more severe learning difficulties will probably benefit from the right kind of help but is unlikely ever to be completely independent.

SPECIFIC LEARNING DIFFICULTIES

A child whose general development is normal for his or her age, but who is 2 or more years below the expected level in one area of learning, is said to have a specific learning difficulty. The difficulty may be with reading and/or writing (sometimes called dyslexia), or with arithmetical ability.

What are the causes?
Specific learning difficulties may be due to impaired hearing or vision or minor brain damage. In most cases, however, the causes of the problems are unknown.

What are the symptoms?
A child with a specific learning difficulty may not show any signs of the problem until the time when speech, language, and arithmetical skills would normally have developed. A child who has a specific learning difficulty may:
• Be slow in developing speech.
• Have difficulty telling left from right.
• Find spatial tasks, such as doing jigsaw puzzles, difficult.
• Have below-average drawing ability.
• Have difficulty telling certain letters apart, such as "p" and "q".
• Read from back to front, and reverse letters or symbols when writing.
• Find spelling particularly hard.
• Have difficulty in counting objects or recognizing numerical symbols.
• Show antisocial behaviour.
If you believe your child has a specific learning difficulty, consult a doctor.

What is the treatment?
Your child's hearing and vision will be tested. Besides receiving any medical treatment that is required, your child may be given specialist educational help and, if he or she has behavioural problems, psychotherapy. To improve your child's confidence, encourage him or her in areas such as woodworking, where reading, writing, and arithmetic are not so important.

What is the outlook?
The outlook depends on the severity of the problem and the age of your child when it was first detected. Children whose learning was delayed as a result of a physical problem, such as impaired hearing, tend to catch up quickly once the problem has been treated. Most children who need special educational help show improvement and a number make good progress. Some children continue to experience difficulties in a particular area throughout their lives.

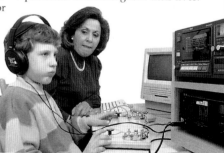

Testing a child's hearing
A child with a learning difficulty is given a hearing test. Sounds of varying pitch and loudness are played into one ear. The child presses a switch to indicate when and in which ear he or she has heard the sounds.

EATING DISORDERS

Most common in adolescents, especially girls, anorexia nervosa and bulimia nervosa are eating disorders in which there is a fear of becoming fat and a preoccupation with body shape. Another type of eating problem is overeating, which may lead to a child being overweight or obese. Obesity (weighing 20 per cent or more than expected for a person's height and sex) is common in developed countries and can lead to serious health problems.

ANOREXIA AND BULIMIA

These disorders may develop because a teenager feels insecure and associates thinness with attractiveness. The desire to avoid growing up by staying thin and undeveloped may also be a cause. Anorexia and bulimia are dangerous illnesses that must be taken seriously.

What are the symptoms?

An adolescent suffering from anorexia or bulimia may:
- Be fussy about food and eat little.
- Binge and purge (a more prominent feature of bulimia than anorexia).
- Feel guilty, anxious, and depressed about his or her eating behaviour.
- Use a large amount of laxatives.
- Exercise excessively.
- Avoid eating with the family.
- Wear clothes that conceal thinness.
- In girls, menstrual periods may fail to begin, become irregular, or stop.

A child with long-standing anorexia becomes thin, weak, and lethargic; fine hair may grow on the face and trunk;

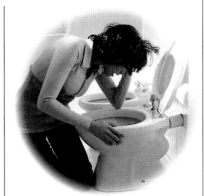

Bingeing and purging
Bouts of overeating followed by self-induced vomiting are the main features of bulimia. These activities are often carried out in secret.

and skin becomes dry. Rarely, a child may starve to death. A child who has bulimia is at risk of dehydration.

Your child should be seen by a doctor if you think that he or she might be suffering from anorexia or bulimia.

What is the treatment?

Treatment consists of a programme of supervised eating and psychotherapy to help modify eating habits. A stay in hospital may be required. Sometimes, long-term psychotherapy is needed.

If treated promptly, most adolescents who have anorexia or bulimia make a full recovery. However, some continue to have eating problems throughout life. A very small number of those with anorexia die, often by suicide.

OVEREATING AND OBESITY

The main cause of obesity is probably a family pattern of overeating, although there may also be a genetic factor. To help your child lose weight, set a good example by eating healthily yourself and encouraging him or her to do the same. Consult a doctor if there is no improvement within a few months.

What is the treatment?

Your child will be measured, weighed, and examined to exclude any physical disorders. The doctor will ask about your child's intake of food at mealtimes and between, and whether there are any emotional or behavioural problems. Treatment consists of a low-calorie diet; behaviour therapy may be considered to help alter a child's eating patterns.

The earlier a child is given treatment, the better the outlook for establishing and maintaining a normal weight.

DEPRESSION

Most people feel sad sometimes. In true depression, however, there are intense feelings of hopelessness, lack of self-worth, and guilt that last longer than a few days. In children, depression most often affects teenagers and is an important cause of suicide.

What are the causes?

The reasons for depression are varied. Grief over the loss of a loved one may develop into depression. Some types of depression run in families, and there may also be a biochemical factor. Stress is sometimes an aggravating factor.

What are the symptoms?

A child who is depressed may:
- Look unhappy most of the time.
- Have frequent bouts of crying.
- Be irritable, listless, and inattentive.
- Complain of feeling anxious, bored, sad, or tired most of the time.
- Perform badly at school.
- Wake very early in the morning.
- Lose weight or gain too much weight.
- Have headaches, or stomachaches and diarrhoea, with no apparent cause.

What can I do to help?

You may be able to end a mild bout of depression by talking to your child and trying to identify the reason for his or her feelings. Offer emotional support and try to remove or limit any sources of anxiety. Taking up a sport or hobby; exercising; or mixing with others may also help lift mild depression.

Should I consult a doctor?

If the depression deepens or persists for more than a few weeks, or if grief over the loss of a loved one has lasted for more than a few months, a doctor should see your child. Treatment may consist of psychotherapy and/or, for severe cases, antidepressant drugs.

Most children improve soon after receiving treatment, although some remain depressed for several months before showing improvement. In a minority, depression recurs or persists, and occasionally leads to suicide.

ANTISOCIAL BEHAVIOUR

Behaviour that has a negative impact on others or their property may be termed antisocial. Almost all children behave antisocially at some point; it is only when the behaviour becomes persistent, recurrent, or extreme that it is a cause for concern.

What forms does it take?
Although characterized by aggression and disobedience at all ages, antisocial behaviour tends to take different forms in different age groups.
Preschool children:
• Physical attacks on other children and/or on parents.
• Deliberately destroying objects.
• Temper tantrums.
Schoolchildren and adolescents:
• Bullying or fighting other children.
• Cruelty to other children or animals.
• Stealing and lying.

• Being disruptive in class.
• Truancy and vandalism (these occur mainly in adolescents).

What are the causes?
Antisocial behaviour often reflects an underlying problem. An undiscovered disability, such as deafness, or desires being thwarted may lead to frustration or anger in young children. At any age, unhappiness at home or at school may be the problem. Aggression is usually learned by example, from parents, the media, or a peer group.

What can I do to help?
Provided temper tantrums are ignored, they almost always stop within a few months. With an aggressive child of any age, be consistent, firm, and loving. Talk with an older child or teenager to find out the causes of the behaviour.

If antisocial behaviour is persistent or severe, you should consult a doctor, who may refer you and your child to a child and family guidance clinic.

What is the outlook?
Antisocial behaviour can be curtailed provided it is dealt with before it has become entrenched. Many children outgrow the behaviour after the age of 15 years. Children whose antisocial behaviour is severe and prolonged are likely to become antisocial adults.

SUBSTANCE ABUSE

The use of a drug or chemical to alter the way the mind works is termed substance abuse. It is rare before adolescence, and more common in boys than girls. Substances most frequently abused are alcohol, tobacco, solvents (such as glue, lighter fuel, or paint thinner, which are inhaled), cannabis (marijuana), amphetamines ("speed", including Ecstasy), and LSD. Abuse of hard drugs, such as heroin or cocaine, does not usually occur in this age group.

What are the causes?
Children experiment with substances in order to have enjoyable, exciting, or new experiences, to "fit in" with their peer group, or to feel grown up. Some may use substances to relieve anxiety and depression caused by problems at school or at home. For a minority of children, the abused substance becomes the focal point of their life: a physical and/or psychological dependence on it develops. Dependence is more likely when a drug is used to relieve emotional problems.

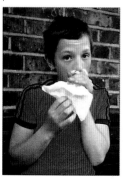

Using solvents
Inhaling solvents is most common among younger teenagers. It can lead to brain, liver, and/or kidney damage.

How can I prevent it?
A child is less likely to drink too much if others in the family do not drink or drink only moderately. If people in the family do not smoke, your child is less likely to take up the habit.

Prohibition of drugs is not helpful. Discuss with your child the drugs he or she may be offered and explain honestly the harm that drugs can cause. Point out the legal risks that may be involved. Your child will almost certainly be less vulnerable to substance abuse if he or she has other interests to occupy his or her time. Spend time with your children so that they know and trust you.

What are the signs?
Alcohol use and cigarette smoking are usually easy to detect. It may be hard to tell if your child is abusing another substance unless he or she is doing so on a regular basis. Although different substances have different effects, there are some general changes in behaviour

that may indicate your child is abusing a substance on a regular basis:
• Changes in sleeping patterns.
• General lack of energy or drowsiness.
• Unusual moodiness, irritability, or aggressiveness.
• Changes in appetite.
• Increased time spent away from home.
• Lies and secretiveness about activities.

What can I do to help?
If you think that your child is abusing a substance, do not overreact. Try to find out why the abuse has taken place so that you can give appropriate help. For example, if your child is taking drugs because of emotional problems, extra attention and support may give your child the self-confidence to stop.

Consult a doctor if you think your child may be becoming dependent on a drug. Advice on support and treatment is also available from many voluntary groups, advice centres, and helplines.

What is the outlook?
Most children who abuse substances do so only occasionally, and after some experimentation, give up altogether. It is very rare for a child to progress to hard drugs. A child who has become dependent on a substance can usually be helped provided that he or she has recognized the problem and positively wants help in giving up the habit.

MOUTH AND TEETH DISORDERS

YOUNG CHILDREN USE THEIR MOUTHS for exploring the world around them. Most of the body is protected by tough skin, but the mouth is more vulnerable: the tongue and lining of the mouth are exposed to infections and are damaged easily by chewing coarse food or other objects. Although a child's first teeth are replaced by permanent teeth, which begin to emerge around the age of 6 years, both sets must be looked after carefully to avoid tooth decay and gum problems.

MOUTH ULCERS

Ulcers, which are open sores, may develop on the lining of the mouth or the margins of the tongue. Aphthous ulcers are the most common type of mouth ulcer; they develop for no known reason and tend to be recurrent. Although they may make your child's mouth very painful, they are not serious and usually heal on their own. Mouth ulcers may also be due to minor injury, for example from a jagged tooth, or, rarely, to an underlying disorder.

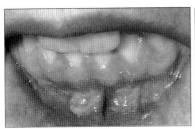

Appearance of an aphthous ulcer
An aphthous ulcer is seen here at the base of the gums of the lower jaw. It has a hollowed-out grey centre, with a raised, paler rim. The area surrounding the ulcer is inflamed.

What are the symptoms?
A child with mouth ulcers may have the following symptoms:
- A single ulcer or a cluster of ulcers inside the cheeks or lips or on the margin of the tongue. Each ulcer has a grey centre with a pale white or yellow rim and a red border.
- Painful, tender mouth, which may make your child reluctant to eat and to brush his or her teeth.

For 1 or 2 days before aphthous ulcers appear, there may be a sore or burning sensation of the lining of the mouth, the insides of the lips, or the tongue.

Most ulcers heal without treatment within 4 to 10 days. Mouth ulcers that are less than 2 mm ($1/12$ in) in diameter heal quickly; other, larger mouth ulcers may take longer to heal.

What can I do to help?
Your child may find that rinsing out his or her mouth with a dilute solution of bicarbonate of soda helps to relieve pain or tenderness. To make up the solution, dissolve ¼ teaspoon of bicarbonate of soda in 100 ml (3.5 fl.oz) of warm water. Another means of relieving discomfort is to apply an anaesthetic ointment or gel (available over the counter) to the ulcers. You may also give your child liquid paracetamol to relieve pain.

Avoid offering food or drinks that are acidic, spicy, hot, or salty, because they may irritate the ulcers. If chewing is very painful, offer your child soft foods or liquidize his or her meals. Drinking through a straw may help because it prevents liquid from bathing the ulcers.

Should I consult a doctor?
If the ulcers are causing your child a great deal of pain, fail to heal within 10 days, or recur frequently, make an appointment to see a doctor. If an ulcer recurs in the same place, your child should be seen by a dentist because a sharp tooth may be the cause.

To help reduce inflammation, ease pain, and speed healing, the doctor may prescribe hydrocortisone (a type of corticosteroid drug) lozenges. The lozenges are placed in the mouth, in contact with the ulcer, and allowed to dissolve slowly. Children over the age of 12 years may be given a tetracycline mouthwash (this treatment should not be given to younger children because it leads to discoloration of erupting teeth). Both of these treatments need to be repeated three or four times daily until the ulcers have disappeared, which is usually within 5 days. The treatments are most effective if they are started as soon as your child has the initial sore or burning sensation in the mouth.

If the doctor thinks that your child's mouth ulcers point to the presence of an underlying disease, he or she may arrange for your child to undergo tests.

What is the outlook?
Attacks of aphthous ulcers are usually infrequent, minor, and short-lived, and cause little distress. In some children, attacks occur frequently or are severe. The outlook is unpredictable, but most children grow out of the problem.

ORAL THRUSH

A yeast infection of the mouth, oral thrush occurs most commonly in babies during the first year of life. The infection is caused by an abnormal growth of the yeast *Candida albicans*, which occurs naturally in the mouth.

Appearance of oral thrush
Here, oral thrush has caused raised, white spots to appear inside the mouth. They occur on the gums and soft palate, and merge to form a foam-like coating on the tongue.

How is it caused?
The amount of *Candida* in the mouth is usually small, but the balance between *Candida* and oral bacteria (which keep it in control) may be upset by a course of antibiotics or by general illness.

What are the symptoms?
The main symptoms of oral thrush are:
• A sore mouth, which may make your baby reluctant to feed.
• Creamy-yellow or white spots on the tongue and the lining of the mouth (see photograph right). Your child should be seen by a doctor within a few days if you think he or she may have oral thrush.

What is the treatment?
The doctor will examine your child and may send scrapings from the mouth for analysis. He or she may prescribe antifungal gel or drops to apply to the inside of your baby's mouth. To help prevent reinfection, make sure you are meticulous when sterilizing feeding bottles and teats. If you are breast-feeding, the doctor may prescribe an antifungal cream, which you can use to treat your nipples.

GINGIVOSTOMATITIS

This rare illness causes painful ulcers to appear in the mouth. It results from a first infection by the herpes simplex virus, which also causes COLD SORES (p.139). Gingivostomatitis occurs most commonly in children between the ages of 6 months and 4 years.

What are the symptoms?
Gingivostomatitis usually starts with a fever and sore mouth. Infants are often irritable, restless, and unwilling to eat or drink anything. The following more distinctive symptoms soon develop:
• Painful, shallow ulcers on the gums, tongue, and palate.
• Red, swollen gums that bleed easily.
• Swelling of lymph nodes in the neck.
A child with these symptoms should be seen by a doctor within 24 hours.

What is the treatment?
If necessary, follow the advice given in the panel: *Relieving a sore mouth* (p.105). To prevent dehydration and provide energy, you should offer frequent, small drinks of milk or rehydrating solution (see panels: *Preventing dehydration in babies*, p.38, or *Preventing dehydration in children*, p.53).

The doctor may prescribe a course of the antiviral drug acyclovir. If the child is very ill or has been refusing fluids, he or she may be admitted to hospital so that acyclovir and rehydrating fluids can be given intravenously.

Without treatment for the infection, full recovery usually occurs in about 10 days. If given acyclovir within 3 days of the onset of severe symptoms, your child should recover more quickly.

GINGIVITIS

Inflammation of the gums is known as gingivitis. It may develop if a child does not clean his or her teeth and gums thoroughly. The condition is caused by the irritant effect of bacteria that live in plaque, a sticky deposit of food debris and saliva that collects on and around the teeth, and at the gum margins.

What are the symptoms?
The main symptoms of gingivitis are:
• Red, swollen, and tender gums.
• Tendency of the gums to bleed when they are brushed.
Gingivitis itself is a minor, reversible problem. However, if it is not checked, it may progress to a serious infection, with the risk that teeth may be lost. Your child should be seen by a dentist if you think he or she has gingivitis.

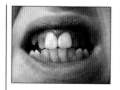
Signs of plaque
Disclosing agents reveal plaque. The stained areas show the places where plaque has accumulated.

What is the treatment?
If the gingivitis is mild, the dentist may just give your child instructions about how to look after for his or her teeth properly (see DENTAL CARIES, opposite, for advice on oral hygiene). For more advanced gingivitis, the dentist may also recommend that your child uses an antibacterial mouthwash to relieve inflammation and tenderness. When the gums are less tender, the dentist may scale (scrape) the teeth to remove plaque and calculus (hardened plaque).

What is the outlook?
With good oral hygiene, your child's gums should return to normal in a few months. Continued attention to proper oral hygiene combined with regular visits to the dentist for check-ups and scaling will help to prevent your child from having a recurrence of gingivitis.

DENTAL CARIES

Also known as tooth decay, dental caries was formerly the most common childhood disease. However, over the past 15 years, its prevalence and severity in children have greatly declined, mainly because of the addition of fluoride to toothpastes. This decline has now come to a halt, and in some areas, especially socially deprived ones, dental caries is becoming more common again. Research has shown that the increase in dental caries is due to the consumption of too much sugary food and drink.

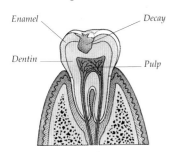

Enamel   *Decay*

Dentin   *Pulp*

Tooth decay
A cavity forms when acids produced by the bacterial breakdown of food erode the tooth's hard outer surface of enamel. The softer layer of dentin beneath is exposed, and as it too is eroded, the cavity gradually enlarges.

How is it caused?
Dental caries results from the action of the bacteria that live in plaque, a sticky coating of saliva and food debris that forms on the surface of the teeth. The bacteria use components of food and drinks (mainly sugars) for energy and, in breaking them down, produce acids. These acids, which are held in close contact with the teeth by plaque, cause calcium and phosphate to be lost from the tooth's enamel (demineralization). If this process continues unchecked, the enamel and eventually the dentin beneath is destroyed (see illustration above). If dental caries is not treated at this stage, the pulp at the centre of the tooth may become infected, resulting in permanent damage to the nerves and blood vessels that it contains.

What are the symptoms?
Early tooth decay does not usually cause any symptoms. The main symptoms of established caries are:
• Sensitivity of the tooth to hot, cold, and/or sweet foods or liquids.
• In very advanced decay, the tooth may be brown, have visible pits or holes in the enamel surface, and may also be very painful.

Should my child see a dentist?
Your child should be visiting a dentist regularly so that tooth decay can be detected at an early stage. However, if any symptoms of tooth decay develop between regular check-ups, you should make an appointment for your child to see a dentist within a few days.

What might the dentist do?
The dentist will examine your child's teeth and may also take X-rays. If the dentist finds signs of early decay, he or she may just clean the teeth and scrape them to remove plaque. This treatment allows the surface of the teeth to come into contact with saliva, which has a natural ability to remineralize enamel. A fluoride gel may also be applied.

For more advanced caries, the dentist may remove the decayed portion of the tooth, using a drill, and then insert a filling. If the nerve of the tooth has been irreversibly damaged or destroyed by infection, it may need to be removed. The entire tooth may need to be taken out if dental caries is very advanced.

How can I prevent dental caries?
A diet low in sugar, good oral hygiene, and regular visits to the dentist are the keys to preventing tooth decay.

The amount of sweet food and drink that your child consumes, and especially the frequency with which he or she has them, should be limited. Discourage sugary snacks and drinks between meals. Frequent consumption of acidic food and drinks, including fruit juice and all fizzy drinks (diet and regular) should also be avoided; ideally, your child should have them only with a meal. Fruit juice should be diluted to half strength with water and preferably drunk through a

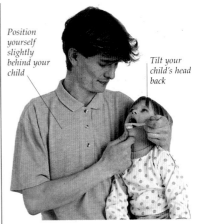

Position yourself slightly behind your child

Tilt your child's head back

Brushing your child's teeth
Until the age of 6 or 7 years, most children cannot brush their teeth effectively. Using a pea-sized amount of toothpaste, gently scrub all surfaces of your child's teeth thoroughly.

straw (as should fizzy drinks). Do not give a baby sweetened drinks in a bottle because the liquid will bathe the teeth and lead to rapid decay. Ask the dentist whether your water supply is fluoridated, and if fluoride treatment is advisable for your child.

Your child's teeth should be brushed twice a day with a fluoride toothpaste, after breakfast and especially last thing at night. If brushing after a meal is not convenient, it is a good idea to chew sugar-free gum, which stimulates the flow of saliva. Saliva neutralizes acid and helps to remineralize tooth enamel.

From the age of about 2½ years, your child should visit a dentist regularly for check-ups as often as the dentist advises, usually once every 6 months.

Visiting the dentist
At your child's routine dental examination, the dentist will examine the teeth for signs of tooth decay. X-rays may also be taken to detect areas of decay that may be hidden in the crevices of the teeth's biting surfaces.

The dentist gently probes the teeth to detect areas of decay

DENTAL ABSCESS

A dental abscess is a collection of pus around the root of a tooth. An abscess results when the pulp (the tooth's sensitive core, containing nerves and blood vessels) is invaded and destroyed by bacteria. Bacteria can enter the pulp cavity only if the tooth has been badly damaged or has become severely decayed.

What are the symptoms?
The main symptoms of an abscess are:
- A persistent and throbbing toothache.
- Severe pain in the tooth when biting or chewing on it, or when consuming hot foods or liquids.
- Tenderness, redness, and swelling of the gum around the affected tooth.
- Occasionally, a discharge of foul-tasting pus through an opening in the gum, after which the pain tends to subside.
- Looseness of the affected tooth.

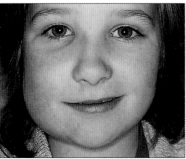

Swelling caused by a dental abscess
Infection that has spread from a dental abscess has caused the right side of this girl's face to swell. There is usually little pain at this stage.

If the infection spreads into surrounding tissue, the face and lymph glands in the neck may swell. Eventually, the child might develop symptoms of general infection, such as fever and headache.

Should my child see a dentist?
You should take your child to see a dentist within a few hours of any of the symptoms appearing.

If possible, the dentist will try to save the affected tooth. He or she will drill into your child's tooth to release the pus and relieve the pressure. The dead and dying pulp is removed, and the cavity washed, dried, and filled, a procedure known as root canal treatment. The dentist may extract the tooth if it is severely affected or if it is a primary ("milk") tooth. A course of antibiotics may be prescribed to clear up any remaining infection.

What can I do to help?
To relieve the pain while waiting to see the dentist, you may give your child liquid paracetamol. A well-wrapped hot water bottle held against the affected side of the face may also provide relief.

How can I prevent a dental abscess?
The tooth decay that sometimes results in a dental abscess can be prevented by good oral hygiene (see DENTAL CARIES, p.177), sensible eating habits (such as avoiding sweet foods), and by regular visits to the dentist every 6 months.

What is the outlook?
Following root canal treatment, a tooth usually functions as well as a healthy tooth. If a tooth has been removed, the other teeth often move into the space.

MALOCCLUSION

A poor fit between the upper and lower teeth when they bite together is called malocclusion. Treatment is necessary only if the teeth are so crooked or out of position that they look ugly or are difficult to clean, which increases the risk of tooth decay (see DENTAL CARIES, p.177) or gum problems (see GINGIVITIS, p.176).

How is it caused?
Malocclusion is most commonly caused by overcrowding of teeth. About two out of three 12-year-old children have overcrowded teeth. The condition is usually inherited and appears as the child's jaws and teeth develop. It may also occur when primary ("milk") teeth are lost early, because of either decay or injury. Early loss of this kind may lead to the remaining teeth moving into the gaps, so that there is insufficient room for the permanent teeth. Teeth that are overcrowded may grow to be crooked, overlapping, or too prominent.

Another, less common, inherited cause of malocclusion is misalignment of the jaws so that the upper or lower set of teeth is too far forwards or too far back.

Should my child see a dentist?
Regular 6-monthly visits to the dentist will allow the growth of the teeth and jaws to be monitored. However, if you are worried about your child's teeth or if your child is concerned about his or her appearance, make an appointment with the dentist as soon as possible. The dentist may recommend waiting to see if the malocclusion corrects itself as the jaws grow. If treatment is needed, your child will be referred to an orthodontist.

What is the treatment?
Orthodontic treatment is usually carried out at 11 to 13 years of age. If the teeth are overcrowded, the orthodontist may remove some of them and/or fit an orthodontic appliance (braces). Braces may be fixed (see photograph below) or removable. The braces exert pressure on the teeth to move them into the right position. In another type of treatment, a device called a bioblock, which the child bites into, is used to guide the growth of the jaws. Orthodontic treatment may take up to 2 years. Misalignment of the jaws may be corrected by surgery.

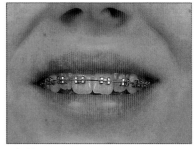

Fixed braces
This type of appliance is used most often to correct malocclusion. Brackets are cemented to the teeth; flexible wires are attached to the brackets and exert pressure to move the teeth.

DIGESTIVE SYSTEM DISORDERS

PROBLEMS AFFECTING THE digestive system are second only to colds and sore throats in frequency as causes of illness in childhood. Infections of the digestive system resulting in diarrhoea and/or vomiting are especially common. Although these symptoms may be upsetting for parent and child, they are rarely persistent enough to be a serious threat to health. Other digestive disorders are less common but some may cause chronic illness that can affect growth if not treated.

APPENDICITIS

The appendix is a small, worm-shaped tube that branches off the first part of the large intestine. It has no known function, yet for no apparent reason, it sometimes becomes infected and inflamed (appendicitis). Appendicitis is a common cause of abdominal pain requiring surgery in children under 16 years old.

What are the symptoms?
The main symptoms are:
- A dull pain in the lower abdomen (see illustration below). Slight pressure on the painful area, movement, or deep breathing increase the pain, and a child with appendicitis often lies still.
- Nausea, which may or may not be accompanied by vomiting.
- Fever.
- Constipation or diarrhoea.

Should I consult a doctor?
If the pain is so severe that it makes your child cry out or if the pain continues for 3 hours, phone a doctor at once. Call an ambulance or take your child to a hospital accident and emergency department if the pain has been continuous for more than 6 hours. If appendicitis is not treated promptly, the appendix may perforate (burst). Pus is then able to pass into the abdominal cavity, causing infection, and leading to a potentially fatal condition called peritonitis (inflammation of the lining of the abdominal cavity). If the appendix perforates, the pain affects the whole abdomen and is present continuously.

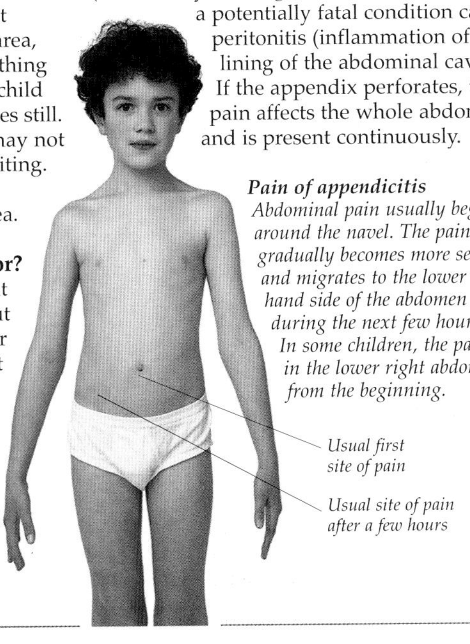

Pain of appendicitis
Abdominal pain usually begins around the navel. The pain gradually becomes more severe and migrates to the lower right-hand side of the abdomen during the next few hours. In some children, the pain is in the lower right abdomen from the beginning.

Usual first site of pain

Usual site of pain after a few hours

What can I do to help?
When an episode of abdominal pain occurs, it may be difficult to know at first whether or not it may be a serious problem. A hot water bottle wrapped in a towel may be held against the site of the pain. You should not give your child paracetamol or other painkillers because they may make the diagnosis more difficult for the doctor. The child should not eat or drink anything in case an operation may be necessary.

What might the doctor do?
The doctor will examine your child. If appendicitis is suspected, your child will be admitted to hospital. If further examinations indicate that appendicitis is likely, an operation to remove the appendix (appendicectomy) will be performed immediately.

Your child will be given painkillers for about 24 hours after the operation. If the appendix was not perforated, your child should be able to go home after 3 to 4 days. If the appendix was perforated, your child will be given antibiotics and will need to stay in hospital until the infection has cleared up, which may take about 7 days.

After leaving hospital your child will be able to eat a normal diet. Sports and strenuous physical activities should, however, be avoided for about a month.

GASTROENTERITIS

Attacks of gastroenteritis (inflammation of the stomach and intestines), causing diarrhoea and/or vomiting, are common in children. Although gastroenteritis is usually a mild illness, it can be serious, especially in infants. The most common cause of the illness in children is infection with viruses that are transmitted through the air or by contact with infected faeces. Bacteria transmitted in food or drinks may also cause gastroenteritis.

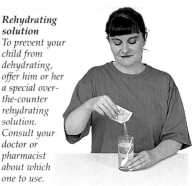

Rehydrating solution
To prevent your child from dehydrating, offer him or her a special over-the-counter rehydrating solution. Consult your doctor or pharmacist about which one to use.

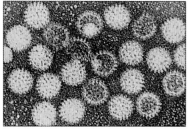

Micrograph of rotaviruses
A group of spherical viruses, rotaviruses are responsible for most cases of gastroenteritis in children aged under 2 years.

What are the symptoms?
Some or all of the following symptoms appear 1 to 5 days after infection:
- Diarrhoea.
- Vomiting.
- Loss of appetite.
- Abdominal pain.
- Lack of energy.
- Fever.

What are the complications?
Dehydration due to diarrhoea and/or vomiting is a serious complication of gastroenteritis. Young babies are at the greatest risk of becoming dehydrated.

Should I consult a doctor?
Phone a doctor at once if your child is under 2 months old and you suspect he or she might have gastroenteritis. You should also phone a doctor at once if your infant or child has any symptoms of dehydration (see *Danger signs*, pp.38 or 52). In other cases, you may try self-help treatment (see "What can I do to help?"). However, if the bout of gastroenteritis has not improved after 24 hours you should phone a doctor, even if the symptoms are mild.

What can I do to help?
To replace fluids lost through vomiting and/or diarrhoea, it is vital to give a child drinks of rehydrating solution (see panel: *Preventing dehydration in babies*, p.38 or *Preventing dehydration in children*, p.53 for quantities to give).

If your baby is entirely breast-fed, give the rehydrating solution first and then breast-feed. Provided that the symptoms subside, you may gradually reduce the amount of solution over a period of about 5 days.

For how to treat bottle-fed babies and older children, see the table below. For a weaned infant, follow the instructions given in the table for a bottle-fed baby. In addition, give no solids on Day 1. From Day 2 to Day 5, give a gradually increasing amount of puréed vegetables and fruit, followed by a light diet. A normal diet may be resumed on Day 6.

What might the doctor do?
The doctor will examine your child and decide whether treatment at hospital or home is needed. If your child is to be treated at home, you will be advised about how to care for him or her.

If your child is admitted to hospital, he or she may be given blood tests to determine how severe the dehydration is. Your child may be given rehydrating solution intravenously, and may not be allowed to eat or drink for 24 hours. After this, oral rehydrating solution will be given, followed by the gradual reintroduction of ordinary food.

How can I prevent gastroenteritis?
Your child cannot be prevented from becoming infected with the viruses that cause gastroenteritis. However, after infection your child will be immune to the particular virus that caused it.

The spread of gastroenteritis due to bacterial infections is prevented more easily. For example, sterilize a baby's feeding utensils and dummies before use, make sure all family members are scrupulous about personal hygiene, and always store food at the correct temperatures. In order to reduce the risk of infection with *Salmonella* bacteria, hardboil eggs for 6 minutes and make sure that chicken is well cooked.

An infected child will be infectious until the faeces return to normal, so you may need to take special care with personal hygiene, particularly with washing hands after going to the toilet.

TREATING BOTTLE-FED BABIES		TREATING OLDER CHILDREN	
DAY 1	Give your baby no milk for the first 24 hours. Instead, give rehydrating solution at regular intervals.	DAY 1	Instead of milk, give your child rehydrating solution; alternatively, give unsweetened fruit juices.
DAY 2	Give your baby a mixture of 2 parts rehydrating solution and 2 parts milk formula at each feed time.	DAY 2	You may add vegetable and unsweetened fruit purée to your child's diet.
DAY 3	Your baby should have recovered completely and may return to his or her normal feeding routine.	DAY 3	You may add chicken and/or soups to your child's diet. You may also reintroduce milk.
		DAY 4	You may add bread, biscuits, eggs, meat and/or fish to your child's diet.
		DAY 5	Your child should have recovered completely and may return to his or her normal diet.

Treating gastroenteritis
This table shows the recommended method for treating bottle-fed babies and older children with gastroenteritis. You may make your own rehydrating solution as shown above right; sachets for making rehydrating solution are also available over the counter.

TODDLER'S DIARRHOEA

Children between the ages of 1 and 3 years may be affected by toddler's diarrhoea. In this form of diarrhoea, a child who is healthy passes watery faeces that often contain recognizable pieces of food, such as raisins, carrots, peas, or beans.

How is it caused?
The cause of toddler's diarrhoea is not certain, but the problem may be due to insufficient chewing of food.

What are the symptoms?
Apart from passing watery faeces with pieces of food in it, your child will probably feel generally well. A constant NAPPY RASH (p.136) may be a problem.

Should I consult a doctor?
Although toddler's diarrhoea is not a cause for concern, your child should be seen by a doctor to make sure that the condition is not the result of an infection or another disorder. The doctor will check whether your child's growth is normal by measuring his or her height and weight. Toddler's diarrhoea does not affect growth, so failure to grow

normally may suggest another disorder. As a precaution, the doctor may send a sample of stool for laboratory analysis.

What can I do to help?
No treatment is necessary for toddler's diarrhoea and no dietary restrictions have any effect on the condition. It may help, however, if you mash or liquidize the foods that your child has difficulty in chewing and digesting.

What is the outlook?
Your child will grow out of toddler's diarrhoea by 3 years of age and will not suffer any lasting adverse effects.

CONSTIPATION

A child who is constipated passes hard, dry faeces infrequently. Infrequent defaecation by itself does not indicate constipation since children differ in their bowel habits: the normal frequency for passing stools may vary from four times a day to once every 4 days. Constipation is usually short-lived but sometimes persists.

How is it caused?
Temporary constipation is commonly caused by dehydration that results from illness involving vomiting and fever. Some medicines may also have a dehydrating effect. From 1 to 2 years of age, the changes that are made in a child's diet (for example, from formula or breast milk to cow's milk) may cause constipation. Insufficient fibre in the diet is the most common cause of constipation in older children.

A child's constipation may become chronic if a painful anal fissure (see illustration above right) develops as a result of passing hard stools. Chronic constipation can also develop if a child deliberately withholds faeces during toilet-training (which is most likely if training is started too early) or because he or she has emotional problems.

What are the symptoms?
The symptoms of constipation include:
• Infrequent defecation.
• Pain on defecation.
• Hard, dry faeces.

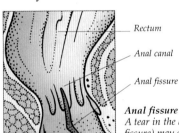

Rectum

Anal canal

Anal fissure

Anal fissure
A tear in the anal canal (anal fissure) may occur if a child strains to pass large, hard, stools. Because the tear makes defecating painful, the child withholds faeces deliberately, leading to chronic constipation.

In chronic constipation, there may be:
• Liquid faeces trickling from the anus, which may soil the underclothes.
• Pain on trying to defecate.
• Loss of appetite.
• Blood on the faeces.

What can I do to help?
Constipation can usually be alleviated and prevented by giving your child plenty of fluids and (if the child is aged 6 months or over) dietary fibre. Whole-grain cereals and bread, vegetables, and fruit are good sources of fibre. If constipation is a problem, a child should not drink more than 500 ml (1 pint) of

milk a day: milk aggravates the problem. Schoolchildren should drink skimmed or semi-skimmed, not full-cream, milk.

Your child should be seen by doctor if constipation persists for more than a week, if there is pain on defecation, or if you suspect chronic constipation.

What might the doctor do?
The doctor will examine your child and ask about his or her diet and any recent illnesses. In most cases, advice about improving diet (see "What can I do to help?") is all that is required.

If your child has symptoms of chronic constipation, the doctor will arrange for X-rays to determine the amount of retained faeces. Your child will be put on a high-fibre diet with plenty of fluids, and laxatives will be prescribed. You will be asked to ensure that your child sits on the lavatory at the same time each day to re-establish a regular bowel habit. After about 3 months, when a regular bowel habit has been regained, the drug dose is gradually reduced. No local treatment is needed for an anal fissure; the softened faeces produced by laxatives allow it to heal on its own, usually within 6 weeks.

If no physical causes can be found for the constipation and laxatives do not relieve it, your child may be sent to a paediatrician or a child psychiatrist.

What is the outlook?
Temporary or chronic constipation in childhood does not increase the risk of bowel problems later in life.

FOOD INTOLERANCE

A child who suffers from food intolerance develops symptoms in response to a particular food or to one of its constituents. Food intolerance differs from food allergy (see ALLERGIES, p.152), which is a rare, adverse reaction to food due to an inappropriate response by the body's immune system. Some of the common types of food intolerance are described below. A child who is thought to have the disorder should be seen by a doctor; a baby should be seen within 24 hours of the onset of symptoms.

COW'S MILK PROTEIN

Many children are intolerant to cow's milk protein. The cause is uncertain, but the problem appears initially in the first year of life, between a week and several months after an infant starts on cow's milk. By the age of 3 years, the intolerance to cow's milk protein usually disappears.

Milk substitutes
Children under 1 year who are intolerant to cow's milk protein may be given a milk substitute, such as a preparation made by breaking down cow's milk protein into smaller, more easily absorbed components.

What are the symptoms?
The symptoms of intolerance develop soon after drinking milk and include:
• Diarrhoea.
• Vomiting.

What might the doctor do?
If the doctor suspects that your child is intolerant to cow's milk protein, he or she will recommend that you exclude all products containing cow's milk from the diet for a period of 2 weeks. If the symptoms disappear, your child will be given a small, trial amount of cow's milk under medical supervision. The diagnosis of intolerance to milk protein is confirmed if symptoms recur.

What can I do to help?
Under the supervision of a dietitian, you will need to give your child a diet free of products containing cow's milk. Children under 1 year may require a milk substitute (see illustration above). The cow's milk trial will be repeated every 3 months, until your child no longer has an adverse reaction to the protein. The amount of milk given can then be increased gradually.

LACTOSE AND SUCROSE

Children are sometimes intolerant to the sugar lactose (found in milk) or to sucrose (a sugar present in many fruits).

How is it caused?
Intolerance occurs when there is a deficiency of the enzyme responsible for breaking down lactose or sucrose in the small intestine. Both types of intolerance may develop as a complication of an infection (see GASTROENTERITIS, p.180) or another intestinal disorder, such as COELIAC DISEASE (p.183), and are usually temporary. Some children with cow's milk protein intolerance are also intolerant to lactose.

Permanent lactose intolerance of genetic origin is common in people of African or Asian descent. In this form of the disorder, children up to the age of 2 or 3 years tolerate an unlimited amount of milk, but when older suffer from diarrhoea after ingesting only a small amount. Sucrose intolerance also occurs occasionally as an inherited, permanent disorder.

What are the symptoms?
Symptoms appear soon after drinking milk or eating foods containing lactose or sucrose and may include:
• Diarrhoea.
• Vomiting.

What might the doctor do?
The diagnosis is made by giving the child a test dose of lactose or sucrose in water and then examining the faeces to see whether an excessive amount of the sugar has passed through the intestines without being absorbed.

If your child is intolerant to lactose, a dietitian can design a lactose-free diet. Milk should not be included in your child's diet, but he or she may be able to tolerate fermented milk products, such as yoghurt. Sucrose intolerance is treated with a sucrose-free diet.

SPECIFIC FOODS

The foods, apart from milk, to which intolerance most frequently occurs in children are shown in the illustrations below. The reason why intolerance to a specific food occurs is not known.

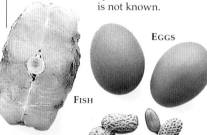

FISH

EGGS

Possible problem foods
Children are most often intolerant to the foods illustrated here. Sometimes a child can tolerate a food when it is cooked, but not raw.

NUTS

What are the symptoms?
Symptoms, which appear soon after a particular food is eaten, may include:
• Diarrhoea and abdominal pain.
• Vomiting.

What might the doctor do?
The doctor will examine your child and may carry out tests to exclude other causes of the symptoms. Your child may be put on a milk-free diet to rule out intolerance to cow's milk protein or lactose. If your child continues to have symptoms, one of two methods may be tried to find out whether he or she is intolerant to another specific food.

One method involves keeping the child under close medical supervision during periods when the suspected food is included and then when it is excluded; symptoms are compared. In another method, the child is put on a "few foods" diet, consisting of several specific foods known to be least likely to induce symptoms. Within 2 weeks, symptoms usually stop. A single new food is then introduced every 3 days until a specific food causes symptoms.

What is the outlook?
In many children, no specific cause can be found for the symptoms. However, the problem often clears up during the course of a "few foods" diet. In others, exclusion of between one and three foods eliminates the symptoms. Most children outgrow food intolerance.

COELIAC DISEASE

This rare but serious disease is caused by an extreme sensitivity of the small intestine to a protein (gluten) present in the cereals wheat, rye, barley, and oats. Eventually, the lining of the small intestine becomes damaged. As a result, absorption of food is impaired, a condition known as MALABSORPTION (below).

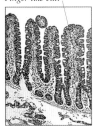 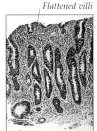

Finger-like villi   *Flattened villi*

NORMAL   ABNORMAL

Damage to the small intestine
The lining of the small intestine has millions of finger-like projections, called villi, which absorb nutrients. In coeliac disease, the villi become flattened and absorption is impaired.

What are the symptoms?
Symptoms occur a few months after a baby starts on solids. They may include:
• Weight loss or failure to gain weight.
• Very pale, floating faeces that have an unpleasant smell.
• Pale skin, breathlessness, and lack of energy due to ANAEMIA (p.145).

Foods containing wheat, such as bread, breakfast cereals, and biscuits, are most likely to cause symptoms.

Should I consult a doctor?
Symptoms usually develop gradually, so your baby is not likely to become ill suddenly. However, if your child has any of the symptoms listed above, he or she should be seen by a doctor.

What might the doctor do?
The doctor will check to see whether your baby's weight is less than would be expected for his or her age and birth weight. Blood tests to look for anaemia and antibodies to gluten may then be carried out. If these tests indicate that coeliac disease is likely, your child may be sent to hospital for a biopsy of the lining of the small intestine. A biopsy involves removal of a minute sample of tissue for analysis. If the biopsy shows changes in the intestinal lining (see micrographs above left), the diagnosis of coeliac disease is confirmed.

What can I do to help?
Keeping to a diet free of gluten is the most important factor for the health of a child affected by coeliac disease. Many specially produced substitute foods are available, including gluten-free bread, biscuits, flour, and pasta. Other foods, such as dairy products, eggs, meat, fish, vegetables, fruit, rice, and corn, can be eaten as normal. You should make sure that everyone concerned with the care of your child knows that he or she can eat only certain foods.

As your son or daughter grows up and becomes increasingly independent, you will need to make sure he or she is aware of the importance of keeping to the diet. Children vary in how they react to renewed exposure to gluten, and you will soon learn how much gluten is likely to cause a reaction and how severe the reaction might be.

The symptoms of coeliac disease will clear up within a few weeks of your child starting a gluten-free diet, and he or she should begin to put on weight.

What is the outlook?
Your child will remain in good health and grow as expected, provided he or she keeps to a gluten-free diet. Your child will, however, have to adhere to a gluten-free diet throughout life.

MALABSORPTION

Failure of the small intestine to absorb adequately nutrients from food is termed malabsorption. The disorder is always associated with an underlying condition, such as COELIAC DISEASE (above), Crohn's disease (see INFLAMMATORY BOWEL DISEASE, p.184), CYSTIC FIBROSIS (p.201), or FOOD INTOLERANCE (opposite).

How is it caused?
Malabsorption sometimes results from damage to the intestinal lining, which interferes with the intestine's ability to absorb nutrients. It may also be due to a deficiency of digestive enzymes, which prevents the breakdown of food into units small enough to be absorbed.

What are the symptoms?
The main symptoms are:
• Very pale, floating faeces that have an unpleasant smell.
• Weight loss or failure to gain weight.
• Listlessness.

In severe cases, malabsorption results in vitamin and mineral deficiencies. These deficiencies may, in turn, lead to malnutrition and ANAEMIA (p.145).

Your child should be seen by a doctor if there are symptoms indicating that he or she might have malabsorption.

What might the doctor do?
Your child will be examined and his or her weight checked. Tests may then be carried out to determine the underlying cause of malabsorption. The doctor may ask a dietitian to assess whether your child's intake of food is adequate.

Malabsorption is treated by attention to the underlying cause and also by modifying or supplementing the diet, which in most cases will ensure that your child grows and gains weight normally. Your child may, however, need to stay on a special diet for life.

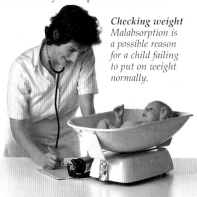

Checking weight
Malabsorption is a possible reason for a child failing to put on weight normally.

INFLAMMATORY BOWEL DISEASE

The term inflammatory bowel disease includes Crohn's disease and ulcerative colitis, both of which cause chronic inflammation of the intestine. Ulcerative colitis and Crohn's disease are rare under the age of 7 years and are more common in adolescents. The causes are unknown, but the diseases tend to run in families.

CROHN'S DISEASE

Once a rare disorder, Crohn's disease is becoming more common. Although it can cause inflammation of any part of the digestive tract, the condition most often affects only the last section of the small intestine (the ileum). As a result of chronic inflammation, the intestinal wall becomes extremely thick, and deep, penetrating ulcers may form. Crohn's disease reduces the ability of the small intestine to absorb nutrients from food (see MALABSORPTION, p.183).

What are the symptoms?

The symptoms of Crohn's disease often develop gradually and consist of:

- Diarrhoea. Occasionally, the faeces contain blood, pus, or mucus if the colon is affected.
- Spasms of abdominal pain.
- Fever.
- Nausea.
- Poor growth and / or delayed puberty.
- Loss of weight and reduced appetite.
- Sometimes, ulceration of the anus.

What are the complications?

Thickening of the intestinal wall may narrow the inside of the intestine to such an extent that the bowel becomes obstructed (see INTESTINAL OBSTRUCTION, opposite). Complications in other parts of the body may include arthritis and inflammation of the eye.

Should I consult a doctor?

Your child should be seen by a doctor if the symptoms persist for more than a few days. Crohn's disease is less likely to be the cause of the symptoms than some other disorder, such as intestinal infection. However, if Crohn's disease is suspected, investigations, which may include barium X-ray and endoscopic examinations of the intestines, will probably be performed in hospital to look for evidence of the disease.

What is the treatment?

If your child has Crohn's disease, anti-inflammatory drugs may be prescribed. As an alternative to drugs, your child may be given a liquid diet containing proteins that have been broken down into smaller components, making absorption easier.

In severe cases, and if your child is badly malnourished, he or she may receive drugs and nutrients intravenously. A blood transfusion may also be needed. If the condition does not improve with medical treatment or if complications occur, damaged parts of the intestine may be removed surgically.

What is the outlook?

Crohn's disease is a long-term condition, and some children continue to suffer from flare-ups of the disease for many years; the symptoms may recur at intervals of a few months or a few years. For others, Crohn's disease may subside after only one or two flare-ups.

ULCERATIVE COLITIS

In this condition, the colon and rectum become inflamed and ulcerated. The initial attack of ulcerative colitis is often the worst, and then the symptoms may fluctuate over a long period of time.

What are the symptoms?

Bloody diarrhoea is the main symptom. It may be accompanied by:

- Abdominal pain and tenderness.
- A feeling of fullness in the bowel.
- Fever.
- Nausea.
- Loss of appetite.
- Poor growth and/or weight loss.
- A general feeling of being unwell.

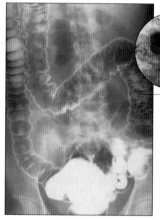

Ulcerated lining of colon

Diseased colon

Ulcerative colitis
In the barium X-ray (left), areas affected by disease are distinguished by loss of the folds found in a healthy colon. In the endoscopic view (above), ulcerated areas of the lining of the colon are seen as whitish patches.

Repeated blood loss may cause ANAEMIA (p.145). Another possible complication is an abnormally enlarged colon, which may become life threatening.

Should I consult a doctor?

Your child should be seen by a doctor within 24 hours if he or she has bloody diarrhoea and abdominal pain. Bacterial infection is the most common cause of these symptoms; but, if ulcerative colitis is suspected, investigations like those for Crohn's disease may be carried out.

What is the treatment?

Anti-inflammatory drugs may have to be taken indefinitely. If drugs do not control the symptoms, or if the colon is badly damaged, the affected part may be removed surgically. If a large part is removed, your child may be left with an ileostomy (an opening through the abdominal wall for passage of faeces).

Ulcerated lining of small intestine

Narrowed area

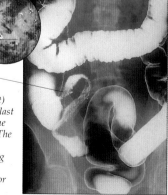

Crohn's disease
The barium X-ray (right) shows narrowing of the last part of the small intestine due to Crohn's disease. The endoscopic view (above) reveals a thickened lining punctuated with ulcers, which appear as yellow or whitish patches.

IRRITABLE BOWEL SYNDROME

An uncommon disorder in children, irritable bowel syndrome consists of recurrent bouts of abdominal pain accompanied by either diarrhoea or constipation and often both. The condition may be triggered by anxiety or, in some cases, intolerance to a specific food, such as cow's milk protein, nuts, or eggs.

What are the symptoms?
The main symptoms are:
- Abdominal pain, which is relieved by a bowel movement or passing wind.
- A persistent sense of fullness and distension of the bowel.
- Wind and diarrhoea or constipation, or bouts of diarrhoea alternating with periods of constipation.
- Sometimes nausea, headache, and general lack of energy.

Your child should be seen by a doctor if you think that he or she could have irritable bowel syndrome.

What is the treatment?
The diagnosis is usually made on the basis of the symptoms and a physical examination. Sometimes investigations are carried out in hospital to exclude another disorder, such as GIARDIASIS (p.187), FOOD INTOLERANCE (p.182), or INFLAMMATORY BOWEL DISEASE (opposite). A high-fibre diet is helpful in many cases, especially if constipation is the predominant symptom. Certain foods may make the symptoms worse, and you may find it helpful to keep a diary of your child's diet so that the problem foods can be identified and avoided. Stress sometimes increases the severity of symptoms. Try to identify situations that may make your child feel anxious, and if they cannot be avoided, give your child additional support.

What is the outlook?
Irritable bowel syndrome is a condition that often persists, and symptoms may recur periodically throughout life.

INTESTINAL OBSTRUCTION

A partial or complete blockage of the small or large intestine is known as an intestinal obstruction. The passage of food through the intestine is blocked, resulting in cramping abdominal pain. Treatment is usually needed for intestinal obstruction. Complete obstruction of the intestine may be fatal without treatment.

How is it caused?
In children under 2 years, obstruction is most often due to a disorder known as intussusception (see illustration right). However, a blocked intestine in infants may be due to a strangulated HERNIA (p.187) or to a congenital abnormality of the intestine. Other possible causes of intestinal obstruction in children of any age include Crohn's disease (see INFLAMMATORY BOWEL DISEASE, opposite) and volvulus (twisting) of the intestine.

What are the symptoms?
The symptoms may include:
- Intermittent attacks of severe pain in the abdomen.
- Attacks of vomiting greenish-yellow fluid, which occur at increasingly frequent intervals.
- Wind and failure to pass faeces. In partial obstruction, passing wind and defecating usually bring temporary relief from pain.
- Blood-stained, jelly-like mucus on the faeces, in cases of intussusception.
- Fever and swelling of the abdomen, if treatment is delayed.

There is a chance that the blocked part of the intestine may rupture, leading to

Intussusception
A condition in which part of the intestine telescopes in on itself, intussusception tends to occur in the area where the large and small intestines meet.

Large intestine

Area shown in detail

Small intestine

Large intestine

Small intestine

Appendix

Telescoped intestine

peritonitis (inflammation of the lining of the abdominal cavity), or that it may die and become gangrenous, which is a potentially fatal complication. Another serious complication that may develop as a result of frequent vomiting attacks is dehydration (see *Danger signs*, p.38, for signs of dehydration).

Should I consult a doctor?
Call an ambulance or take your child to to the nearest accident and emergency department, if you think that he or she might have an intestinal obstruction. A doctor will examine your child and fluids may be given intravenously to prevent dehydration. To confirm the diagnosis and to find out the cause of the obstruction, an X-ray examination may be performed. If intussusception is suspected, a special X-ray examination that involves the use of a barium or air enema may be carried out. Pressure exerted by the enema often forces the displaced intestinal tissue back into the right position. If the enema does not correct the problem, an operation is carried out. Other types of intestinal obstruction require surgical treatment, which sometimes involves removing the obstructed part of the intestine.

What is the outlook?
Normal growth and development can be expected once the obstruction has been treated or if only a short section of bowel has been surgically removed. However, if the intestinal obstruction was due to an underlying condition (such as Crohn's disease), the blockage may recur unless the disorder that caused it is being effectively treated.

GASTRO-OESOPHAGEAL REFLUX

Usually starting a few weeks after birth, gastro-oesophageal reflux is a common problem in the first year of life. The contents of the baby's stomach pass back into the oesophagus because the muscle at the entrance to the stomach is weak. In most cases, gastro-oesophageal reflux is a temporary problem.

What are the symptoms?
The main symptoms of reflux are:
- Persistent vomiting; the vomit may be bloodstained.
- Regurgitation of feeds, which may dribble continuously from the mouth.
- A cough, if regurgitated milk or feed is breathed into the lungs.
- Crying and irritability.
- Failure to gain weight, if the reflux is prolonged and severe.

Phone a doctor at once if your baby's vomit is bloodstained. Otherwise, you should make an appointment for your baby to be seen by a doctor.

What might the doctor do?
The doctor will examine your baby. In addition, he or she may send samples of urine and blood for testing so that any other cause of the vomiting, such as GASTROENTERITIS (p.180) or PYLORIC STENOSIS (below), may be ruled out.

What is the treatment?
Altering your baby's normal sleeping position may help to reduce reflux (see illustration right). If he or she is old enough, your child should also spend more time sitting in a baby chair. If the symptoms of reflux are severe, making your baby's feed thicker with carob seed powder or cornflour may help. If your baby is eating solids, you should reduce the amount of liquid in his or her diet and introduce more solids. You should try to avoid giving your child anything to drink without solids.

If the reflux does not improve within about 6 weeks, the doctor will probably prescribe a drug that helps to prevent the problem by increasing the muscular activity of the oesophagus. The doctor may also prescribe a drug that reduces the amount of acid in the stomach. Most babies outgrow reflux by the age of 1 year with or without treatment.

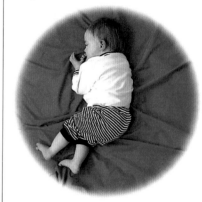

Treating gastro-oesophageal reflux
Your baby should sleep on his or her side with the head higher than the feet. This position will help to reduce gastro-oesophageal reflux.

PYLORIC STENOSIS

An uncommon condition that occurs in babies aged less than 2 months, pyloric stenosis is narrowing of the outlet (pylorus) from the stomach into the small intestine. A severely narrowed outlet allows only a small amount of food to enter the intestine; the rest is vomited, causing the baby to lose weight.

Narrowed pylorus
In pyloric stenosis, the pylorus is narrowed as a result of thickening of the surrounding muscle. The cause of the thickening is not known, but it is more common in boys.

Stomach

Small intestine

Normal width of muscle

Area shown in detail

Pylorus

Thickened muscle

What are the symptoms?
The main symptoms of pyloric stenosis usually appear between 2 and 6 weeks after birth. They are:
- Persistent projectile vomiting (vomit that is produced forcefully, reaching some distance from the baby).
- Constant hunger: the baby often accepts another feed immediately after vomiting.
- Infrequent bowel movements.
- Weight loss and listlessness if symptoms have been present for more than a few days.

Your baby may become dehydrated from persistent vomiting. Phone a doctor at once if your baby has any of the symptoms listed above or if there are any signs indicating that he or she might be dehydrated (see *Danger signs*, p.38). Until you are able to see the doctor, feed your child small amounts frequently, so that there is not too much undigested food in his or her stomach.

What might the doctor do?
The doctor will examine your baby's abdomen, while the baby is feeding, to feel for a swelling in the area of the pylorus. If pyloric stenosis seems likely, your child will be admitted to hospital. In hospital, he or she will have another physical examination, and an ultrasound examination will probably be carried out to confirm the diagnosis.

Intravenous fluids are given if your baby is dehydrated. The obstruction is relieved by a minor surgical operation to widen the pylorus. Your baby can probably leave hospital the next day.

After the operation, the amount of your baby's feeds should be gradually increased until feeding is normal again (usually within 48 to 72 hours).

What is the outlook?
Once pyloric stenosis has been treated, the condition will not recur and there are no permanent ill effects.

HERNIA

Protrusion of a part of the intestine through the abdominal wall is termed a hernia. Umbilical and inguinal hernias are the most common types of hernia in children. In an umbilical hernia, the intestine bulges through the muscle wall at or above the navel (umbilicus). In an inguinal hernia, the intestine protrudes into the inguinal canal (the passage in the groin through which, in boys, the testis descends into the scrotum before birth).

UMBILICAL HERNIA

This type of hernia occurs as result of a gap in the muscles of the abdominal wall and usually appears a few weeks after birth. In most cases, an umbilical hernia disappears without treatment before 2 years of age but it may persist up to the age of 5 years.

What are the symptoms?

Appearing as a soft swelling, usually at the navel, an umbilical hernia:
• Is often not present in the morning but may reappear during the day.

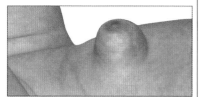

Umbilical hernia
Usually, an umbilical hernia is at the navel (umbilicus); sometimes, it appears just above.

• May increase in size if the child cries or tenses the abdominal muscles.
• Is painless.
Your child should be seen by a doctor if the hernia is particularly large or if it has not disappeared by the time the child has reached the age of 5 years.

What is the treatment?

A minor operation may be required to replace the intestine in the abdominal cavity and stitch together the gap in the muscles of the abdominal wall. Hernias above a child's navel more often require surgery. An umbilical hernia is unlikely to recur after it has been treated.

INGUINAL HERNIA

Boys under the age of 1 year are most commonly affected by inguinal hernia. The hernia occurs when the inguinal canal, which normally closes shortly after birth, remains open, forming a space through which a loop of intestine can pass into the groin or scrotum.

What are the symptoms?

An inguinal hernia appears as a soft swelling just above the groin crease or in the scrotum. The hernia:
• Is often not present in the morning but may reappear during the day.
• May increase in size if the child cries.
A strangulated hernia is a complication that occurs when a loop of intestine becomes trapped in the canal so that its blood supply is reduced or cut off. If a hernia is strangulated, the swelling in the groin or scrotum will become hard, tender or painful, and discoloured, and your child may vomit.

If there is a painless swelling in the groin or scrotum, your child should be seen by a doctor within 24 hours. If the swelling is painful or tender, however, you should call an ambulance or take your child to the nearest accident and emergency department.

What is the treatment?

An inguinal hernia will not disappear without treatment, so an operation is always required. If the hernia is painful or tender, your child may be admitted to hospital immediately for emergency surgery. The intestine is replaced in the abdominal cavity and the inguinal canal is stitched closed. An inguinal hernia is not likely to recur once your child has had surgery to reposition the intestine and close the inguinal canal.

GIARDIASIS

Swallowing food or water contaminated with the single-celled parasite *Giardia lamblia* can lead to giardiasis, an infection of the small intestine. Once confined to the tropics, giardiasis now also occurs in temperate countries, where it affects mainly preschool children.

What are the symptoms?

About two-thirds of children who are infected have no symptoms. When they do occur, the symptoms start 1 to 3 days after the parasite has entered the body. The symptoms of giardiasis are:
• Violent attacks of diarrhoea accompanied by wind.
• Very pale, floating, unpleasant-smelling faeces, resulting from MALABSORPTION (p.183).
• Abdominal discomfort and cramps.
• Swollen abdomen and nausea.

What is the treatment?

The majority of cases of giardiasis are mild and clear up on their own within 2 weeks. A doctor should see your child if he or she has been suffering from diarrhoea for more than 2 weeks or from severe diarrhoea for over 48 hours. Samples of faeces will be sent to the laboratory for microscopic

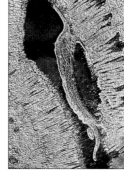

Lining of the intestine

Parasite

The cause of giardiasis
The parasite Giardia lamblia *clings to folds in the lining of the intestine and absorbs nutrients from the fluid in the intestine.*

examination. If *Giardia lamblia* is found, the doctor will prescribe a week-long course of an antiparasitic drug.

You should make sure that your child drinks plenty of fluids to replace those he or she has lost through diarrhoea.

Being scrupulous about handwashing after going to the toilet and before preparing food will help to prevent the disease from spreading to other members of your family.

THREADWORMS

The most common parasitic worms in temperate countries, threadworms (pinworms) live in the intestines. The thread-like parasites primarily affect children. Often, several members of the household are infested at the same time (although some may have no symptoms), so all the family should be treated together.

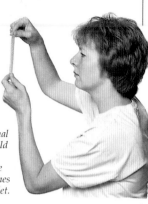

Collecting worms' eggs
Eggs may be collected for microscopic examination by pressing a piece of sticky tape to your child's anal area. You should do this in the morning before your child bathes or uses the toilet.

How is infestation caused?
Children catch threadworms by sucking objects or eating food that has been contaminated with worms' eggs. The swallowed eggs develop into adults in the intestine. The female worms emerge from the rectum at night to lay their eggs on the skin around the anus.

What are the symptoms?
The main symptoms of infestation are:
• Itching in the anal region, especially at night when the worms lay eggs.
• An itchy vulva in girls.
• Inflammation of the anus as a result of constant scratching.
Sometimes, tiny white worms can be seen wriggling in faeces.

Should I consult a doctor?
Your child should be seen by a doctor if you suspect he or she has threadworms. The doctor may ask you to collect some eggs for microscopic examination (see photograph right). The doctor will treat the whole family with one of three antiparasitic drugs – two are taken in a single dose; the third is taken daily for a week. One course should cure your child, but to prevent reinfection, the family may be treated again in 2 weeks.

HEPATITIS

The most common cause of hepatitis (inflammation of the liver) is viral infection. Several strains of virus can cause the infection. The hepatitis B virus causes some cases among newborn babies, who may be infected during birth if their mothers are carriers of the virus. However, most babies who are thought to be at risk are immunized against hepatitis B. The strain that most often causes hepatitis in children is the hepatitis A virus.

How is it caused?
The hepatitis A virus is usually caught by swallowing water or food that has been contaminated with infected faeces. Immunization against the hepatitis A virus may be recommended if you and your family are planning to visit one of a number of developing countries where the disease is most prevalent.

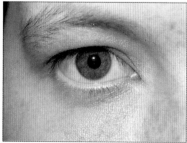

Jaundice
In hepatitis, a build-up in the blood of the waste product bilirubin may cause jaundice, yellowing of the whites of the eyes and skin.

What are the symptoms?
In preschool children, most hepatitis A infections are mild and do not produce any symptoms. Older children usually do have symptoms. The symptoms are rarely severe, and may include:
• Flu-like symptoms of fever, headache, and weakness.
• Poor appetite.
• Nausea and vomiting.
• Tender upper right abdomen (where the liver is located).
About a week after the other symptoms have appeared, your child may develop jaundice (see photograph left), often accompanied by dark urine and pale faeces and, sometimes, by diarrhoea. Jaundice may last for up to 2 weeks.

Should I consult a doctor?
Make an appointment to see a doctor within 24 hours if your child has any symptoms of hepatitis. Hepatitis A cannot be treated with drugs, but the doctor will advise you on how to care for your child at home. Rarely, an attack may be serious enough for your child to be admitted to hospital, where he or she can be monitored closely.

The doctor may recommend that all family members should be immunized against hepatitis to prevent the spread of the disease. A child with hepatitis A is infectious for 2 weeks before and for 1 week after the onset of jaundice.

What can I do to help?
Your child should be allowed to stay in bed if he or she wants to. While your child is vomiting or his or her appetite is poor, small volumes of rehydrating fluid (see panel: *Preventing dehydration in children*, p.53) flavoured with fruit juice should be given hourly during the day. As the jaundice increases, your child's appetite should improve and he or she may be given a fully mixed diet.

The spread of the hepatitis A virus between members of the family can be prevented by scrupulous handwashing and by boiling food utensils.

What is the outlook?
Your child should feel well enough to go back to school from 2 to 6 weeks after the onset of symptoms.

Hepatitis A rarely causes permanent damage to the liver and, after the first attack, your child should be immune to further attacks of the disease.

HORMONAL DISORDERS

HORMONES IN THE BLOOD CONTROL growth, production of energy, biochemical activities, such as digestion, and sexual development and function. They also help the body deal with stress, danger, and fatigue. A fault in the production of hormones may affect physical and/or mental development.

HYPOTHYROIDISM

The thyroid gland manufactures hormones that are essential for normal physical and mental development. Hypothyroidism (underactivity of the thyroid gland) is a condition that results in insufficient production of hormones by the gland. If hypothyroidism is not treated, it may adversely affect a child's growth and learning abilities.

How is it caused?
Hypothyroidism may be present from birth, usually as a result of a small thyroid gland. The condition may also develop later as a result of disease of the thyroid gland or underactivity of the hypothalamus or pituitary gland (both of which stimulate the thyroid gland to produce thyroid hormones).

What are the symptoms?
All babies have their blood tested for hypothyroidism within a week of birth. If your child has an underactive thyroid gland, treatment for the disorder will be given before any symptoms appear.

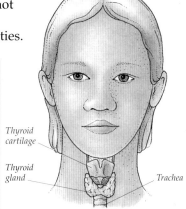

Thyroid cartilage

Thyroid gland

Trachea

Location of the thyroid gland
The thyroid gland is located at the base of the neck in front of the trachea. The gland helps to regulate the body's energy levels and growth.

The symptoms in older children who develop hypothyroidism are:
• A noticeable reduction in the child's growth rate.
• LEARNING DIFFICULTIES (p.172).
• Lack of energy, poor appetite, and weight gain.
• Goitre (enlarged thyroid gland).

Should I consult a doctor?
Your child should be seen by a doctor. The doctor will probably take a sample of your child's blood to measure his or her hormone levels. A synthetic form of thyroxine (the principal hormone produced by the thyroid gland) will be prescribed if the tests confirm that your child has hypothyroidism.

What is the outlook?
Provided a baby who is born with the condition or a child who develops it is treated promptly, physical and mental development will probably be normal. However, the child will have to take thyroxine for the rest of his or her life.

GROWTH HORMONE DEFICIENCY

In order to grow normally, children and adolescents need growth hormone, which is produced by the pituitary gland at the base of the brain. A congenital fault in the pituitary gland, disease of the pituitary gland, or a head injury may lead to a deficiency of the hormone, resulting in a slow rate of growth.

What are the symptoms?
Growth hormone deficiency in a child is usually indicated by:
• Slow rate of growth (see GROWTH CHARTS, pp.17–21).
• Short stature and chubbiness.
• Delayed development of sexual characteristics in older children.

Make an appointment for your child to be seen by a doctor if you are worried about his or her rate of growth.

What might the doctor do?
Your child's height will be measured at regular intervals and plotted on a chart. If the doctor finds that your child's rate

of growth is slower than normal, your child will probably be sent to a hospital for tests. If growth hormone deficiency is diagnosed, the doctor may prescribe synthetic growth hormone. You will have to inject your child with growth hormone once a day, 5 days a week, until the end of puberty.

What is the outlook?
Treatment improves a child's growth rate. However, your child may reach the normal adult height expected for your family only if treatment begins by about the age of 6 years.

DIABETES MELLITUS

In childhood diabetes, cells in the pancreas suddenly stop making insulin, a hormone that enables body cells to use and store the sugar glucose. The lack of insulin causes a build-up of glucose in the blood and a disturbance of the body's chemical processes. The unused glucose is passed out in large volumes of urine, causing frequent urination and thirst. People with diabetes mellitus need to have insulin injections daily throughout their lives.

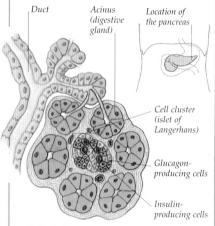

Duct

Acinus (digestive gland)

Location of the pancreas

Cell cluster (islet of Langerhans)

Glucagon-producing cells

Insulin-producing cells

Cells in the pancreas
The pancreas, a digestive gland, has several types of cell arranged in clusters. Some cells secrete insulin to lower the blood glucose level; others secrete glucagon to raise it. In diabetes mellitus, insufficient insulin is produced.

What are the symptoms?
In diabetes that has not been treated or that is poorly controlled, the amount of glucose in the blood is greatly raised (hyperglycaemia). In addition, because the cells are not able to use glucose for energy, the body has to use fats and protein as alternative energy sources. This upset of internal biochemical processes typically produces:
• Frequent passing of urine (which sometimes causes bed-wetting in children previously dry at night).
• Excessive thirst.
• Tiredness and lack of energy.
• Poor appetite.
• Losing a large amount of weight.
In more severe cases of biochemical upset, there may also be:
• Vomiting.
• Abdominal pain.
• Abnormally fast breathing.
• Drowsiness and confusion, which, without treatment, may be followed by loss of consciousness and coma.

What are the complications?
People with diabetes mellitus, especially those in whom the disease is not well controlled, are at risk of developing complications that affect the heart and circulation, the kidneys, the eyes, and the nervous system. Complications do not appear during childhood; typically, they develop about 10 to 15 years after the onset of the disease.

Should I consult a doctor?
Phone a doctor at once if you think that your child might have diabetes mellitus.
If your child has been diagnosed as having diabetes mellitus, you should consult the doctor if you ever have any worries about your child's condition. You should consult the doctor without delay if your child has an infection or an attack of gastroenteritis, because these conditions may make it difficult to control the blood glucose level.

What might the doctor do?
If the doctor suspects that your child might have diabetes mellitus, he or she will arrange for a sample of urine to be tested for the level of glucose. Blood may also be tested for the glucose level. If the level of glucose is abnormally

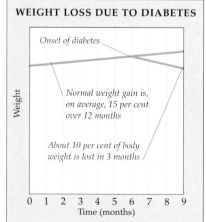

WEIGHT LOSS DUE TO DIABETES

Onset of diabetes

Normal weight gain is, on average, 15 per cent over 12 months

About 10 per cent of body weight is lost in 3 months

Weight

0 1 2 3 4 5 6 7 8 9
Time (months)

high, the doctor will probably arrange for your child to be admitted to hospital immediately. Usually, several days' stay in hospital is necessary at this time for investigation and for the start of insulin treatment. The length of your child's stay in hospital will depend on his or her age and condition. If your child is dehydrated from passing large amounts of urine, intravenous rehydrating fluids may be given as well as insulin.
The long-term control of your child's diabetes mellitus will be carried out under medical supervision. The aim of treatment is to provide sufficient insulin to keep your child's blood glucose level within the normal range, so that he or she is able to lead a normal life. Keeping the blood glucose level normal requires eating regular, balanced meals and having injections of insulin twice and, sometimes, three times a day.
Your child's blood glucose level may sometimes fall too low, resulting in a hypoglycaemic attack. Hypoglycaemia may be triggered by too high a dose of insulin, missing a meal, or a sudden burst of exercise. You will be told how to recognize hypoglycaemia and what action you should take if your child has an attack (see "What should I do if my child has a hypoglycaemic attack?"). The doctor will prescribe glucagon, which can be injected to stop an attack.

What can I do to help?
You will need to learn how to test for the amount of glucose in your child's blood, and how to record the results. The measurements obtained from the tests allow adjustments to be made to the amount of insulin your child is to be given by injection. You will also need to learn how to give injections, and how to store and dispose of used insulin bottles and syringes.
Another important aspect of caring for a child with diabetes mellitus is to make sure he or she has the right kind of diet. A dietitian will be available to give you advice. Meals will need to be planned with extra care and to be served at regular times. Your child should eat a normal, balanced diet that

Example of severe weight loss
A typical symptom of diabetes is rapid and severe weight loss. A child may lose as much a 10 per cent of his or her total body weight over a period of just 3 months.

contains consistent proportions of fats, protein, and carbohydrates. The daily energy intake should be constant. For a child over 5 years of age, just over a third of the diet should be made up of fats, about 15 per cent should consist of protein, and the remainder should be carbohydrates. Children younger than 5 years may eat more fats. Your child's diet should also be high in soluble and insoluble fibre. Soluble fibre is found in baked beans and oat-based dishes, such as porridge; foods containing insoluble fibre include wholemeal breads, pasta, and cereals. You do not have to make special meals for a diabetic child. A similar healthy, well-balanced diet will benefit all members of the family.

If your child has a poor appetite for any reason, it is important that he or she gets the same amount of energy in the form of glucose drinks as he or she would be gaining from a healthy diet. Make sure that you give your child the normal amount of insulin.

Exercise can trigger a hypoglycaemic attack, so your child's diet and dosage of insulin may need adjustment if he or she is participating in a sports event or will be doing strenuous exercise. Ask the doctor who is supervising your child's treatment for advice.

Your child should carry a medical identification card or bracelet indicating that he or she has diabetes mellitus and showing the medication that he or she is taking. It is essential that everyone

involved in caring for your child, such as teachers, knows what to do if the child has a hypoglycaemic attack.

As your child gets older, he or she should be encouraged to take as much responsibility as possible for control of his or her own diabetes mellitus. In fact, even quite young children can soon learn to inject themselves, to test and record their own blood glucose levels, to understand the need to eat regularly, and to watch for and treat symptoms of hypoglycaemia.

What should I do if my child has a hypoglycaemic attack?
The main signs of hypoglycaemia are abdominal pain, sweating, dizziness, and/or confusion. If your child shows any of these signs, give a sweet drink or sweet food, such as chocolate or a biscuit, immediately. If your child will not eat or drink, or blood glucose drops so low that he or she becomes drowsy or even loses consciousness, give an injection of glucagon in order to bring the glucose level back to normal.

What is the outlook?
A well-controlled blood glucose level should allow your child to live a normal life, with a normal amount of exercise, and should reduce the chance of any complications developing. However, your child will need to monitor his or her blood glucose level and to have injections of insulin daily for life.

TESTING FOR GLUCOSE
Blood glucose levels can be checked by two methods. For each method, a finger is pricked (which can be done using an automatic device) to obtain a drop of blood. The blood is applied to a special strip that chemically reacts with glucose.

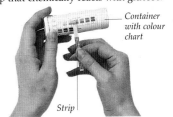

Container with colour chart

Strip

Colour-match method
The strip changes colour and is compared with a colour chart provided on the side of the strip container. The blood glucose level is given underneath the relevant colour.

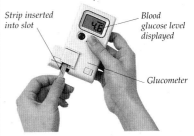

Strip inserted into slot

Blood glucose level displayed

Glucometer

Glucometer method
In this more precise method, the strip does not change colour, but the chemical reaction can be read automatically by a glucometer, which displays the blood glucose level on a screen.

DIABETES INSIPIDUS

The main symptoms of diabetes insipidus – the passage of large amounts of urine frequently and excessive thirst – are similar to those of diabetes mellitus (opposite). However, diabetes insipidus is due to a deficiency of an entirely different hormone and has nothing to do with the sugar glucose, or with energy use.

What are the causes?
In most cases, diabetes insipidus is the result of failure of the pituitary gland to secrete antidiuretic hormone (ADH). ADH normally acts on the kidneys to cause them to concentrate the urine and thus restrict the amount of fluid that is excreted from the body. Failure of the pituitary gland to produce ADH may be the result of injury to the gland or, less commonly, a tumour.

In rare cases, diabetes insipidus occurs because the kidneys fail to respond to normal levels of ADH.

What are the symptoms?
The symptoms of diabetes insipidus are:
• Excessive thirst.
• Frequent passing of large quantities of very pale, weak urine.
Dehydration can occur as a result of the excessive fluid passed as urine.

Should I consult a doctor?
Phone a doctor at once if your child has any of the symptoms listed above or if he or she has any of the following signs of dehydration: sunken eyes; abnormal drowsiness; or weight loss.

What might the doctor do?
The doctor will arrange for a sample of urine to be analysed. If the urine is not adequately concentrated, diabetes insipidus is a possibility. Further tests will probably be carried out in hospital to confirm the diagnosis and determine the cause. If the pituitary gland is not producing ADH in sufficient quantities, your child will need to take synthetic ADH. If your child's kidneys are failing to respond to normal levels of ADH, the treatment is a low-sodium diet and, paradoxically, a diuretic drug.

What is the outlook?
A damaged pituitary gland may return to normal. In other cases, the condition is lifelong. However, treatment enables the person to live a normal life. There are no long-term complications.

URINARY AND GENITAL DISORDERS

URINARY TRACT INFECTIONS are common in childhood, but they affect many more girls than boys. Most of these infections clear up quickly with treatment, but all urinary infections and any other disorders affecting the kidneys, the bladder, or the genitals require investigation to check for a possible structural defect present from birth. Serious kidney disorders are today mainly treatable, including the most common childhood kidney cancer, Wilms' tumour.

ENURESIS

Bed-wetting (enuresis) is a common problem. The age at which children become dry at night is extremely variable. Few children can control their bladder function before they are 3 years old. Reliable control day and night may be gained any time between the ages of 3 and 7 years. There is usually no cause for concern unless your child is still bed-wetting after 7 years of age or has started bed-wetting after a prolonged dry period (6 to 12 months).

How is it caused?

In most cases, enuresis probably results from delayed maturation of the parts of the nervous system that control the bladder. Enuresis may also occur if a child has a URINARY TRACT INFECTION (opposite) or is anxious (see ANXIETY AND FEARS, p.170). Rarely, a congenital defect of the urinary tract or DIABETES MELLITUS (p.190) is responsible.

Should I consult a doctor?

Make an appointment to see a doctor if you are concerned about your child's bed-wetting, especially if he or she is aged 7 years or over. Your child should also be seen by a doctor if the problem starts after your child has been dry at night for a prolonged period. The doctor will examine your child and will test a urine sample for infection or diabetes. If a physical cause for the enuresis is identified, treatment will be given; for example, antibiotics may be prescribed to treat a urinary tract infection. If no physical reason can be found, follow the advice given here (see also panel: *Toilet-training tips*, p.63).

What can I do to help?

Bed-wetting may be less likely to occur if a child gets into the habit of passing urine at regular times during the day and just before going to bed.

Do not punish your child if he or she does wet the bed; you may increase his or her anxiety and make the problem worse. You should always give praise for dry nights. A chart on which your child can stick a star after each dry night may provide motivation (see photograph right). Some children become completely dry after using a star chart for a few weeks without having any other treatment. However, if your child becomes discouraged because the chart reflects poor results, the method should be discontinued.

If methods involving praise and encouragement are not successful, you could try using an enuresis alarm. This device has a detector (which is placed under the bottom sheet) that activates a buzzer when urine is passed. The alarm wakes the child, who stops the urine stream, and gets up to go to the toilet. The amount of urine passed before the child wakes becomes less and less. After a few months, most children wake up before the alarm starts or sleep through the night without wetting the bed. If your child has been dry at night for 6 weeks, you may remove the alarm. If bed-wetting recurs, however, the alarm may be used to treat your child again.

What is the outlook?

Most children stop bed-wetting without treatment. Those who are treated often improve within a few months. The older a child is, however, the longer it may take for the condition to improve.

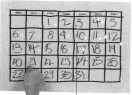

| Chart made
by the child

Star chart

Sticking a star on a chart after each dry night is a satisfying way for your child to mark progress. The chart also allows family members to see how well the child is doing and to give praise for good results.

URINARY TRACT INFECTIONS

Infections of the urinary tract are common in children, especially in girls. However, newborn male babies are more susceptible to urinary tract infections than female babies. An infection may affect the urethra (urethritis), the bladder (cystitis), and/or the kidneys (pyelonephritis). Prompt treatment of urinary tract infections is important to prevent scarring of the kidneys, which is most likely to occur in children under 5 years of age.

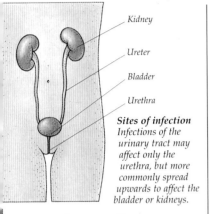

Kidney

Ureter

Bladder

Urethra

Sites of infection
Infections of the urinary tract may affect only the urethra, but more commonly spread upwards to affect the bladder or kidneys.

How are they caused?

Urinary tract infections are most often caused by bacteria from the rectum that enter the urethra. Bacteria sometimes spread to the urinary tract through the bloodstream. Girls are more prone to infections of the urinary tract than boys because they have shorter urethras.

Children who have urinary reflux are especially vulnerable to infection. In this congenital condition, when the bladder empties, some urine passes backwards towards the kidneys. Children who have congenital malformations of the urinary tract that prevent the free flow of urine, or who have kidneys scarred from previous infection, are also more susceptible to infection.

What are the symptoms?

Children under the age of 2 years tend to have symptoms of general infection, which may include the following:
• Fever.
• Diarrhoea.
• Vomiting.
• Lack of energy or irritability.
In older children, symptoms are usually more specific, and may include:
• Burning sensation on passing urine.
• Passing urine increasingly often.
• Pain affecting the lower back or one side of the abdomen.

• Bed-wetting after being dry at night.
• Urine that is red, pink, or smoky in colour, due to the presence of blood.
• Fever.
Scarring of the kidneys from recurrent infections may lead to high blood pressure or kidney failure in adult life.

Should I consult a doctor?

Your child should be seen by a doctor within 24 hours if there are symptoms of a urinary tract infection.

What might the doctor do?

The doctor may collect a urine sample from your child or may ask you to do so (see "What can I do to help?"). A baby may be seen at hospital in order to have urine withdrawn from the bladder via a hollow needle passed through the skin. The urine is tested to rule out an underlying disorder and to confirm that infection is the cause of the symptoms.

If infection is confirmed, the doctor may prescribe oral antibiotics. A seriously ill child may be treated in hospital with intravenous antibiotics. The antibiotics may be given for up to a week. About a week after treatment for infection has ceased, your child's urine will be tested again. If infection is still present, he or she may be given another course of antibiotics.

Further investigations may be carried out to see if your child has scarred kidneys or a structural abnormality of the urinary tract. Special tests for urinary reflux may be performed in some children. Because children with these conditions are often prone to recurrent infections, they may be prescribed antibiotics for several years, as a preventive measure.

What can I do to help?

If the doctor asks you to collect a urine sample, you will be supplied with a sterile container and an adhesive bag (for an infant). The sample should be collected after your child has had a bath or after washing the genital area with plain water. For an infant, a urine sample can be caught in the container, without letting the container touch the child (to prevent contamination). Alternatively, apply the adhesive bag around the genitals, and pour a small amount of the sample into the container.

After washing the genitals, an older child should collect a mid-stream sample by passing some urine, stopping, and starting again, directing the stream into the sterile container. The child should stop when the container is full and then complete emptying the bladder. If you are unable to take the urine sample to the doctor right away, you may keep it in the main compartment of your refrigerator for up to 48 hours.

While your child has an infection, he or she should drink plenty of fluids. A high fluid intake dilutes the urine, easing pain and discomfort when passing urine, and helps to get rid of bacteria.

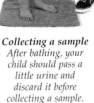

Collecting a sample
After bathing, your child should pass a little urine and discard it before collecting a sample.

How can the infections be prevented?

Children should pass urine at least every 4 hours or before each meal, and before going to bed. After using the toilet, your child's bottom should be wiped from front to back. Your child should have a bath or shower every day, avoiding the use of irritants, such as scented soaps or bubble bath, and should be dried thoroughly afterwards.

What is the outlook?

Recurrences of urinary tract infections are common, but prompt treatment should prevent permanent damage to the kidneys. Any scars of the kidneys become smaller as your child grows. A tendency to reflux usually disappears without treatment by 9 years of age.

GLOMERULONEPHRITIS

Inflammation of the glomeruli, the filtering units in the kidneys, is known as glomerulonephritis. The condition usually affects both kidneys. The inflamed glomeruli are not able to process wastes efficiently, resulting in decreased urine production and loss of blood and protein into the urine. Usually, the cause of glomerulonephritis is not known. Sometimes, the condition may follow an infection by streptococcal bacteria or by viruses.

What are the symptoms?
In post-infective glomerulonephritis, the symptoms begin about a week after the infection. Whatever the cause, the main symptoms are:
- Urine that is red, pink, or smoky in colour, caused by the presence of blood (see photographs right).
- Passing a smaller amount of urine than usual.
- Sometimes, a headache. Fluid may accumulate in the tissues, leading to swelling, particularly of the face and legs. High blood pressure is a rare complication.

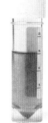

NORMAL URINE **ABNORMAL URINE**

Blood in urine
The presence of blood gives urine an abnormal appearance. It looks darker and cloudier than normal clear, pale-yellow urine.

Should I consult a doctor?
You should phone a doctor at once if you suspect that your child might have glomerulonephritis. Your child will be examined by the doctor and will probably be admitted to hospital for diagnostic tests. A sample of urine will be examined, and your child's intake and output of fluid may be measured.

What is the treatment?
If the diagnosis is confirmed, your child will need to stay in hospital for treatment. He or she may be put on a diet that is low in sodium and protein, and his or her intake of fluids may be restricted. This regimen alleviates the strain on the kidneys and prevents the accumulation of fluids. Your child does not need to stay in bed if he or she feels like walking around.

Your child may be given antibiotic drugs if the glomerulonephritis was caused by a bacterial infection. If he or she has high blood pressure, this condition may be treated for several days until it returns to normal.

With treatment, glomerulonephritis usually clears up within a week.

What is the outlook?
In most cases, glomerulonephritis does not have any lasting effect on a child's kidneys and does not often recur. Very rarely, it may be followed by NEPHROTIC SYNDROME (below), a chronic disease that may require prolonged treatment.

NEPHROTIC SYNDROME

In this condition, a large amount of protein is lost through the kidneys from the bloodstream into the urine. Reduced levels of protein in the blood lead to oedema (accumulation of excess fluid in body tissues). Nephrotic syndrome is an uncommon disorder, mainly affecting children aged between 1 and 6 years.

What are the symptoms?
The main symptoms are:
- Swelling of parts of the body (see photograph right), usually developing gradually over several weeks.
- Reduction in the quantity of urine.
- Weight gain.
- Sometimes, diarrhoea, loss of appetite, and unusual tiredness.

Children who have nephrotic syndrome are susceptible to infections and to the formation of blood clots in veins.

Should I consult a doctor?
Your child should be seen by a doctor within 24 hours if parts of his or her body are swollen. The doctor will examine your child and test his or her urine for protein. If the results suggest nephrotic syndrome, your child will be admitted to hospital for further tests. If

Swelling around the eyes

Pale, puffy face

Distended abdomen

Swollen scrotum

Swollen legs (particularly ankles)

Effects of nephrotic syndrome
In nephrotic syndrome, little fluid is passed in the urine. Instead, the fluid collects in body tissues, causing them to swell.

the diagnosis is confirmed, your child will be treated in hospital. Treatment includes corticosteroids and antibiotics. Within 10 days, as the excess fluid in the body is excreted by the kidneys, there should be an improvement in the oedema, which coincides with a rapid fall in weight. Your child will probably be kept in hospital until tests show that there is no protein in the urine, which may take up to 6 weeks.

What can I do to help?
After your child leaves hospital, you may be asked to test a sample of his or her urine every day, using strips that change colour when protein is present. If the test shows that there is protein in the urine, phone the doctor for advice.

What is the outlook?
Your child may make a full recovery from nephrotic syndrome and have no further problems. However, some children have one or more relapses. If your child suffers from frequent relapses, he or she may be prescribed corticosteroids for a year or more.

WILMS' TUMOUR

This rare malignant (cancerous) tumour of the kidney may be present at birth or develop during the first 4 years of life. In most cases, Wilms' tumour affects one kidney; only very rarely does the tumour develop in both kidneys.

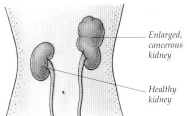

Enlarged, cancerous kidney

Healthy kidney

Kidney affected by Wilms' tumour
Wilms' tumour is usually very large. It is roughly spherical in shape and often grows from the top part of the kidney.

What are the symptoms?
The main symptoms of the tumour are:
• Swollen abdomen.
• Abdominal pain.
• Urine that is red, pink, or smoky in colour, due to the presence of blood.

Should I consult a doctor?
Your child should be seen by a doctor within 24 hours if his or her abdomen is swollen and/or if there is blood in the urine. If the doctor suspects your child has a tumour, he or she will be sent to hospital for investigations. Ultrasound scanning and other imaging techniques will be used to confirm the diagnosis and to provide information about the nature of the tumour.

What is the treatment?
The cancerous kidney will be surgically removed. Chemotherapy and, in some cases, radiotherapy may be used before the operation to reduce the size of the tumour; they may be used after surgery to kill any remaining cancer cells.

Your child will make a full recovery as long as the affected kidney is removed before the tumour spreads. The kidney that is left will be able to carry out the function of both kidneys.

VULVOVAGINITIS

Inflammation of the vulva and vagina is called vulvovaginitis. The problem is common in young girls and is usually minor. Vulvovaginitis may be caused by irritation of the delicate genital tissues (for example, by bubble baths) and, in this case, usually clears up with self-help treatment. Sometimes, the cause is a bacterial or yeast infection, and medical treatment is required. Frequently, however, vulvovaginitis has no obvious cause.

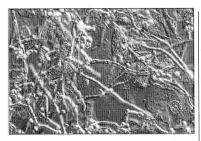

Micrograph of Candida yeast
The yeast Candida albicans *is responsible for the infection known as thrush. Although* Candida *normally lives in the vagina, an overgrowth of the yeast causes vulvovaginitis.*

How is it caused?
Common causes of irritation include poor hygiene, tight clothing, bubble baths, or scented soap. In some girls, there may be no obvious cause for the symptoms; the vulva and vaginal lining are just particularly sensitive.

Bacteria from the rectum may infect the vulva and vagina if your child's bottom is wiped from back to front after a bowel movement. Less often, a bacterial infection may be due to the presence of a foreign body (such as a crayon or a forgotten tampon) in the vagina. A possible cause in young girls may be an infestation by THREADWORMS (p.188). After puberty, thrush (see micrograph left) is a common cause.

What are the symptoms?
The symptoms of vulvovaginitis are:
• Inflammation, soreness, and itchiness affecting the genital area.
• Pain on passing urine.
• Greenish or greyish-yellow vaginal discharge, if bacterial infection is the cause. The discharge may be smelly if the infection is caused by a foreign body in the vagina.
• Thick, white vaginal discharge, if thrush is the cause.

Should I consult a doctor?
If your daughter is very uncomfortable, has a vaginal discharge, or experiences pain when she passes urine, she should be seen by a doctor within 24 hours. Consult a doctor if other symptoms have persisted for more than 2 weeks.

The doctor will examine your child. If it is likely that a foreign body is in the vagina, your child will be sent to hospital; if an object is found, it will be removed under a general anaesthetic. A vaginal swab may be taken to check for infection. If bacterial infection is found, an antibiotic cream or oral antibiotics may be prescribed. An antifungal cream or pessaries (which are inserted into the vagina) may be used for thrush.

For persistent irritation when there is no infection, the doctor may prescribe an oestrogen cream, which thickens the skin of the vulva and the vaginal lining.

What can I do to help?
Vulvovaginitis that is not caused by an infection usually clears up with self-help treatment. Twice a day for a week, your child should sit in a bath to wash the area, without using scented soaps or bubble baths. After washing, a barrier cream (for example, zinc cream) may be applied. Your child should wear loose-fitting cotton underwear, which should be changed daily. If possible, the genital area should be exposed to the air for a little while each day.

To keep the vulva and vagina free of irritating faecal material, make sure that your child's bottom is wiped from front to back after a bowel movement.

PENIS AND TESTIS DISORDERS

Disorders of the penis affecting boys include a tight foreskin, paraphimosis (a tight foreskin stuck in the retracted position), balanitis (inflammation of the head of the penis and foreskin), and hypospadias (an abnormally positioned urethral opening). The most common disorders of the testis in young boys are a hydrocele (an abnormal collection of fluid around a testis) and an undescended testis. Adolescent boys are prone to the painful disorders of testicular torsion (in which the testis twists around in the scrotum) and orchitis (inflammation of the testis).

TIGHT FORESKIN

In the first year of life, a boy's foreskin cannot usually be pulled back over the head of his penis (glans). You should never attempt to retract the foreskin by force. You are likely to injure the tissues, resulting in bleeding and the formation of scar tissue. In most boys, retraction becomes possible during the second year of life, but in some boys may not occur until the age of 4 years. After this age, inability to pull back the foreskin over the glans is abnormal.

Should I consult the doctor?

Your child should be seen by a doctor if he is older than 4 years and his foreskin cannot be retracted and/or he is having problems with passing urine.

The doctor will examine your son. If your son has phimosis, the doctor may recommend circumcision, an operation to remove the foreskin. If the foreskin is attached to the glans and the outlet is of normal diameter, the tissues may be separated surgically. Both operations are performed under general anaesthesia.

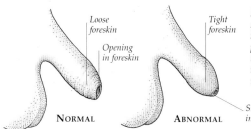

Loose foreskin

Opening in foreskin

NORMAL

Tight foreskin

ABNORMAL

Small opening in foreskin

Phimosis
An abnormally small opening in the foreskin is known as phimosis. The condition makes the foreskin tight and hard to retract over the glans. Passing urine may also be difficult.

What are the causes?

A tight foreskin may simply be due to persistence of the strands of tissue that attach it to the glans at birth. It may also be due to phimosis, a narrowed outlet in the foreskin (see illustrations above). Phimosis may be congenital, or is sometimes due to scarring caused by recurrent balanitis or by forceful attempts to retract the foreskin.

What are the symptoms?

The only symptom may be difficulty in retracting the foreskin. If phimosis is present, the narrowed opening may cause the following symptoms:
• Ballooning of the foreskin when the child passes urine.
• A narrow stream of urine.
A boy with phimosis is at increased risk of URINARY TRACT INFECTIONS (p.193).

PARAPHIMOSIS

Forcible retraction of a foreskin that is affected by phimosis may result in a condition known as paraphimosis. In this disorder, the retracted foreskin is stuck behind the glans and constricts the penis, causing swelling and pain.

Should I consult a doctor?

If your child's retracted foreskin has become stuck, you should take him to the nearest accident and emergency department at once. Your son will be sedated or anaesthetized, after which the doctor gently compresses the penis and returns the foreskin to its normal position. In some cases, the doctor may make an incision in the foreskin to free it. Paraphimosis will probably recur unless circumcision is performed to correct your son's phimosis.

BALANITIS

Infection by bacteria or fungi, usually as a result of inadequate cleaning of the penis, is the most common cause of balanitis. Phimosis tends to make cleaning difficult and so may increase the likelihood of balanitis occurring. Balanitis may appear as a reaction to chemicals in detergents or soaps or to irritating materials such as wool.

What are the symptoms?

The main symptoms of balanitis are:
• Swelling of the glans and foreskin (in uncircumcised boys).
• Pain or itching.
• White discharge from the penis.
• Genital area may be red and moist.

What can I do to help?

In most cases, balanitis clears up with improvements in hygiene. You should make sure your son washes his penis and genital area twice daily. After the inflammation has disappeared, the penis should be washed thoroughly every day to prevent recurrence.

If the balanitis is due to irritation, make sure that your son wears cotton underwear and that his clothes are thoroughly rinsed after washing. He should avoid using scented soaps.

Should I consult a doctor?

If balanitis does not clear up with self-help treatment within 3 days, make an appointment to see a doctor. He or she will probably prescribe an antifungal or antibiotic cream or oral antibiotics, which usually clears up the infection within a week. If your son suffers from recurrent attacks of balanitis, the doctor may recommend circumcision.

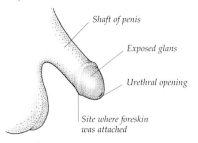

Shaft of penis

Exposed glans

Urethral opening

Site where foreskin was attached

Penis after circumcision
Circumcision involves removing the foreskin, so that the glans is exposed. The operation may be recommended if the foreskin is tight or a boy suffers from recurrent infections.

HYPOSPADIAS

In this congenital abnormality, affecting about 1 in 300 male babies, the opening of the urethra is located on the underside of the penis rather than at the tip. The opening is usually on the glans, but may be anywhere along the shaft of the penis. The lower half of the foreskin may be absent, and the upper half may form a hood over the end of the penis. In some babies, the shaft curves downward. Hypospadias is detected during the routine physical examination that is done on all newborn babies.

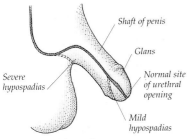

Degrees of hypospadias
In mild hypospadias, the urethral opening is on the glans. The opening may also be on the shaft of the penis; in the most severe cases, it is located well back towards the scrotum.

What is the treatment?

Hypospadias is usually corrected by an operation that is performed before a boy is 2 years of age. The surgeon may construct an extension for the urethra out of a tube of skin (made from the foreskin) so that it is able to reach the tip of the penis. A curved penis shaft is straightened during the same operation. A child should not be circumcised before hypospadias has been surgically repaired because the foreskin is needed at the operation.

What is the outlook?

Once your son has received treatment for hypospadias, his penis should look normal and he should not have any difficulties with passing urine, or, in adult life, with sexual intercourse.

HYDROCELE

This painless swelling of the scrotum occurs when fluid accumulates in the space around a testis. Hydroceles are common in newborn babies, and they usually disappear without treatment by the age of 6 months. The sudden appearance of a hydrocele in an older boy may be the result of an injury.

Should I consult a doctor?

Your child should be seen by a doctor if a scrotal swelling persists beyond the age of 6 months, or if it makes its first appearance after this age. In these cases, the hydrocele may be associated with an inguinal hernia (see HERNIA, p.187), and will require surgical treatment. A hydrocele that suddenly appears in an older boy should also be assessed by a doctor. It is likely to be caused by an injury and will probably get better without treatment. However, tests, including ultrasound scanning, will be done to exclude damage to the testis.

UNDESCENDED TESTIS

Sometimes one or, less frequently, both testes fail to descend into the scrotum before birth. All newborn male babies are examined to determine whether the testes have descended normally. If not, a further examination is carried out at 3 months because descent often occurs naturally up to this age. If the testis has still not descended, an operation will probably be performed to move the testis into the scrotum, usually when your child is 2 or 3 years old.

What is the outlook?

As long as the operation is carried out at the right time, your child's sexual development and fertility should not be affected. There may, however, be a slightly increased risk of testicular cancer developing later in life.

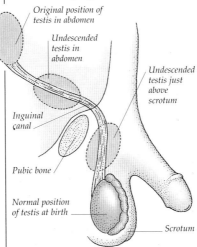

Possible sites of an undescended testis
The testes normally move down the inguinal canal into the scrotum before birth. A testis that fails to descend may stop anywhere, from high in the abdomen to just above the scrotum.

TESTICULAR TORSION

This condition occurs when a child's spermatic cord (the cord from which the testis is suspended) becomes twisted, cutting off or reducing blood supply to the testis. Testicular torsion causes acute pain. If the torsion is not corrected within hours, the affected testis may be permanently damaged.

What are the symptoms?

The main symptoms of torsion are:
- Sudden, severe pain in the abdomen.
- Severe pain in the testis.
- The affected testis may be noticeably higher than normal in the scrotum.
- Possibly, nausea and vomiting.
- After a few hours, the scrotum may become swollen, red, and tender.

If your son has pain in a testis, you should call an ambulance or take him to the nearest hospital accident and emergency department immediately.

What is the treatment?

An operation is carried out to untwist the spermatic cord and both the testes are stitched to the scrotum to prevent torsion recurring. A testis that has been irreversibly damaged is removed.

What is the outlook?

Provided treatment is carried out in time, your child's testis should function normally. If a testis has been removed, the remaining testis should ensure that your son's sexual development and fertility are not affected.

ORCHITIS

This inflammation of a testis most often occurs as a complication of mumps. Orchitis is also occasionally caused by a bacterial infection. It is not serious, and usually disappears within a week.

What are the symptoms?

The main symptoms of orchitis are:
- Pain in the testis.
- Sometimes, fever.

If your son has not had mumps within the past 2 weeks, call an ambulance or take him to an accident and emergency department immediately in case he has testicular torsion (above). If your son has had mumps recently, he should be seen by a doctor within 24 hours.

What is the treatment?

Give your child paracetamol to relieve the pain. If there is a bacterial infection, the doctor may prescribe antibiotics.

GENETIC DISORDERS

ALL THE INFORMATION that the embryo needs for growth and development is carried on around 100,000 genes packaged in 23 pairs of chromosomes. Abnormalities of these genes (or of whole chromosomes) may cause birth defects, or symptoms that may not appear until later. Genetic analysis allows couples with a family history of an inherited disease to estimate their chances of having an affected child. Tests during pregnancy can reveal whether a fetus is affected.

DOWN'S SYNDROME

The most common chromosomal abnormality, Down's syndrome affects about 1 in every 700 babies. Children with the condition have a characteristic physical appearance combined with slow mental development. The diagnosis is usually suspected at birth. The risk of giving birth to a Down's syndrome baby increases sharply in women over 37 years old; a third of all babies with Down's syndrome are born to women in this age group. The risk is also greater in women who have already had an affected child.

What are the symptoms?

The characteristics of children affected by Down's syndrome include:

• Upward-sloping eyes, which have prominent skin folds at the inner corner of the eyelids.

• Small, round face and full cheeks.

• Large tongue that tends to protrude.

• Flat back to the head.

• Floppy limbs.

• Slow physical development.

• LEARNING DIFFICULTIES (p.172).

• Short stature.

What are the complications?

Many children with Down's syndrome are born with a heart defect, and some have an intestinal abnormality. Down's syndrome children are at greater than average risk of developing an under-active thyroid gland and acute LEUKAEMIA (p.146), and have an increased frequency of instability of the neck joints (which may mean restricting some sports activities). They may have hearing problems and tend to be susceptible to infections.

What might the doctor do?

The doctor will examine your child for typical features of Down's syndrome. He or she will arrange for chromosome analysis of blood samples to confirm the diagnosis. Most parents are offered genetic counselling to discuss the risks of further children being affected.

Ultrasound examination of the heart may be performed in hospital to look for defects, and X-rays of the abdomen may be taken if an intestinal defect is suspected. Surgery may be required to correct any defects that are found.

Follow-up care from specialists, such as speech and occupational therapists, and special educational help will be arranged for your child.

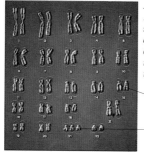

Abnormal chromosomes
In the usual form of Down's syndrome, body cells have an extra chromosome 21. Each cell normally has 22 pairs of identical chromosomes and two sex chromosomes.

Normal pair of identical chromosomes

Extra chromosome 21

What can I do to help?

You may wish to contact a support group for Down's syndrome to obtain advice and details of pamphlets and books. Your child's therapists and teachers may suggest ways to stimulate and help your child to develop his or her capabilities as much as is possible.

How can Down's syndrome be prevented?

Pregnant women who have already had an affected child or who are over the age of 37 years will be offered chorionic villus sampling (removing a sample of tissue from the edge of the placenta) or amniocentesis (removing a sample of the fluid surrounding the fetus). Fetal cells in these samples are analysed for chromosomal abnormalities. If the test results indicate the fetus has Down's syndrome, the parents may opt for a termination of the pregnancy.

Pregnant women of all ages should be offered a blood test that determines whether they are at increased risk of having a baby with Down's syndrome. Women shown to be at increased risk are offered amniocentesis.

What is the outlook?

Many children with Down's syndrome survive into early middle age, but up to 20 per cent die before they reach the age of 5 years, usually because of severe heart problems. Adults with Down's syndrome are susceptible to Alzheimer's disease and atherosclerosis (hardening of the arteries). As a result of advances in educational methods, the outlook for the achievement of maximum potential is now better than in the past.

FRAGILE X SYNDROME

This inherited chromosomal abnormality is a relatively common cause of LEARNING DIFFICULTIES (p.172) and also results in a slightly abnormal physical appearance. It affects about 1 in 1,000 boys and 1 in 2,500 girls. A woman with no symptoms can carry the defective chromosome and pass it on to some of her children.

What are the symptoms?
Features of fragile X syndrome include:
- Above-average height.
- Relatively large head.
- Delay in mental development, which is usually slight in girls and moderate to severe in boys.
- Delayed speech development, which is usually more severe in boys.
- Features of AUTISM (p.171).
- Square prominent jaw, long face, large ears, and large testes in boys after they reach puberty.

Fragile X syndrome may be suspected only after puberty, when the physical features become more apparent. By this time, your child will probably already be receiving special education. Consult your doctor, however, so that a definite diagnosis of the disorder can be made.

What might the doctor do?
The doctor will examine your child and assess his or her learning ability. If the doctor suspects fragile X syndrome, he or she will arrange for   omosome analysis of a blood sample. If the tests show that your child has the defective chromosome, you will be referred for genetic counselling to discuss the risks of further children being affected.

There is no specific treatment. If your child is not already receiving special help for speech or learning difficulties, the doctor may refer him or her to a speech therapist and/or psychologist. Fragile X syndrome was identified only recently and is being researched further.

SICKLE-CELL ANAEMIA

Most commonly affecting people of African descent, sickle-cell anaemia is a serious, inherited blood disease in which red blood cells become distorted into a sickle shape. The "sickle" cells can block narrow blood vessels. The cells are also destroyed more easily than normal red blood cells, producing ANAEMIA (p.145).

How is it caused?
The distortion of red blood cells occurs because the cells contain an abnormal type of haemoglobin (oxygen-carrying pigment) known as haemoglobin S. If a child inherits the abnormal gene from each parent, the child will have sickle-cell anaemia. If a child inherits the abnormal gene from one parent and a normal haemoglobin gene from the other, the child will have sickle-cell trait. Children with sickle-cell trait have no symptoms but are able to pass on the abnormal gene to their children.

What are the symptoms?
The main symptoms are:
- Lack of energy and breathlessness.
- Episodes of jaundice (yellowness of the skin and whites of the eyes).
- Attacks of severe pain in the bones, chest, or abdomen, resulting from blockage of narrow blood vessels (which reduces the oxygen supply to tissues). Dehydration, cold, or severe infection makes attacks more likely.

Children who have sickle-cell anaemia are at increased risk of pneumococcal pneumonia. Occasionally, blood supply is reduced to the kidneys, spleen, or brain, causing damage to these organs.

Should I consult a doctor?
Many affected babies are identified by blood tests at birth. Consult a doctor if you are unsure whether your child might be at risk or if he or she has any of the symptoms listed above.

The diagnosis can be confirmed by blood tests. Treatment includes folic acid supplements to reduce the severity of anaemia, penicillin given regularly to prevent infections, immunization against pneumococcal infection, and painkillers to be taken as necessary.

What can I do to help?
In order to reduce the likelihood of painful attacks, you should make sure that your child drinks plenty of fluids (to prevent dehydration) and that he or she does not become chilled.

Phone a doctor at once if your child has a painful attack accompanied by: a fever; sudden paleness; persistent vomiting or severe diarrhoea; difficult or fast breathing; abnormal drowsiness; or lack of energy. You should call an ambulance if your child has severe abdominal pain or tenderness.

Your child may need to be admitted to hospital for pain relief and treatment of dehydration or any infection.

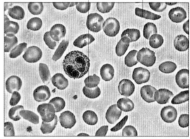

Normal red blood cell   Sickle cell

Red blood cells in sickle-cell anaemia
Seen through a microscope, blood taken from a person affected by sickle-cell anaemia shows distorted, sickle-shaped red blood cells.

How can sickle-cell anaemia be prevented?
People at risk of sickle-cell anaemia are advised to have a blood test to find out whether they have the abnormal gene. A couple who both have the abnormal gene should have genetic counselling before starting a family. Tests can be carried out during early pregnancy to find out whether a fetus has sickle-cell anaemia; if the fetus is affected, the parents may opt for termination.

What is the outlook?
With good medical care, most affected children survive into adulthood. If symptoms are severe, a child with sickle-cell anaemia may be considered for bone marrow transplantation if a suitable donor is found. If successful, a transplant provides a complete cure.

THALASSAEMIA

An inherited form of ANAEMIA (p.145), thalassaemia occurs most commonly among people of Mediterranean, African, and Asian origin. There are two types: thalassaemia major is a serious disorder that, untreated, causes slow growth and deformity of the skull; thalassaemia minor does not usually cause symptoms.

How is it caused?
Thalassaemia results from a defect in the gene that codes for the production of haemoglobin (the oxygen-carrying pigment in red blood cells). A child who inherits the faulty gene from both parents has thalassaemia major, which causes an inability to produce normal haemoglobin. Red blood cells are small and fragile and are rapidly broken up, leading to severe anaemia. If the faulty gene is inherited from only one parent, the result is thalassaemia minor. Red cells are slightly smaller than normal.

What are the symptoms?
Children with thalassaemia major have symptoms of anaemia, beginning in infancy. These symptoms include:
• Pale skin.
• Chronic tiredness.
• Shortness of breath.

If your child has symptoms of anaemia, you should make an appointment for him or her to see a doctor.

What is the treatment?
Thalassaemia is diagnosed by blood tests. Thalassaemia major is treated by monthly blood transfusions, from the age of a few months. Frequent blood transfusions may, however, eventually cause damage to internal organs, such as the heart and the liver, because they become overloaded with iron. This problem can be prevented by regular infusions of a compound known as desferrioxamine. Thalassaemia minor does not require any treatment.

How can thalassaemia be prevented?
The parents or other close relatives of a child with thalassaemia, and any prospective parent with thalassaemia

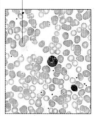 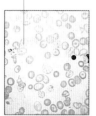

Healthy red blood cell   *Pale red blood cell*

NORMAL   ABNORMAL

Blood cells in thalassaemia major
A microscopic view of blood from a person with thalassaemia major shows abnormally pale red blood cells. The cells are fragile and rapidly broken up, causing severe anaemia.

may benefit from genetic counselling to establish the risk of having an affected child. Prenatal tests are available in specialized centres. Parents may opt for termination if the fetus is affected.

What is the outlook?
Children with thalassaemia major who receive regular blood transfusions and desferrioxamine have a good prospect for normal growth and development, and many survive into middle age.

HAEMOPHILIA

A genetic disorder that causes episodes of spontaneous bleeding, haemophilia affects about 1 in 10,000 boys. The condition is due to deficient activity of factor VIII, a clotting factor in the blood. Girls who carry the haemophilia gene have no symptoms, but some of their sons may be affected by the disorder.

What are the symptoms?
The symptoms of haemophilia include:
• Prolonged bleeding after an injury or even a minor surgical operation, such as tooth extraction.

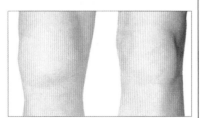

Swollen knee joint
Bleeding due to haemophilia has caused this child's right knee to become swollen. Joints can become damaged and painful as a result of recurrent episodes of internal bleeding.

• Painful swelling of muscles and joints as a result of internal bleeding.
The extent and frequency of bleeding in haemophilia vary greatly from one person to another. Some people suffer from only occasional episodes of minor bleeding. When the condition is severe, there is a risk of damage to muscles and joints from recurrent internal bleeding.

Should I consult a doctor?
If your child has any signs of abnormal bleeding, he or she should be seen by a doctor. The doctor will ask about your son's symptoms, and if he or she thinks that haemophilia is a possibility, will arrange for blood tests to assess the blood's ability to clot. The results of the tests confirm the diagnosis.

What is the treatment?
Treatment may consist of injections of factor VIII, given by parents, to treat bleeding episodes. Severe bleeding may require admission to hospital. If bleeding episodes are frequent, factor VIII can be given regularly by parents via a drip in order to prevent bleeding. Factor VIII in current use is free of viruses, such as HIV (the AIDS virus).

How can haemophilia be prevented?
Women who have a family history of haemophilia can be tested to find out if they have the haemophilia gene and can seek genetic counselling to assess the risk of having an affected child.

What is the outlook?
Children with haemophilia are advised to avoid hazardous activities, such as contact sports. As long as factor VIII is given promptly when bleeding occurs, or regular infusions are given, muscles and joints may not be damaged, and life expectancy should be normal.

PHENYLKETONURIA

In this inherited condition, a defect in body chemistry causes a build-up of phenylalanine (a constituent of protein) in the blood. Untreated, phenylketonuria causes brain damage. The disorder affects about 1 baby in 10,000. Babies are routinely screened for phenylketonuria by a blood test soon after birth.

What are the symptoms?
At birth, affected babies show no signs of abnormality. If phenylketonuria is not treated, however, the child may develop the following symptoms:
• Severe LEARNING DIFFICULTIES (p.172).
• A tendency to have seizures.
• A characteristic mousey odour.
• Rash like that of ATOPIC ECZEMA (p.135).

What is the treatment?
Phenylketonuria is treated by a special diet. Phenylalanine, which is present in most protein foods, must be restricted while ensuring that the child receives sufficient protein for growth. The diet is mainly vegetarian; supplements may also be prescribed. A baby needs to be given special milk substitutes.

How can phenylketonuria be prevented?
If a couple have an affected child, there is an increased risk that further children will also be affected. Prenatal diagnosis is available, and the parents may opt for termination if the fetus is affected.

What is the outlook?
The majority of children with treated phenylketonuria attend normal schools and have normal intelligence. A small proportion have behavioural problems and learning difficulties. It is usually recommended that the diet should be continued throughout life.

CYSTIC FIBROSIS

A serious inherited disease, cystic fibrosis causes recurrent chest infections and inability to absorb nutrients from the intestines (see MALABSORPTION, p.183). The repeated chest infections result in progressive lung damage. Although cystic fibrosis is present from birth, the condition sometimes goes undetected for many months or years, during which time damage to the lungs may have begun. Cystic fibrosis affects about 1 in 2,000 children.

How is it caused?
Cystic fibrosis is caused by a defective gene. For a child to have the disorder, the faulty gene must be inherited from both parents (who are carriers, but have no symptoms of the disease). The defective gene results in the secretion of sticky mucus that cannot flow freely through the air passageways, leading to recurrent chest infections. The faulty gene also causes deficient secretion of pancreatic enzymes (which help in the digestion of food), leading to diarrhoea.

What are the symptoms?
The main symptoms are:
• Failure to grow normally and to gain a normal amount of weight.
• Persistent coughing.
• Chronic diarrhoea, typically with pale, oily, strong-smelling faeces.
You should see a doctor if your child has any of these symptoms.

What might the doctor do?
If the doctor thinks that cystic fibrosis is a possibility, your child will be sent to a paediatrician for tests. A sample of your child's sweat will be analysed in the laboratory; in cystic fibrosis, the salt content of sweat is higher than normal. Genetic tests may also be performed. If the tests confirm that your child has cystic fibrosis, the doctor will prescribe pancreatin (a replacement pancreatic enzyme preparation) for your child to take with meals so that food is digested properly. A diet high in energy and protein is recommended, and vitamin supplements will be prescribed. The doctor will prescribe antibiotics and will recommend regular physiotherapy for treatment of chest infections and to help prevent chronic lung disease.

What can I do to help?
After tuition from a physiotherapist, you should start giving your child regular chest physiotherapy as soon as possible (see photograph right).
It is vital that you contact your doctor at the first sign of any illness so that appropriate treatment can be given quickly. When your child is ill with a chest infection, you will need to carry out physiotherapy more often than usual. To help your child to absorb enough nutrients for normal growth, encourage him or her to take high-energy snacks.

How can cystic fibrosis be prevented?
Genetic counselling may be offered to any prospective parent who already has a child with cystic fibrosis or who is a carrier. Prenatal testing can be carried out, and termination may be considered if the fetus is affected.

What is the outlook?
There is no cure for the disorder, but the outlook has improved greatly due to earlier diagnosis and new methods of treatment, and most sufferers now survive well into adulthood. A few severely affected children have had a lung or heart-lung transplant, which has improved their quality of life and increased their life expectancy.

Chest physiotherapy
To help loosen the thick mucus in the lungs, clap your child's back with a cupped hand. Physiotherapy should be performed twice a day, and more often when your child is ill.

First Aid & Nursing a Sick Child

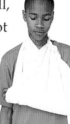

Occasionally, a parent may have to deal with an emergency. The first-aid section provides a quick guide to treating some of the most serious

FIRST AID FOR BURNS

or life-threatening injuries. The techniques shown have been validated by the British Red Cross. Do not wait for an emergency before studying these pages – familiarize yourself with the techniques now. Bear in mind, however, that first aid is a practical skill, and reading a book cannot replace practical training. The Red Cross runs a wide variety of first-aid courses, some of which are specifically on first aid for children.

ARM SLING

PRINCIPLES OF FIRST AID

The **Airway–Breathing–Circulation** check – called the **ABC** of resuscitation – is the most important principle of first aid. If there is breathing and a pulse, treat other problems in the following order: bleeding and shock (p.208); burns (p.209); fractures (pp.210–211); other injuries. An unconscious child should be put in the recovery position (opposite).

ABC OF RESUSCITATION: BABIES

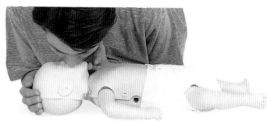

Airway
To open the airway of an unconscious baby, tilt the head back slightly and lift the chin with one finger. Check for breathing; if breathing is evident, hold the baby in the RECOVERY POSITION (opposite).

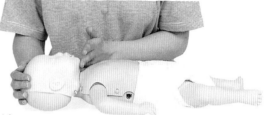

Breathing
If your baby is not breathing, give ARTIFICIAL VENTILATION (p.205). If your breaths do not go in, your baby's airway may be obstructed (see CHOKING, p.204).

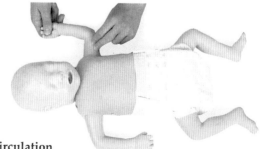

Circulation
Check the pulse by placing two fingers on the inside of the upper arm, and your thumb on the outside. If there is no pulse, give CARDIOPULMONARY RESUSCITATION (p.206).

WARNING
IF THERE IS A SPINAL INJURY
- Do not move your child unless: you or your child are in danger; your child's breathing is obstructed; or you must perform cardiopulmonary resuscitation on your child.
- Do not tilt your child's head to give breaths; just lift the chin gently.

ABC OF RESUSCITATION: CHILDREN

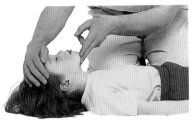

Airway
To open the airway of an unconscious child, tilt the head back and lift the chin with two fingers. Check for breathing; if evident, place the child in the RECOVERY POSITION (right).

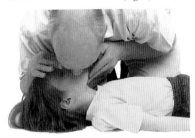

Breathing
If your child is not breathing, carry out ARTIFICIAL VENTILATION (p.205). If your breaths do not go in, your child may have an obstructed airway (see CHOKING, p.204).

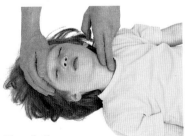

Circulation
Check your child's pulse by pressing on the groove of the neck, in front of the large muscle at each side. If there is no pulse, give CARDIOPULMONARY RESUSCITATION (p.207).

RECOVERY POSITION

Any unconscious child who is breathing and who has a pulse should be placed in the recovery position while you wait for the ambulance. This position allows fluids to drain out of the child's mouth so they are not inhaled. Check your child's breathing and pulse frequently (see ABC OF RESUSCITATION, opposite or left) and give artificial ventilation (p.205) or cardiopulmonary resuscitation (pp.206–207) if necessary. If your child has a fracture, support the injury.

A child with a spinal injury should be turned only if the breathing is obstructed. Keep the child's head, neck, and back aligned at all times.

BABIES

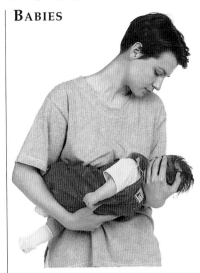

Hold your baby
An unconscious baby should be held securely, with his or her head tilted back slightly to keep the airway open, while you wait for an ambulance.

CHILDREN

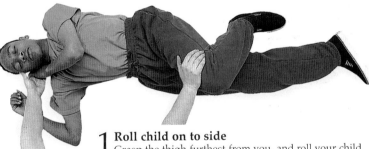

1 Roll child on to side
Grasp the thigh furthest from you, and roll your child over by pulling the bent leg towards you. As you roll, keep your child's hand held against his or her cheek.

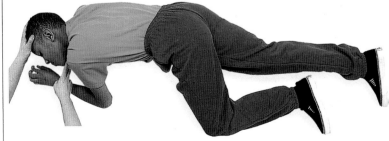

2 Position child
Bend the top leg at a right angle and adjust the position of the bottom arm to prevent your child rolling forwards. Tilt the head back to keep the airway open.

CHOKING

You may not realize that your child is choking. Initially, he or she may cough and gasp or make high-pitched squeaking noises, and then lose the ability to speak or breathe. A baby's face may turn red and then blue, and he or she may seem to have difficulty breathing or appear to cry without making any noise. If the back slaps and thrusts do not remove the obstruction at first, keep trying, since methods that are not initially successful may work eventually.

UNCONSCIOUS BABY OR CHILD
Call an ambulance immediately. If you can see an object in your baby's or child's throat, remove it carefully, but never poke a finger down blindly. Open the airway, check for breathing, and try to give breaths (see artificial ventilation, opposite). If breaths do not go in, give back slaps and chest thrusts (see below), check the mouth, and try to give breaths. Repeat until breaths go in, your baby or child breathes, or the ambulance arrives.

BABIES

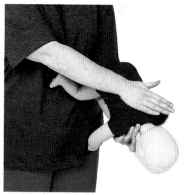

1 Give 5 back slaps
Lay your baby face-down along one arm with the head lower than the rest of the body, and support the chin between your fingers. Give 5 sharp slaps on the middle of your baby's back with the heel of your hand.

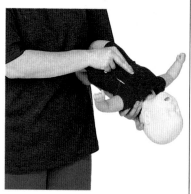

2 Give 5 chest thrusts
Turn your baby over, with the head low. Put two fingers on the breastbone, just below an imaginary line between the nipples, and give 5 downward thrusts. If an object is visible in the mouth, remove it carefully. Continue steps 1–2 until your baby can breathe.

CHILDREN

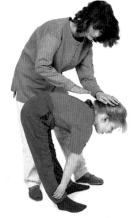

1 Give 5 back slaps
Make your child lean over. Give 5 sharp slaps between the shoulder blades with the heel of your hand. If the child is small, you can lay him or her across your lap, the head lower than the body, to do the back slaps.

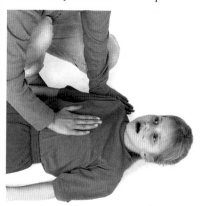

3 Give 5 abdominal thrusts
If your child is still unable to breathe, place the heel of your hand just below the edge of your child's ribs and give 5 upward thrusts.

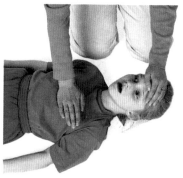

2 Give 5 chest thrusts
If the airway is still blocked, lay your child on the ground. A small child can be laid across your lap with his or her back on your thigh. Give 5 sharp downward thrusts on the breastbone with the heel of your hand.

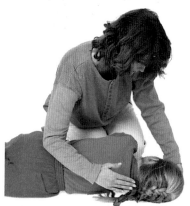

4 Repeat slaps and thrusts
Roll the child towards you on the ground to perform the back slaps. Continue the cycle of slaps and thrusts until your child can breathe.

ARTIFICIAL VENTILATION

If your child stops breathing, you must breathe for him or her, using a technique known as artificial ventilation. This technique is effective because even the air that you exhale contains enough oxygen to sustain your child's vital organs until medical help is obtained. The first aid is slightly different for babies and children due to their different sizes.

BABIES

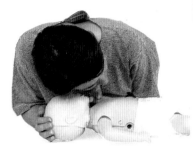

1 Open airway, check breathing
Tilt your baby's head back very slightly with one hand and lift the chin with a finger of the other hand. Look, listen, and feel for breathing.

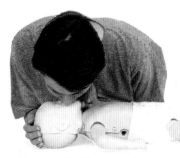

2 Give artificial ventilation
If your baby is not breathing, seal your lips over the mouth and nose. Give 5 breaths, taking a fresh breath yourself after each one.

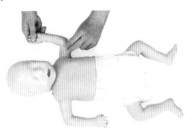

3 Check for pulse
If your baby has a pulse, give 20 breaths, one every 3 seconds. Call an ambulance. Continue giving breaths until help arrives, checking for a pulse and breathing after every 20 breaths.

CHILDREN

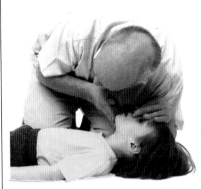

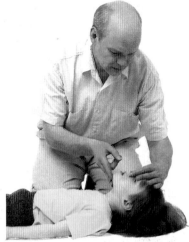

1 Open airway, check breathing
Tilt your child's head back slightly with one hand and lift the chin with two fingers of the other hand. Look, listen, and feel for breathing.

2 Pinch nose shut
If your child is not breathing, pinch the nose tightly shut. Keep the child's airway open by lifting his or her chin with two fingers.

3 Give artificial ventilation
Seal your lips over your child's mouth. Give him or her 5 breaths of artificial ventilation, taking a fresh breath yourself after each of the ventilations.

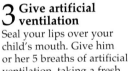

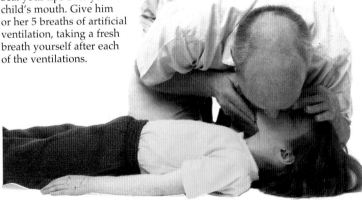

4 Check for pulse
If your child has a pulse, give 20 breaths, one every 3 seconds. Call an ambulance. Continue giving breaths until help arrives, checking for a pulse and breathing after every 20 breaths.

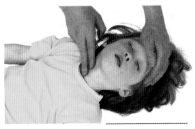

CARDIOPULMONARY RESUSCITATION (CPR)

A child who is not breathing and does not have a pulse must receive cardiopulmonary resuscitation (CPR) in order to keep the vital organs supplied with oxygen until treatment can be given in hospital. Cardiopulmonary resuscitation is the combination of artificial ventilation, to deliver air into your child's lungs, and chest compressions, to distribute the oxygenated blood throughout the body. If your child is a baby – under one year old – and the pulse is less than 1 per second (60 per minute), you should perform CPR because the baby's heart is not beating strongly enough to deliver oxygen throughout the body.

BABIES

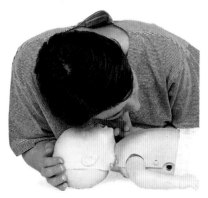

1 Open airway, check breathing
Lay your baby down on a flat surface. Tilt the head back very slightly with one hand and lift the chin with one finger of the other hand. Look, listen, and feel for breathing.

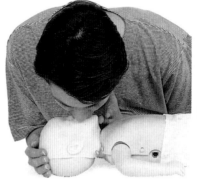

2 Give artificial ventilation
If your baby is not breathing, seal your lips over his or her mouth and nose. Give 5 breaths, taking a fresh breath yourself between each breath of the artificial ventilation.

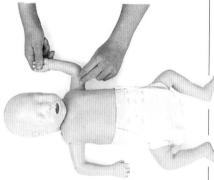

3 Check for pulse
Feel for a pulse on the inside of the upper arm for 5 seconds. If your baby has no pulse, or the pulse is less than 1 per second, you will need to give CPR (steps 4 and 5).

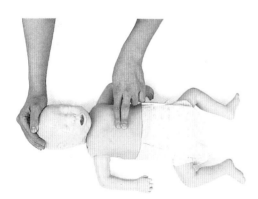

4 Give compressions
Place your index and middle fingers along your baby's breastbone, just below an imaginary line connecting the nipples. Press down sharply with your fingertips, 5 times within about 3 seconds, to a depth of approximately 2 cm (¾ in). Keep your other hand on the baby's head.

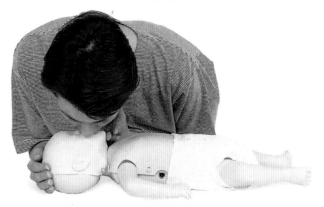

5 Give artificial ventilation
Seal your lips over your baby's mouth and nose, and give one breath. Repeat the compressions and breaths for about 1 minute (10 cycles). Call an ambulance; if you have no helper, take your baby with you to the telephone. Continue CPR (steps 4 and 5) until the ambulance arrives.

CHILDREN

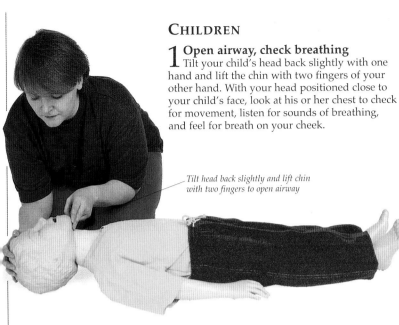

1 Open airway, check breathing

Tilt your child's head back slightly with one hand and lift the chin with two fingers of your other hand. With your head positioned close to your child's face, look at his or her chest to check for movement, listen for sounds of breathing, and feel for breath on your cheek.

Tilt head back slightly and lift chin with two fingers to open airway

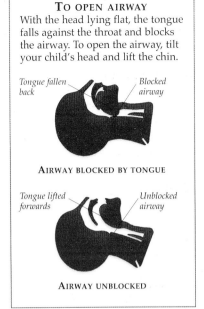

TO OPEN AIRWAY

With the head lying flat, the tongue falls against the throat and blocks the airway. To open the airway, tilt your child's head and lift the chin.

Tongue fallen back   *Blocked airway*

AIRWAY BLOCKED BY TONGUE

Tongue lifted forwards   *Unblocked airway*

AIRWAY UNBLOCKED

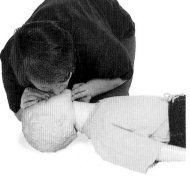
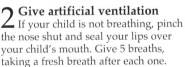

2 Give artificial ventilation

If your child is not breathing, pinch the nose shut and seal your lips over your child's mouth. Give 5 breaths, taking a fresh breath after each one.

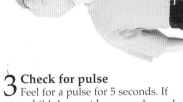

3 Check for pulse

Feel for a pulse for 5 seconds. If your child does not have a pulse and is not breathing, you will need to give CPR (steps 4–6).

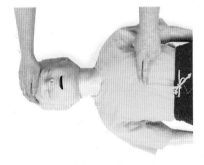

4 Find position on breastbone

Place your middle finger at the spot where your child's ribs meet, and put your index finger on the breastbone just above this.

6 Give artificial ventilation

Seal your lips over your child's mouth, and give one breath. Repeat the compressions and breaths for about 1 minute (10 cycles). Call an ambulance, then continue CPR (steps 4–6) until the ambulance arrives.

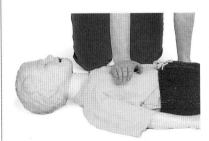

5 Give compressions

Place the heel of your other hand on the breastbone next to your fingers. Press down to a depth of 3 cm (1¼ in). Do this 5 times within 3 seconds.

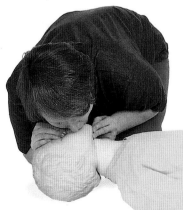
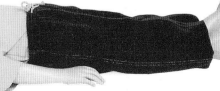

BLEEDING

In most cases bleeding stops quickly. However, if it is profuse, you may need to control it to prevent shock (below). If an object is embedded in the wound, do not remove it because you might cause further bleeding and damage. Use disposable gloves to reduce the risk of infection, or avoid touching the wound and wash your hands before and after treatment.

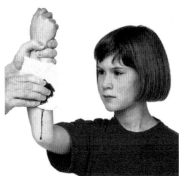

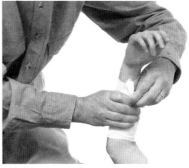

1 Press on wound
Raise the affected limb and press on the wound with your hand, over a clean pad or handkerchief. Press until the bleeding stops. Treat your child for SHOCK (below), if necessary.

2 Secure pad
Fasten the pad firmly in place. Support the injury in a raised position, for example with an elevation sling (see BROKEN COLLARBONE, p.210), and take your child to hospital.

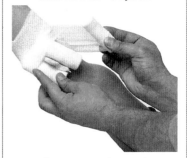

EMBEDDED OBJECT

Cover the wound lightly with a piece of gauze to prevent infection. Surround it with bandage rolls built up to the same height as the protruding object, and secure them in place by bandaging above and below the wound. Take your child to hospital or call an ambulance.

This technique can also be used if your child has a broken bone that has pierced the surface of the skin (an open fracture). Take care not to push the bone into the wound.

SHOCK

Shock is a dangerous reduction in the amount of blood, and therefore of oxygen, flowing to the body's tissues. It can be caused by blood loss (as a result of either internal or external bleeding), dehydration, or severe burns. The first signs of shock may be skin that is pale grey, cold, and sweaty; a rapid pulse that becomes weaker; and shallow, fast breathing. Later signs include unusual restlessness or aggression, thirst, and yawning or gasping for air. Shock may lead to a loss of consciousness. If your child has any of the signs, you should call an ambulance immediately, and then perform the necessary first aid for any specific injuries.

Lay your child down
Put your child on a blanket and raise the feet to a height of 20–30 cm (8–12 in) on several pillows. Cover your child with another blanket if he or she is cold. Reassure your child, but do not give anything to eat or drink. If your child loses consciousness, monitor his or her breathing and pulse, and perform artificial ventilation (p.205) or cardiopulmonary resuscitation (pp.206–207) if necessary.

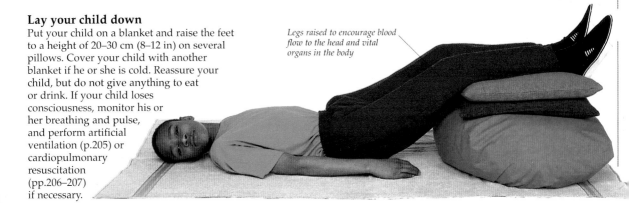

Legs raised to encourage blood flow to the head and vital organs in the body

BURNS

Whether the cause of a burn is heat or fire, electricity, or a chemical, the first aid is basically the same: your first priority is to cool the burned area by flushing with cold water. If your child's clothes are on fire, wrap him or her tightly in a rug or blanket until the flames go out. After performing first aid, take your child to hospital or call an ambulance.

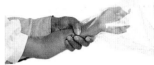

ALTERNATIVE TREATMENT:
BURNED HAND OR FOOT

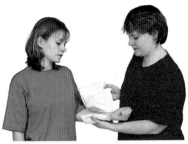

If your child burns a hand or foot, hold it under cold running water for at least 10 minutes, then enclose it in a clean plastic bag. Secure the bag with a plaster wrapped around the bag, not on your child's skin. Take your child to hospital.

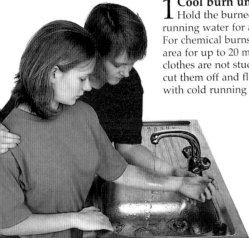

1 Cool burn under running water
Hold the burned area under cold running water for at least 10 minutes. For chemical burns, rinse the affected area for up to 20 minutes. If your child's clothes are not stuck to the burned skin, cut them off and flush the area again with cold running water.

2 Cover burned area
Place a clean bandage, pillowcase, or some other non-fluffy material over the burned area to prevent it from becoming infected. Treat your child for SHOCK (opposite) if necessary. Take your child to hospital or call an ambulance.

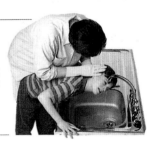

EYE WOUND

A child whose eye has been injured will be frightened and in intense pain. Movement of the wounded eye may increase the injury, so tell your child to look straight ahead. It will help if you calm your child and hold the head still as you cover both eyes. After the eyes are bandaged, either call an ambulance or take your child to hospital.

CHEMICAL IN EYE
Flush the eye for 10 minutes under gently running cold water. Keep it from splashing on to your child's face or into the unaffected eye. Bandage the injured eye (below), then take your child to hospital.

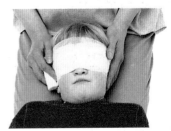

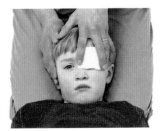

1 Cover injured eye
Use a pad to cover the injured eye. If an object is embedded, take care not to push it further into the eye.

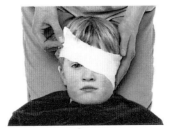

2 Bandage pad in place
Use a clean bandage to secure the pad firmly in place. Wrap the bandage around your child's head.

3 Cover both eyes
Place a clean bandage across both eyes. A child who cannot see at all is unlikely to move the injured eye.

BROKEN LEG

If your child breaks a leg, you should support it to prevent further injury while you are waiting for an ambulance. Do not attempt to straighten the leg. A broken knee should be supported with particular care in the position in which your child fell down by placing padding under and around the knee. Do not give your child anything to eat or drink.

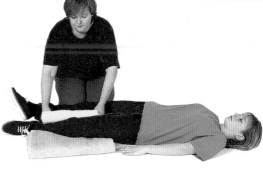

1 Place padding
Put plenty of padding, such as rolled-up towels or blankets, or folded newspaper, on both sides of the injured leg. Call an ambulance.

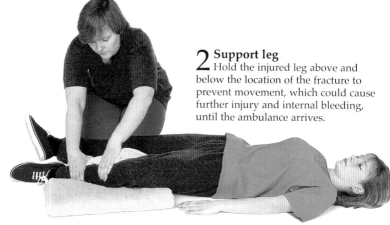

2 Support leg
Hold the injured leg above and below the location of the fracture to prevent movement, which could cause further injury and internal bleeding, until the ambulance arrives.

OPEN FRACTURES
If the broken bone has pierced the skin, the injury should be treated as an embedded object (see BLEEDING, p.208). Control the bleeding and bandage the wound before you continue with the first aid for a broken leg (right).

BROKEN COLLARBONE

A broken collarbone should be immobilized, by tying an elevation sling around the arm on the affected side, before you take your child to hospital. An elevation sling can also be used for a broken, bleeding, or bruised hand because it minimizes swelling by raising and supporting the injury.

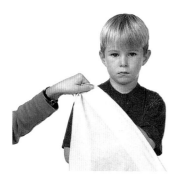

1 Place triangular bandage
Put the fingertips of the hand on the injured side on the other shoulder. Hold one end of the bandage at your child's fingertips, and drape the long edge down the body. The point should be below the elbow on the injured side.

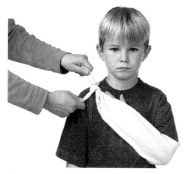

2 Gather bandage, tie sling
Take the bandage under the child's elbow so that it supports the arm on the injured side. Bring the bandage across the child's back. Tie it on the uninjured side with a reef knot, making sure that a few fingers are visible.

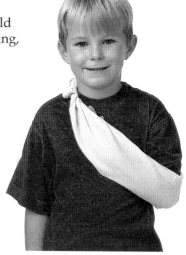

Finished sling
The excess fabric at the elbow has been tucked in behind the sling; it could also be pinned to the front of the sling. Keep checking your child's fingers; if they become pale, cold, or numb, the sling should be loosened.

BROKEN ARM

A broken upper or lower arm bone or wrist and a dislocated shoulder should be immobilized with an arm sling before your child is taken to hospital in order to prevent further injury and lessen pain. Do not use a sling, however, if the fracture is near the elbow, but lay your child down and call an ambulance.

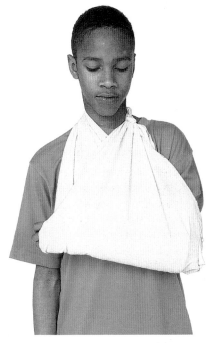

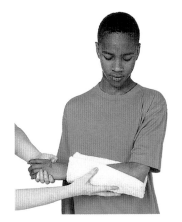

1 Pad injury
Gently place your child's injured arm across his or her chest. Arrange a generous layer of padding, such as a folded towel or newspaper, around the injury, while supporting the injured arm with your other hand.

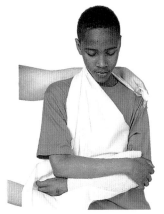

2 Place triangular bandage
Drape a bandage between your child's chest and the injured arm so that its long side extends down from the shoulder of the uninjured arm, and the other corner is positioned at the elbow of the injured arm.

Finished sling
The lower corner of the bandage has been brought up over the forearm and around the neck. The two ends have been tied on the injured side. Extra material at the elbow has been twisted and pinned to the front of the sling.

SWALLOWED POISONS

A child who swallows poisonous leaves or berries, a chemical, alcohol, or someone else's medicine needs immediate medical attention. Identify the substance that was swallowed and determine how much might have been consumed. If your child is unable to give you this information, you may need to look around for telltale signs, such as an open medicine container or bottle of alcohol, and check the mouth for unswallowed material. Phone your doctor or the accident and emergency department of a hospital before attempting to treat your child.

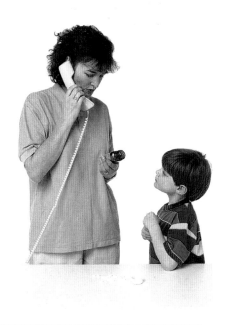

WARNING
IF YOUR CHILD SWALLOWS A POISON
• Do not try to make your child vomit. Some substances, such as bleach, can cause more harm if the child vomits.
• Do not give your child anything to drink, since this may disperse a drug more quickly around the body.

Determine what was swallowed
Ask your child or look for evidence. If the lips are burned, rinse gently with water. Place an unconscious child in the RECOVERY POSITION (p.203). Monitor breathing and pulse (pp.202–203), and perform ARTIFICIAL VENTILATION (p.205) or CARDIOPULMONARY RESUSCITATION (pp.206–207) if needed.

NURSING A SICK CHILD

Most illnesses do not require any specialized nursing care. You should, however, make sure that your child does not become dehydrated, especially if he or she has a fever or diarrhoea, or has been vomiting. A sick child may not have much of an appetite; small helpings of favourite foods may be tempting but you should not force your child to eat. If bedrest is not essential, your child may prefer to rest and read or play quietly in a room where other family members are present.

TAKING A TEMPERATURE

If your child seems unwell and you suspect a fever, you should take his or her temperature. Any of the three types of thermometer (below) can be used. A child over the age of 7 years can hold a mercury or digital thermometer under the tongue but you should never place a mercury thermometer into a younger child's mouth. The easiest way to take a younger child's temperature is with a mercury or digital thermometer in his or her armpit, or a temperature strip on the child's forehead. Bear in mind that the temperature measured in the armpit or on the forehead is about 0.6°C (1°F) less than the actual body temperature so this amount should be added to the reading to obtain the accurate body temperature.

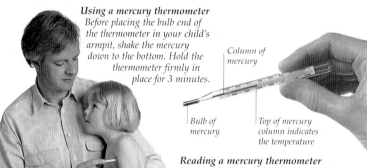

Using a mercury thermometer
Before placing the bulb end of the thermometer in your child's armpit, shake the mercury down to the bottom. Hold the thermometer firmly in place for 3 minutes.

Column of mercury

Bulb of mercury

Top of mercury column indicates the temperature

Reading a mercury thermometer
Remove the thermometer from under the arm, and rotate it until you can see the mercury column next to the scale; then read off the temperature. A fever is a temperature of 38°C (100°F) or above. If the temperature is high, measure it every 2 or 3 hours until it returns to normal. Always wash the thermometer in cool water and dry it after use.

TYPES OF THERMOMETER

The three types of thermometer available over the counter are mercury, digital, and temperature strip models. Although relatively expensive, digital thermometers are easy to use and give a quick and accurate reading, making them ideal for young children. Temperature strips and digital thermometers return to normal automatically, but a mercury thermometer must be shaken down with a quick flick of your wrist to return the mercury to the bulb, below 36°C (96.8°F).

MERCURY THERMOMETER

98.3°F

DIGITAL THERMOMETER

| °F | 95 | 96.8 | 98.6 | 100.4 | 102.2 | 104 |
| °C | 35 | 36 | 37 | 38 | 39 | 40 |

TEMPERATURE STRIP

GIVING MEDICINE

Liquid medicine should be measured carefully to ensure that the correct dose is given. Shake the bottle before every use and follow the storage directions carefully; some liquid medicines must be stored in a refrigerator to prevent deterioration. Use a syringe (below) to give medicines to young children as it avoids spillage and ensures that the proper dose is given. A medicine tube or 5-ml (0.18-fl.oz) plastic spoon can be used to give medicine to older children.

Children find it difficult to swallow tablets, so a type that dissolves or that can be crushed and mixed with fruit juice or honey is preferable.

An antibiotic course should always be completed, even if your child seems to be better, to prevent a recurrence of the infection.

Filling a syringe
The adapter is fitted into the bottle, and the syringe pushed into the adapter. With the bottle upside-down, the plunger is pulled out slowly until the syringe contains the dose.

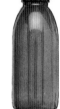

UNIVERSAL ADAPTER   SYRINGE   MEDICINE BOTTLE

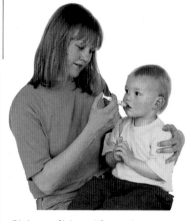

Giving medicine with a syringe
Remove the syringe containing the medicine from the adapter. Place the tip of the syringe in your child's mouth so it points towards the cheek and slowly press the plunger. Aiming the syringe at the throat may cause choking.

INDEX

Page numbers printed in **bold** type indicate the symptom charts. Page numbers printed in *italics* direct you to boxes or illustrations that explain self-help measures, first-aid techniques, or assessments.

ACKNOWLEDGMENTS

The author would like to thank his teachers, Dr. H.V.L. Finlay and Dr. R.J.K. Brown, whose experience and wisdom are reflected in these pages. He is indebted to Dr. Jackie Bucknall and Dr. Warren Hyer, his senior registrars, who checked the symptom charts and made several helpful comments. He thanks Dr. Robert Youngson for writing the articles on eye and vision problems, Dr. Bryan Lask and Dr. Sarah Benton for writing the articles on behavioural and emotional problems, and David P. Cocker, BDS for checking the information regarding teeth disorders. He also thanks Dr. Tony Smith, who has encouraged him in medical writing over many years and who has reviewed and enhanced this manuscript.

DORLING KINDERSLEY WOULD LIKE TO THANK:
Additional medical advice: Ursula Arens, British Nutrition Foundation; Tam Fry, Child Growth Foundation; Prof. John A. Henry MB FRCP, St. Mary's Hospital; Joanna Tempowski, National Poisons Information Service; Dr. Frances Williams
Additional editorial assistance: Dr. Amanda Jackson; Zak Knowles; Ruth Midgley; Cathy Shilling
Additional design assistance: Nicola Webb
Project photography: Andy Crawford
Photographer's assistant: Gary Ombler
Other photography: Mike Good; Steve Gorton; Dave King; Philip Powell; Susanna Price; Jules Selmes; Stephen Shott
Picture research: Christine Rista
Index: David Harding
Models: George Allen; Hugo Allen; Freda Belle; Charles Wilson Barnard; Emma Barnard; Rae Chen; Jane Cunningham; Max Cunningham; Anita Eade; Sally Evason; Lily Blawat Farr; Emma Foa; Lia Foa; Karen Good; Keiran Good; Olivia Grosvenor; Nicola Hampel; Jason Haniff; Ellen Harris; Joseph Lauder; Rebecca Lauder; Mary Lindsay; Michelle Papadopoulos; Nina Papadopoulos; Francesca Pritlove; Angela Rollinson;

Joe Rollinson; Archie Walker; Aidan Walls; Mark J. Wilde; Amelia Wooding; Sally Wooding.

Growth charts are based on information and charts supplied by the Child Growth Foundation, which are subject to copyright. Originals of the growth charts can be purchased from Harlow Printing, Maxwell Street, South Shields NE33 4PU, UK.

The first-aid information in this book has been validated by Anita Eade, first-aid training manager for the British Red Cross.

PICTURE CREDITS
Abbreviations: t=top; c=centre; b=bottom; l=left; r=right.
Heather Angel 152; **AVS Imperial College School of Medicine at St. Mary's** 31bl, 200bl; **Biophoto Associates** 31br, 79tc, 79cl, 120bl, 120cr, 134br, 139cr; **Collections**/Anthea Sieveking 79cr; **Sally Greenhill** 177br; **KeyMed** 184cr; **Medical Slide Library** 79cc, 122tl, 130cl, 135cl, 136cl, 163bl, 165tc, 166bc, 178cl; **National Medical Slide Bank** 79tr, 118, 121cr, 132bc, 139cl, 141bl; **Dr. Price, Northwick Park Hospital** 183tl; **John Radcliffe Hospital, Oxford** 200tr; **Science Photo Library** 137bc, 180cl, 184cc, 187cl, 200tl/Alex Bartel 178br; Biophoto Associates 146bll; Biozentrum 148bl; Oscar Burriel/Latin Stock 173; Chris Bjornberg 155bc; Scott Camazine 15ccl, 15cr/John Durham 146bl; CNRI 159bl, 184bc, 187br, 198; Eric Grave 199; John Heseltine 174; London School of Hygiene and Tropical Medicine 124tr; Dr. P. Marazzi 31cr; 119tl, 119bl, 137cl, 138bl, 140, 142bl, 151tr, 169cr, 175bl, 176tr; Will and Deni McIntyre 160br; Hank Morgan 172br; NIBSC 125, 151bc; Omikron 123; David Parker 141tc; John Radcliffe Hospital, Oxford 143tc; Dept. of Clinical Radiology, Salisbury District Hospital 128cr; David Scharf 153cl; Garry Watson 88bl; Western Ophthalmic Hospital 166tr; **J. Sorrell** 184bl; **Dr. Bernard Valman** 79tl, 147tcr, 158bc; **C. James Webb** 143bl; **Timothy Woodcock Photolibrary** 176bc/Steve Horsted 172tc; **Mike Wyndham Picture Collection** 15bl, 15br.